Enid Blyton

Sneezing Powder

...and other stories

BB Bounty
Books

Published in 2015 by Bounty Books,
a division of Octopus Publishing Group Ltd,
Carmelite House
50 Victoria Embankment,
London EC4Y 0DZ
www.octopusbooks.co.uk

An Hachette UK Company
www.hachette.co.uk
Enid Blyton ® Text copyright © 2011 Chorion Rights Ltd.
Illustrations copyright © 2015 Award Publications Ltd.
Layout copyright © 2015 Octopus Publishing Group Ltd.

Illustrated by Ray Mutimer.

ISBN: 978-0-75373-055-3

A CIP catalogue record for this book is available from the
British Library.

Printed and bound by CPI Group (UK) Ltd, Croydon, CR0 4YY

CONTENTS

Sneezing
Powder

Once upon a time there lived a brownie called Smarty. He kept a little shop in Hallo Town, in which he sold jars of honey, fine yellow lemons, and big yellow pills that helped to cure colds.

In the wintertime Smarty did a fine trade, for anyone who had a cold came to buy his honey, his juicy lemons, and his cold-pills. Then they would go home, squeeze the lemons into a glass, put in hot water and sugar and a spoonful or two of Smarty's golden honey, take a cold-pill, and go to bed – and lo and behold, next morning they were cured!

But in the summertime nobody seemed to have a cold at all. It was most annoying for Smarty. Instead of thinking of selling something else, such as ice creams or cool lemon drinks, Smarty still went on hoping that people would have colds and buy his cold-cure. So he wasn't quite as smart as his name, was he?

He was quite smart enough to think out a naughty trick, though!

"If only I could make people think they had a cold, they would come and buy my honey and lemons and pills," thought Smarty. "If only they would sneeze or cough just as they passed my shop, it would be so easy for me to say, 'Dear me! You are getting a cold! Buy my cold-cure before you are very bad!' But nobody ever sneezes outside my shop."

Smarty sat and thought for a bit, and then he grinned all over his sly little face. He slapped his knee in delight. He had thought of a wonderful idea!

"I'll go and buy some sneezing powder from old Dame Flap!" he said to himself. "And I'll put some into my pepperpot and shake it out of my bedroom window whenever anyone passes! Then they will sneeze hard and perhaps come and buy my goods."

So off he went to buy the sneezing powder. He paid Dame Flap a silver coin

6

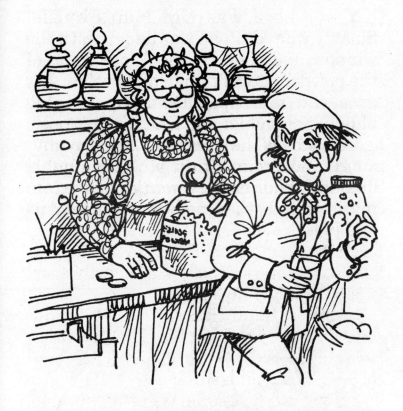

for a boxful and she wrapped it up for him. It was a strange powder, rather like fine green flour, and it had a strange smell.

Smarty ran home with it. He emptied some into his pepperpot and slipped upstairs to his bedroom window, which was just over his shop. He leaned out in excitement. Was anybody coming?

Yes – here was Old Man Shuffle! Smarty waited till he was underneath the window and then he shook out some of the powder. It went on Old Man Shuffle's nose, and he stopped. He took out his big blue handkerchief and held it to his nose.

"Whooosh!" he sneezed. "A-whoosh!"

"Hi, Old Man Shuffle, you've got a dreadful cold!" called Smarty. "Come into my shop and get some honey and lemons and pills!"

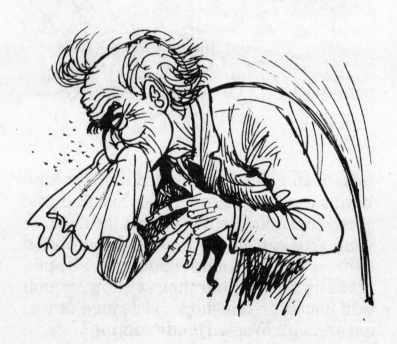

So in shuffled the old fellow, thinking it was very lucky that he should be outside Smarty's shop just when his cold had begun. He bought a jar of honey, two lemons, and a box of yellow pills. Smarty grinned. He ran up to his bedroom again.

"Ah! Here are Mr Twiddle and his wife!" chuckled Smarty. He shook his pepperpot over them. They stopped and fumbled for their hankies.

"Er-tish-oo!" said Mr Twiddle loudly.

"Ish-ish-ish!" sneezed Mrs Twiddle politely into her handkerchief.

"ER-TISH-OOO!" went Mr Twiddle.

"Not so much noise, Twiddle," said Mrs Twiddle. "Ish-ish-ish-ish! Dear me! We are beginning colds, I think. Look, let's buy some honey and lemons, and maybe we'll stop our colds from getting worse."

So into Smarty's shop they went and bought what they wanted, much to Smarty's delight. As soon as they had gone, he popped upstairs again with his pepperpot full of sneezing powder.

He made Twinkle the pixie sneeze and buy honey and pills. He made Mr Meddle sneeze so strongly that his hat flew on to the roof and he had to get a ladder to fetch it. He made Dame Winks sneeze twelve times, and at the end her bonnet was right over her nose and she couldn't see where she was going at all.

Oh, Smarty had plenty of fun that day, and he made plenty of money too! But when everyone found that they had no cold at all when they got home, and didn't need the honey and lemons, they were rather puzzled. They talked about it to one another, and they found that all of them had begun their sneezing fits outside Smarty's shop.

"Very nice for Smarty!" said Mr Meddle. "Let us go along and see what we can see."

So they all went back toward Smarty's shop, and peeped round the corner. And they saw Smarty leaning out of his bedroom window, pepperpot in hand!

"Aha!" Old Man Shuffle said angrily. "So that's his trick, is it! Come along everybody!"

They all went into Smarty's shop. Smarty hurried down to serve them. Mrs Twiddle was waiting for him. She snatched the pepperpot out of his pocket

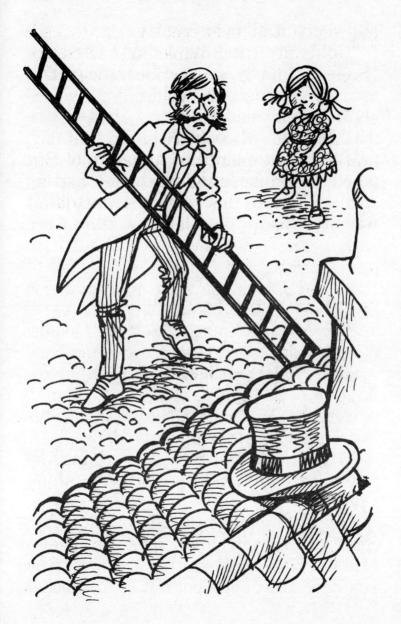

and shook it all over Smarty.

"Colds are catching today!" she said. "Sneeze, Smarty, sneeze! Dear, dear! You must have caught our colds."

"Whoosh!" said Smarty. "Atish-o! Ish-ish-ish! Osha-whoosh! Tish-oo!"

Mrs Twiddle emptied all the sneezing powder over him. My goodness, Smarty simply could not stop sneezing! It was dreadful!

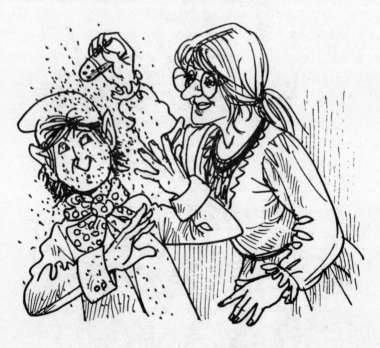

"By the time you've finished I guess you'll want to buy a pot of your own honey, a dozen lemons, and a box of pills!" said Mr Twiddle, laughing. "Goodbye, Smarty. It serves you right!"

They all went out, giggling and chuckling, and they could hear Smarty's sneezes all the way down the road.

Poor Smarty! He sneezed all that day and all that night, and by that time his nose and throat and eyes were so sore that he had to take two jars of honey, six lemons, and two of his own pills to cure himself!

Now he has shut up his shop and gone out selling ice creams. And a very much better idea, too, in the summer – don't you think so?

You're
Late!

"Bessie, the words I say to you more often
than any others are – 'You're late!'" said
Mother. "Why must you always be late?
Are you lazy, or slow, or what is it?"

"I don't know," said Bessie.

"You're late for breakfast, and if I didn't
hurry you off each day for school, you'd be
late there, and you're always home late
for lunch and tea," said her mother.

"Why bother about her?" said Granny.
"Why not let her be late? You don't need
to wait breakfast or lunch or tea – and
surely her teacher at school can punish
her if she's late. Why bother?"

"Well – that doesn't seem a bad idea!"
said Mother. "I'm getting so tired of
saying 'You're late, you're late, you're
late!' I hate nagging. I won't say it any
more. Bessie, you can be as late as you

14

like, but we just shan't wait for you,
that's all."

Bessie thought it would be nice not to
be grumbled at any more. She ate her tea,
and then went to do her homework.

"When you've done that, would you like
to catch the bus with me?" asked Granny.
"I've got a new book at home for you,
and you can fetch it and then catch the
bus back."

"Oh yes, Granny," said Bessie, pleased.
Granny always chose lovely books for her.
Perhaps it would be an adventure story –
or a book about the Faraway Tree. Lovely!

"I'll start at six o'clock," said Granny,
and didn't say any more. Bessie finished

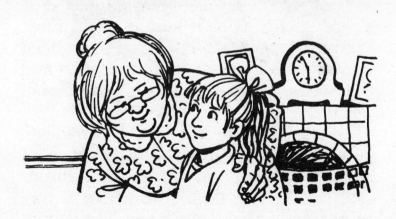

her homework. It was twenty to six. Lots of time before Granny went.

She went into the garden to play with Spanker the dog. They had a fine game, and then Bessie went indoors again. There was no sign of either her mother or Granny.

She pulled on her coat and ran into the street. The bus was at the corner – and there was Granny getting into it!

"Wait, wait!" shouted Bessie. But the

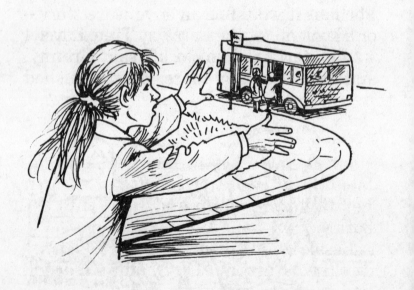

bus didn't wait. Mother waved goodbye to Granny and then turned to go home. She almost bumped into Bessie.

"Oh, Mummy, why didn't you tell me it was getting late!" said Bessie, almost in tears.

"Well, you know I'm not going to bother you any more," said her mother. "Now don't cry about it. It's not my fault or Granny's. It's your own."

Bessie was very upset. She wanted to catch the next bus, but Mother said no. So she had to go home.

When she went up to bed, her mother kissed her goodnight, but she didn't say "Now, hurry up" or "Don't be late for breakfast." She just said, "Sleep well, dear."

Bessie dawdled as usual. Nobody shouted up to her to hurry or she'd be late to bed. But after about half an hour her father came up and went into the bathroom.

Bessie hadn't had her bath. She went into the bathroom. "Oh Daddy – I haven't had my bath yet."

"Why not?" said Father. "You've been

up here for ages! I want the bathroom now. You will have to go without your bath. Sorry!"

"Bother!" said Bessie, and went to bed without the warm bath she loved.

Mother tapped on her door in the morning, "Half past seven, Bessie!"

Bessie turned over and went to sleep again. Her mother didn't come and rout her out as she usually did. She didn't even call up the stairs. So Bessie slept on.

She didn't get up until half past eight. Breakfast was at eight o'clock, so you can see how late she was. She flung on her clothes, forgot to wash, or to clean her teeth, drew a comb through her hair and ran downstairs. There was no breakfast on the table! The cloth was off, and the pot of flowers stood in the centre. What had happened?

"Mummy! Where's breakfast?" cried Bessie. "I'm in an awful hurry."

Her mother didn't say "You're late." She just put her head into the dining-room and said, "Breakfast? Oh, we had that at eight o'clock. I've cleared it away now. I can't start cooking again. If you want anything, cut yourself some bread and butter."

"But it's time I went to school," said Bessie, almost crying.

"I'm sorry, dear," said Mother. "But it's not my fault. I'm quite determined not to keep nagging you about being late."

Bessie had to cut herself some bread and butter, and put some marmalade on it. That was all she had for her breakfast. Then she rushed off to school. But she was late, of course.

"Bessie! Stay in at playtime," said Miss

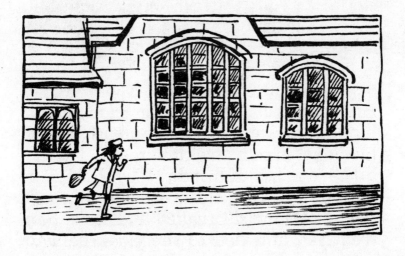

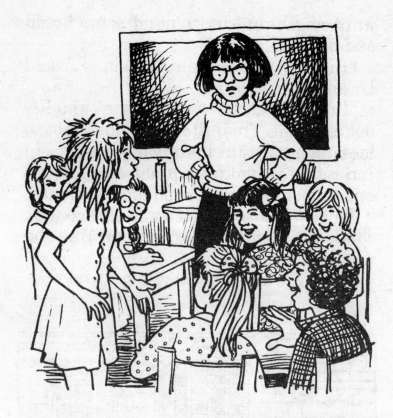

Brown, crossly. "And good gracious, child, haven't you washed or done your hair this morning? Go to the cloakroom at once. You are a dreadful sight. Why, half your buttons are undone. I'm ashamed of you."

The other girls giggled at Bessie. She went red and fled to the cloakroom to wash and do her hair. She had to stay in at playtime and write out *I must not be late* fifty times.

On the way home to lunch she saw some men laying some big drainpipes at the side of the road. She stopped to watch them. Then she saw some exciting looking puzzles in the toyshop and spent ten minutes making up her mind which one to buy next time she had any money.

Well, Bessie always did dawdle home, so this was nothing new. She was always late for lunch, and Mother usually greeted her with "You're late, Bessie!"

But this time she didn't. She was sitting having her lunch, all by herself, reading a book. She had some stewed apple and custard on her plate. She looked up as Bessie came in.

"Hello, Bessie. Have a good morning, dear?"

"Not very," said Bessie, rather sulkily. "I was late for school. Miss Brown was very cross, and I had to stay in at playtime."

"Well, I expect you will tomorrow, too," said her mother. "Still, you'll probably get used to it, won't you."

21

"I shan't be late tomorrow," said Bessie. "I won't have the girls laughing at me again as they did this morning. Horrid things!"

"Sit down and have some apple and custard," said Mother.

"Where's the meat?" asked Bessie, in surprise. "I thought you said that we were going to have cold meat and potatoes in their jackets and tomatoes today for our lunch."

"Yes, I did have that," said Mother. "But I didn't wait for you. I didn't know how late you would be. I had mine at quarter past one as usual. It's nearly quarter to two now. The first course is all cleared away."

"Am I only to have my pudding, then?" asked Bessie, ready to burst into tears. "I hardly had any breakfast!"

"I'm sorry, dear – but it wasn't my fault," said her mother. "Eat up your apple and custard. I told you I wasn't going to nag at you, or wait for you any more. You must come in as late as you please, but don't expect me to keep things hot for you."

Bessie ate her pudding, and sniffed miserably. Mother took no notice. She looked at the clock once, but she didn't say a word to Bessie. Bessie had a music lesson at a quarter past two. Well, well – she must be late for it, that's all!

And she was! She was ten minutes late, and when she got there she found her music teacher in a great rage, for he was a hot-tempered man.

"You have kept me waiting for ten

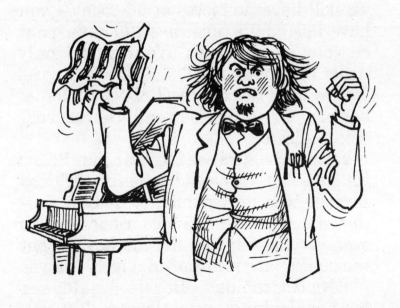

minutes, ten whole minutes!" he almost shouted at her when she went into the room. "What impertinence! I shall report you to the headmistress. Why did your mother not send you in time?"

Bessie said nothing. She could not tell this angry music teacher that her mother was tired of telling her to hurry up or she would be late. She went red and looked down.

"You cannot even say you are sorry, I suppose?" said the music teacher. "Now we will have no pieces at all today – you have wasted the time we could have spent on your pretty pieces. We will have only scales and arpeggios!"

How dull! But the teacher would not let her play anything else at all. He was very cross indeed.

You will be surprised to hear that Bessie got home in very good time for tea! You see, she was so very hungry by that time that she simply flew home for her tea. She even laid the table for her mother, so that she could have it more quickly.

"Good gracious, Bessie!" said her mother, looking quite pleased, "you are

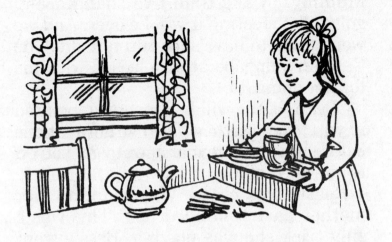

home nice and early – and it's such a help if you lay the table."

Bessie felt happier. She ate an enormous tea, and then actually helped to wash up. Then she did her homework. She looked at the clock. There was a Girl Guide meeting at six. She was a guide, and she wanted to go.

But at six she hadn't even changed into her Guide uniform! There she was, reading hard. Mother didn't say a word. She just went on with her knitting.

At half past six Bessie looked at the clock. "Gracious! Look at the time! Oh,

Mummy, by the time I've changed and got to the meeting it will be over. And we were going to have such fun tonight. The Captain won't be at all pleased with me for not going."

"I expect she will be most disappointed in you," said Mother. "You've always gone before because I've managed to get you off in time. What a pity!"

Bessie was cross. Why couldn't her mother have reminded her? This was a silly trick she was playing. Bessie went out into the garden and sat down in the shed. Now she had missed the meeting. Bother, bother, blow!

She began to mess about in the shed. She heard the supper bell ring, and began to tidy up all the things she had muddled. Then she found a flower catalogue and couldn't help looking at it. Oh, what lovely flowers people could buy for their gardens! When she was old enough she would buy this – and that – and that...

"Gracious! I forgot about supper!" she said suddenly, and tore indoors. She popped her head in at the dining-room. Father was there, having his supper with

Mother. Bessie took a hurried look at the table. Poached eggs! Ooooh!

She flew upstairs to wash her hands, do her hair and put on a clean dress. Alas, when she got down again, supper was over and Mother was clearing away. Bessie burst into angry tears.

Her father spoke to her sternly.

"If you want to make a scene and a noise, you can – but not down here. Go

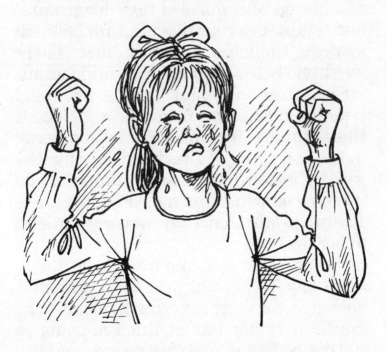

27

and howl in your bedroom. It's your own fault if you've missed your supper. You heard the bell. You'll probably miss breakfast tomorrow, too, and no doubt have to go without a bath again. Well, Mummy and I are just not going to hurry you up any more. Go and think about it a little."

Bessie went upstairs crying. She sat down on the bed. She had wanted to yell and stamp and make a fuss downstairs, just to upset her mother. But up here, all alone, it would be silly to do that. There was nobody to see, nobody to mind at all.

She sat and thought hard. A few tears trickled down her face again. "I don't think Daddy and Mummy love me any more," she said. "They're tired of me! I wonder if they'll like me any better if I do try to be punctual and help a bit more. I'm always so late that I can never even help to lay the table."

She dried her eyes and went down-stairs. "Mummy," she said, in a forlorn kind of voice, "I don't think you like me very much, or Daddy either. But I'm going to try and be better. Please love me again!"

"My dear child, of course we love you," said her father. "But I can't say I have liked you very much lately. Weshall always love you – but it would be so nice to like you, too. We shall, if you try to help in every way you can."

"Then I will," said Bessie. "I really will. And I'll begin by hurrying up when I go to bed, so that I can have a bath before you

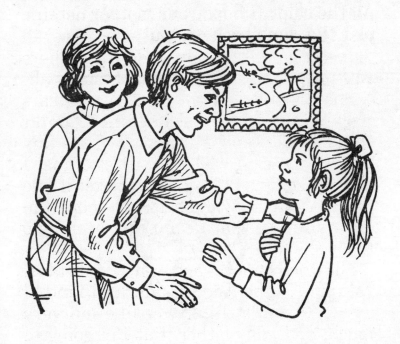

want to get into the bathroom, Daddy!"

And you'll hardly believe it, but Bessie really was different from that very evening. Down to breakfast in time, off to school early, back home early, and never once did her mother say again "You're late, Bessie!"

You know, it was really a very good idea of her granny's to tell her mother to stop saying hurry up, she was late, wasn't it? All the same, I hope your mother doesn't play the same trick on you!

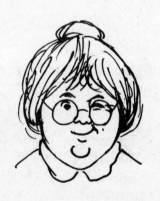

The Runaway Hen

"I'm just going to take Diana Susan for a ride in her pram, Mummy!" called Beth. "I won't be long. I'm only going down the end of the lane and back again."

"Well, post this letter for me, darling," said her mother, and Beth took it and slipped it under Diana Susan's pillow. Then off she went, out of the gate and down the lane.

She heard the cluck-luck-lucking of Mrs Dawkins' hens next door, and wondered if one of them had laid an egg. What a lot of cackling was going on! She peeped through the hedge to see why.

Goodness – there was a dog chasing the hens – and one hen was racing up the garden as fast as she could go with the dog after her. It was only a puppy, and meant to have a game, but the hen didn't know that! It fled out of the gate and ran down the lane.

"Puppy! Stop that!" shouted Beth. "What's your name now? I've forgotten. Oh yes – Tinker. Come here, Tinker. It's very, very bad to chase hens. You'll get into trouble if you do things like that. Go home!" and she pointed sternly down the road.

Tinker put his tail down and ran off at once. He knew quite well he had done wrong.

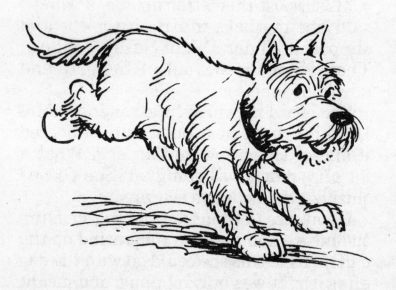

"It's all right, hens, he's gone!" Beth called through the hedge. Then she remembered the hen that had run down the lane. Had she better tell Mrs Dawkins about it? No, perhaps she had better see if she could find the hen. So down the lane she went, wheeling Diana Susan in her lovely blue pram, keeping her eyes open for the hen.

She couldn't see it anywhere. Whatever could have happened to it? Then she saw it, still running fast, going towards the main road. Beth called to it.

"Hen! Don't go there! There are cars whizzing along at sixty miles an hour! Come back, hen!"

But the hen took no notice at all. It was quite lost, it was afraid that the puppy was still chasing it, and it meant to run and run and run!

"Oh, you silly little hen," said Beth, pushing her pram as fast as she could. "If only you'd come back this way I could get behind you and shoo you home."

The hen still ran on and on, and at last came to the main road. A car whizzed by so quickly that the poor hen had quite a shock. She thought it must be a very big puppy.

Then another car came by, saw the hen and hooted at it.

The hen scuttled into the hedge. Yes, that must have been another puppy, because it said "parp-parp", and sounded very like the puppy's barking. The hen peered out of the hedge, wondering if it could make a dash for the other side of the road. Perhaps it would find the other hens there. It really didn't know where it was at all!

Just as Beth came up to where the lane met the main road the hen made a dash across it. A car whizzed by at the same moment, just avoiding the hen, but frightening it very much indeed. It sank down at the side of the road and drooped its head on to its chest. Beth left her pram and hurried over to the hen.

"Are you hurt?" she said. "Or just very frightened? Oh, you poor creature, you do look ill! Can you walk? If you can, I'll guide you home."

But the hen couldn't walk. It had had such a scare that it couldn't even stand. It

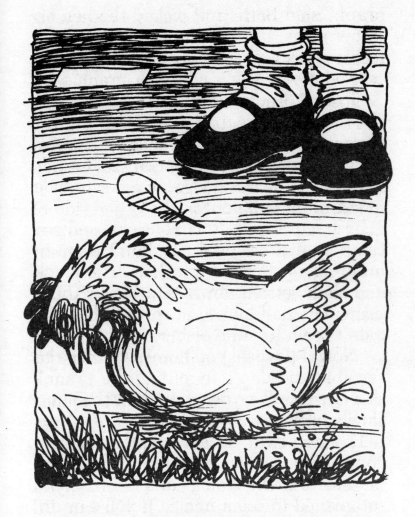

just lay there, looking very feathery and floppy, its eyes half closed.

"I'll carry you safely across, back to my

pram," said Beth, and picked the hen up in her arms. It felt quite heavy. It gave a feeble cluck and then lay quite still. Beth carried it over the road to her pram.

"I don't know what to do with you," she said. "You can't walk. And I can't carry you all the way home and wheel my pram too. Well – I hope my doll won't mind, but I'm afraid you'll have to ride in the pram too, hen!"

Beth moved her doll to one side and put the hen into the pram. It didn't seem to mind at all. It gave another little cluck and then settled down in a big feathery heap. The doll looked surprised, but she didn't seem to mind either.

"Now, I'll wheel you home, so please be sensible and don't fly out of the pram," said Beth, and she began to push the pram slowly back down the lane.

The hen shut its eyes and seemed to go to sleep. A man came hurrying by on his way to catch the bus and he was most astonished to see a hen in a doll's pram. He simply couldn't understand it, but he didn't say anything about it because he was already late for the bus.

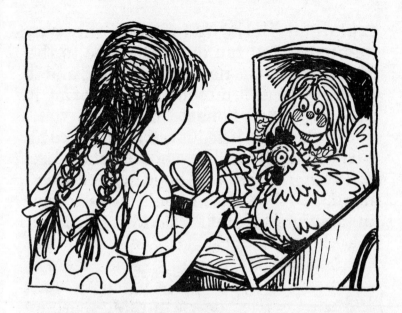

When Beth came near to her own front gate she saw her mother there talking to Mrs Dawkins, who had just come back from doing her shopping in the village.

"Oh, there you are, Beth," said her mother. "Have you had a – why ... good gracious me! *Whatever* have you got in your pram, Beth?"

"A hen!" said Mrs Dawkins. "And it looks like one of mine. Well I never! Do you usually take my hens for rides in your pram, Beth?"

"Oh no. But a puppy chased the hens,"

explained Beth. "And this one was frightened and ran down the lane to the main road. A car nearly ran over it and it felt ill, so I put it into my pram to bring it back home. I do hope it isn't hurt."

Mrs Dawkins lifted it out and looked at it carefully. It suddenly opened its wings and flung itself out of Mrs Dawkins' arms. It ran to join the others. "Not much wrong with it," said Mrs Dawkins,

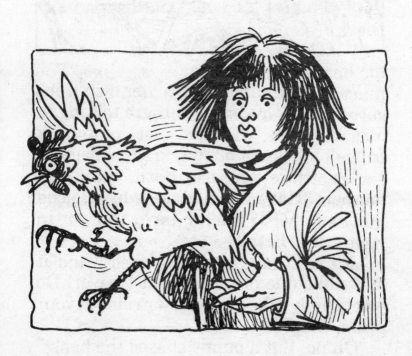

laughing. "Well, you are kind, Beth, to bring my hen home."

"Did you post my letter, dear?" asked Beth's mother.

"Oh dear – no!" said Beth. "The hen made me forget." She groped under the doll's pillow for the letter, and then gave a squeal of surprise. "Here's the letter – and something else as well. Oh *look*!" And she brought out a big brown egg and the letter too. How her mother and Mrs Dawkins laughed.

"Well! It wanted to give you a present for helping it," said Mrs Dawkins. "You must have that for your breakfast. I'm sure it will taste very good!"

It did, and Beth enjoyed it very much. It was nice of the hen, wasn't it? It sometimes lays an egg under the hedge between Mrs Dawkins' garden and Beth's and then Mrs Dawkins says Beth must have it, because she is sure that the hen means it for her. I expect she does, too!

Aha,
Mister Rat!

Mister Rat was a horrid fellow, cruel and cunning. He was always hungry, and he loved to find the nests of the birds and eat their eggs or young ones; he loved to sniff out the nests of the little dormice and gobble up their babies; he would even pounce on a young rabbit if it was all alone.

Mowdie the mole walked along the bottom of the ditch, weeping. She did not often walk above ground, for she loved to tunnel below the earth – but this morning she forgot about burrowing and scuffed along in the ditch.

"What is the matter?" asked Bobtail the rabbit, putting her pretty head out of a hole nearby.

"Oh, oh, Mister Rat has found my nest in the field," wept Mowdie the mole. "And he has eaten all my new little babies, he hasn't left me even one!"

"The wicked fellow!" said Bobtail, her nose woffling up and down. "It is time he was punished!"

"He should be eaten up himself!" said Spiky the hedgehog, uncurling himself where he lay at the bottom of the ditch. "I would eat him myself if I could find him! Yes, I would!"

There came the sound of a laugh in the hedge and all three creatures stiffened with fear. They knew that squealing laugh – it was the snicker of the rat himself!

"So you would eat me yourself, would

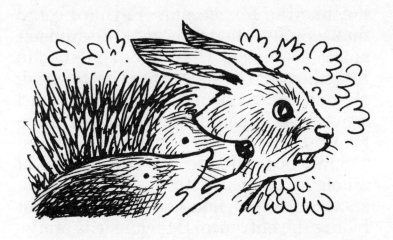

you?" said Mister Rat, putting his long nose out of the hedge. "Come along then, Spiky – come and eat me – or you, Bobtail – or you, Mowdie Mole! I'm here!"

Bobtail the rabbit disappeared down her hole. Mowdie the mole dug a tunnel in the ditch and sank into it as quick as lightning. Spiky the hedgehog curled himself up tightly and lay there quite still. The rat ran out and sniffed at him.

"You would not be so bold if you hadn't your armour of prickles!" he said to the hedgehog. "I will go and tell the fox to come and get you!"

He ran off. Spiky was full of fear. He did not like the fox, because Reynard could make Spiky uncurl by making himself smell so horrid that, in disgust, the hedgehog felt he must crawl away! And, as soon as he uncurled himself to crawl away from Reynard's dreadful smell, the fox would seize him!

Spiky hurried away and hid himself in a hole in the bank. It was only just big enough for him, and had a ferny curtain hiding the entrance. He felt safe there.

Mister Rat snickered softly to himself as

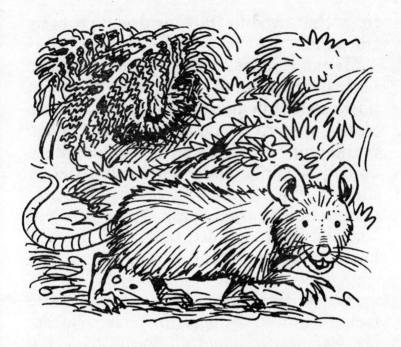

he ran about the hedge and slunk over the fields. He was king of the countryside! He was lord of all the creatures of the hedge and ditch! Soon there would be dozens more rats, for in nests here and there young ones were growing up. Aha! Mister Rat would teach them how to hunt for the nests of young mice, for the soft-spined young hedgehogs, for the nestlings in the hedges, for the lizards that darted about the sunny side of the bank and even for the frogs that lived in the long green grass by the pond.

Mister Rat was very fond of eggs. He had sucked dozens that he had found in nests in the hedgerow. He knew how to glance upwards as he ran along the hedge bank, and spy nests cleverly hidden here and there. Then up he would climb, stick his sharp grey nose into the nest and gobble up the eggs there. Many a robin, thrush, and blackbird had come back in haste to her nest and had found all her eggs gone.

Mister Rat even went down to the farm and stole the eggs in the hen-house. He had many ways of doing that. He would slink in to the house through a hole he knew well, and suck an egg in the nesting box. He would perhaps take one away with him too, to store it in his hole. How he managed to get it out of the nest without breaking it was marvellous! Then he would roll it over and over to the hole he had entered by. He would push it through this hole and then roll the egg to his nest. Sometimes two rats stole the eggs together. Then one would turn on

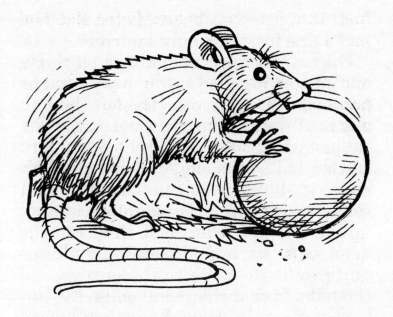

his back and hold the egg, and the other would pull him along. Ah, Mister Rat was the cleverest creature in the kingdom!

But one day he made a great mistake.

He was looking out for eggs as usual. He had eaten two belonging to the hedge-sparrow. They were as blue as the sky, but very small. The rat swallowed them but still felt hungry. He wondered if there were any eggs hidden in the ash tree that stood at the corner of the field. He knew it was partly hollow inside. Once a squirrel

45

had nested there. Then Mister Rat had had a fine feast of young squirrels!

Once a woodpecker had nested there, and Mister Rat had eaten every egg she had laid, till, in despair, she left the tree and flew away to the pinewood on the hill.

Yes – Mister Rat would see if any bird had nested in the ash tree this year! He ran to it, slinking along in the nettles that grew in the ditch. He climbed nimbly up the trunk. It was night-time, but the moon was out, and Mister Rat could see quite well. He came to the entrance of the hole. He sat there and sniffed.

Yes! Some bird was nesting there! The nest smelled of bird. Mister Rat caught sight of something white in the hole. An egg. He slipped down and got it. It was good! But only one egg! How disappointing! Never mind, perhaps there would be others in a day or two.

There were! In two days there was another egg. Mister Rat ate that. In a week's time there was another. Mister Rat ate that! Four days after that there was another – and Mister Rat had that too.

Now the bird who owned the hole in the

ash tree that year was a little owl. She was puzzled to find that her eggs disappeared so mysteriously. She was a young little owl and had never laid eggs before. She told her mate about it, and he hissed solemnly.

"Someone has been stealing them," he said. "Maybe it is the grey squirrel. He is a robber. Or maybe it is the thieving jackdaw. He loves other birds' eggs. We will find out."

It was the dormouse who told the little owl who the robber was.

"It is Mister Rat," said the quivering

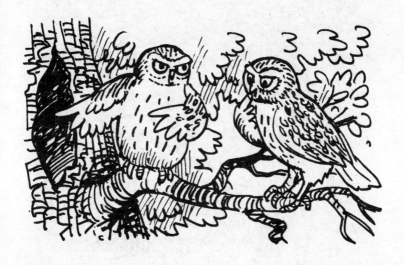

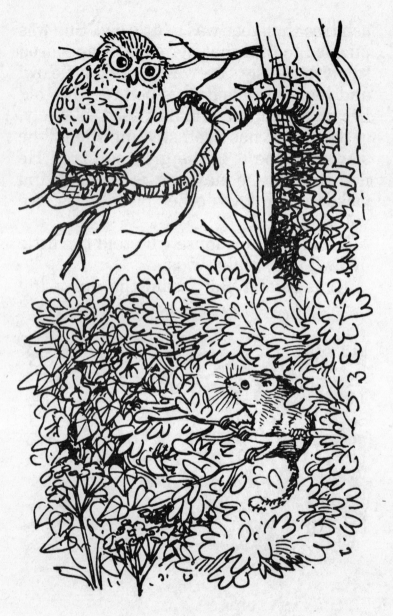

dormouse, from the shelter of the hedge. "Do not catch me, little owl, for I came to warn you of the robber. He stole my own little ones before they even had their eyes open. No one is safe – not even you, little owl!"

The little owls hissed angrily. So that was the robber who had stolen their eggs. This must be seen to.

"Are there many rats here?" said the owls.

"Oh, very many," answered the frightened dormouse. "His families are all growing well now – soon there will be a hundred and more rats running about here and we will all have to flee away. But they will follow us, so we shall be no better off!"

The owls hissed again and flew away. They knew what they were going to do. They flew to the big wood five miles away. Here many little owls nested and brought up their young ones – but lately there had been too little food for them, because the weasels had been about and eaten much of the food that the little owls wanted for their youngsters.

The two little owls called their friends. "Wee-oo, wee-oo, koo-wee-oo!" they called. "Koo-wee-oo!"

"Tvit, tvit!" answered their friends, and from far and near the little owls flew down to the tree where sat the two who had come from the faraway wood.

"Wee-oo, wee-oo!" said the two owls. "We come to tell you of much food in a wood far off. Bring your little ones there as soon as they are grown. There are rats by the score in the wood we know."

"We will come!" cried the owls. "Tvit, tvit!" And in three weeks' time, when the young rats were half grown, and were filling the countryside with fear and panic, a great flock of little owls came to the wood nearby. With them they brought their half-fledged youngsters, still downy – but with claws that could shut like a trap!

"Wee-oo, wee-oo!" called the little owls, as they flew about the wood. They saw the grass move a little in the pale moonlight – down swept an owl, and fixed a young rat in its claws. The rat squealed but could not get away. Another owl dropped like a

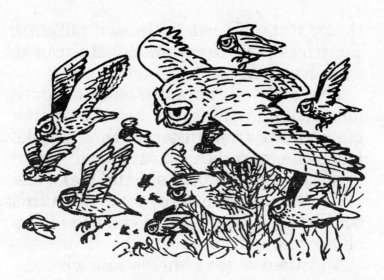

stone on to a full-grown rat and it had not
even time to squeal.

"Tvit, tvit! We have feasted well!" cried
the owls that night, as they flew to trees
to hide away for the daytime.

Mister Rat was scared to find that so
many owls were about. But he said to
himself, "Am I not king of the countryside,
and lord of the hedgerow? I am afraid of
nobody!"

He had a fine wife, and she had a litter
of seven small rats that Mister Rat was
proud of. His wife would only let him peep
at them, for she was afraid he might eat

51

them. Rats did eat their own children sometimes, she knew. Mister Rat ran to warn her to keep close-hidden.

The next night a little owl saw a movement in the grass near the pond. He pounced – and there was a scuffle! He had caught the mother-rat – and nearby in the hole he could hear the little ones squealing! He hooted to his comrades and they flew down and ate up all the young rats.

And then it was Mister Rat who ran along the ditch wailing and weeping for his lost family. But no one heeded him or

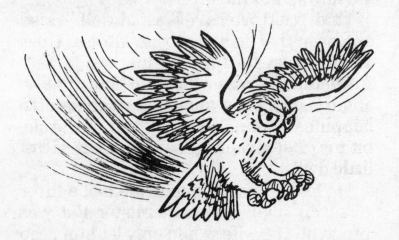

comforted him. The rabbit was glad. The mole laughed. The hedgehog grunted and said to himself, "Do as you would be done by, Mister Rat! You are being served in the same way as you served us!"

There was a squeal in the night. A little owl had caught Mister Rat himself! Ah, Mister Rat, that's the end of you!

"So it was you who ate all my eggs, was it!" cried the little owl, as she held Mister Rat in her sharp claws.

"Let me go and I'll never do such a thing again!" squealed the frightened rat.

"You will never do such a thing again anyhow!" said the owl, eating him up.

That was the end of Mister Rat – and as for the few rats that were left they fled from that part of the country in terror. And now the rabbit, the mole, the mice and the hedgehogs go about in peace and happiness. Aha, Mister Rat, you were a bit too clever when you ate the eggs of the little owl!

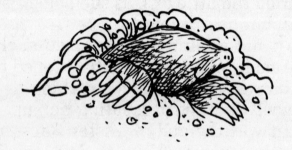

The Big
Humming-Top

Once upon a time there was a big humming-top. It was as tall as the biggest doll in the nursery, and as fat as two teddy bears put together – so you can guess what a big one it was!

It was shining silver, with a handle of red wood. When the handle was pressed down two or three times the top spun round and round on the floor, making a most wonderful humming noise – like this – Ooooomooooooooomoooooom!

The humming-top had a great friend, and that was Whiskers the cat. None of the other toys liked Whiskers because he could walk so quietly on his velvet pads that he very often made them jump. Also one day he had scratched the monkey, quite by mistake.

So the toys thought that the humming-top was wrong to make friends with Whiskers, and they didn't have very much to do with him. This hurt his feelings rather, because he was a friendly top and liked to talk to others. But it is very hard to talk to people who turn their backs on you and whistle when you speak to them – and that is what the rude monkey often did when the humming-top spoke to him.

One night an awful thing happened. A gnome came into the playroom through the window, and what do you think he did? He went straight to the toy sweet-shop and stole a bottle of little

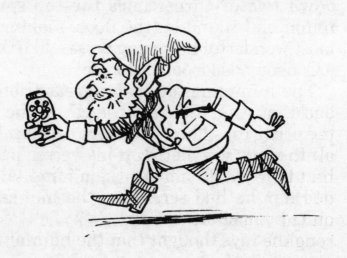

sweets! Yes, he did – took it right off the shelf, and ran off with it!

Well, the toys were very shocked and very angry. They all gathered together and talked about it.

"When Jane and Leslie come into the playroom tomorrow morning, they will see that one of their bottles of sweets is gone, and they will perhaps think that one of us toys took it!" said the big doll.

"How dreadful!" cried everyone, looking quite pale with horror. "Let's think what we can do to stop the gnome stealing any more!"

But, you know, they simply couldn't think of any way to stop him. The humming-top tried to speak once or twice, but the toys wouldn't listen to him. They just turned their backs on him as usual.

Now the next night the gnome came back again – and he took a little bottle of peppermints! Fancy that! Yes, in spite of all the toys rushing at him to stop him, he managed to get it and run off with it! He pushed the monkey over and trod on the biggest doll's toes. Oh, he was a rough fellow!

The toys were in tears. This was dreadful. Whatever were they to do?

The humming-top spoke loudly.

"If you will allow me to tell my friend Whiskers, the cat, I think perhaps I can find some way of frightening that robber gnome," he said.

"Pooh!" said the toys scornfully. "If we can't think of an idea, a cat won't be able to, that's certain."

"But Whiskers is very clever," said the top. "He might even come and hide here in the playroom at night."

"That wouldn't be any good!" said the monkey. "You know quite well that the gnome would smell him as soon as he got to the window! Gnomes have noses as sharp as dogs!"

The humming-top said no more – but when the gnome came again and took a third bottle of sweets, he made up his mind to talk to Whiskers at once.

Whiskers listened patiently, and when he heard how the gnome had taken the bottles he swung his tail from side to side angrily.

"It's no good me hiding in the room,"

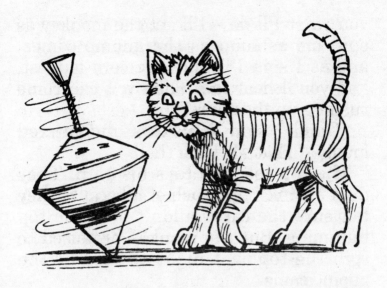

he said, "because the gnome would smell me there. If only there was some way of letting me know as soon as the gnome appears! I sleep in the kitchen, but as soon as I knew the gnome was in the playroom it wouldn't take me two seconds to come flying up the stairs to catch him!"

The top thought for a moment, and then he had an idea.

"Could you hear me hum if I hummed in the playroom and you were in the kitchen?" he asked.

"Easily!" answered the cat.

"Well!" said the top, eagerly, "I'll tell

you what I'll do – I'll get the monkey to spin me as soon as the gnome comes, and as I spin I'll hum my very loudest, and you'll hear me. Then you can come rushing up the stairs!"

"Good!" said Whiskers and purred loudly. "That's settled then."

The top told the toys his plan. They didn't think very much of it because they felt sure the cat wouldn't hear the top humming. But the monkey promised to spin the top that night as soon as the gnome came.

"We'll shut the sweet-shop up tight, and turn it round towards the wall," said the top. "The gnome will take a minute or two more trying to get the sweets then – and that will give Whiskers just time to come up the stairs!"

"He won't wake up, you'll see!" said the big doll.

Well, that night all the toys waited for the robber to come. They didn't have to wait long. Suddenly he appeared at the window, and jumped lightly down to the floor. He ran over to the toy sweet-shop.

At the same moment the monkey

took the big humming-top and pressed the handle up and down three times to make him spin. He spun – and dear me, you should have heard him hum! OOOOOOOM OOOOOOOMOOOOOOOM!

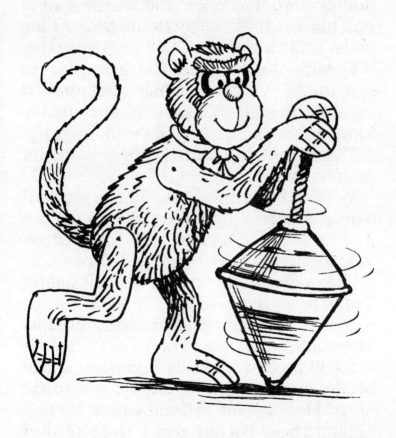

He hummed more loudly than he had ever hummed in his life – and Whiskers the cat, lying asleep in the kitchen, heard the humming and sprang to his feet. In a second he ran up the stairs and burst into the playroom. The gnome had just got the sweet-shop door open and was reaching out his hand for a bottle of pear-drops when he saw the cat.

Goodness me, what a shock he got! He ran to the window at once and jumped up on to the sill. Whiskers pounced after him. Out of the window he went, and the cat went out too. All the toys watched in delight.

What a noise there was in the garden! The cat hissed and spat at the gnome and he shouted at her. The toys longed to know what had happened. Presently Whiskers jumped in at the window again, looking very pleased with himself. In his mouth were the three missing bottles of sweets!

"Mew!" said Whiskers, dropping the bottles by the humming-top. "I made that nasty little gnome tell me where he had hidden these bottles and I went to find

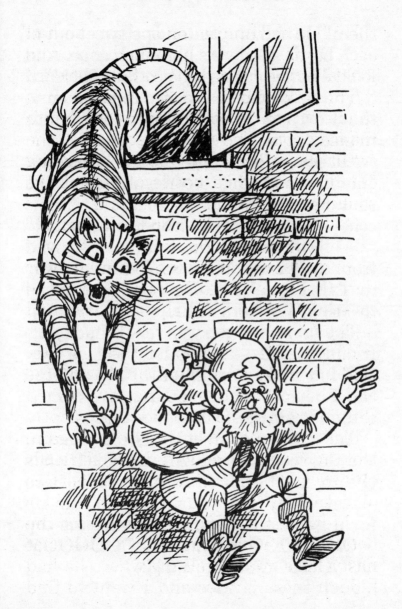

them! He had only eaten one sweet out of each bottle so there's not much gone. And look! I pulled his red coat off his back!"

The cat dropped a ragged red coat on to the floor, and the toys clapped their hands in glee.

"It serves him right," said Whiskers. "He had no right to come and steal like that. I scratched his shoulder and tore his coat – and I'm sure he won't come again!"

Well, of course, he didn't. He moved from the garden and went five miles away in Tall-Tree Wood. He was so afraid of meeting Whiskers again!

The humming-top was very proud of his friend the cat – and as for the toys they couldn't make enough of the top and the cat. They patted the top and stroked the cat, and said all sorts of nice things.

And now, of course, Whiskers sleeps in the playroom every night with his friends the toys. They love to have him there – and when they want to wake him up for a game they spin the humming-top – OOOOOOOOOOMOOOOOOOOOOM OOOOOOOOOOOOMMM!

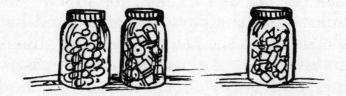

The Little
Sugar House

Mrs Biscuit kept a cake shop in Tweedle Village. All the boys and girls liked her shop because she had such exciting things in the window – gingerbread men, pastry cats and dogs, chocolate horses, and delicious iced cakes.

Mrs Biscuit would have been a very nice woman if only she hadn't told so many stories. She really didn't seem to know how to tell the truth.

"Was this cake baked today?" a customer would ask. "Is it quite fresh?"

"Oh yes, madam, it's just new," Mrs Biscuit would answer, knowing quite well that the cake was stale and dry.

Mrs Biscuit was mean, too. She never gave anything away if she could help it, not even broken bits of stale cake. She made those into puddings for herself.

The Little Sugar House

Now one day she thought she would make a very fine iced cake and put it right in the middle of her window.

"If they come and look at my iced cake they will see my buns, my biscuits, and other things," thought Mrs Biscuit, "and perhaps they will buy them."

So she made a beautiful iced cake with pink roses all round the edge. But she didn't know what to put in the middle.

"I think I'll make a little sugar house," she said to herself. "It shall have windows and a door and two chimneys. Everyone will be delighted to see it."

So she made a wonderful little house all out of sugar. She gave it two red chimneys, four windows, and a little brown door made of chocolate. She put pink sugar roses on the walls, and when it had set hard she popped it on the very top of her big cake. Then she put it into the window.

At first everyone came to look at it but after a little while they thought it was boring.

"Why don't you put someone into your house?" asked a little girl. "Houses are meant to be lived in, aren't they, even

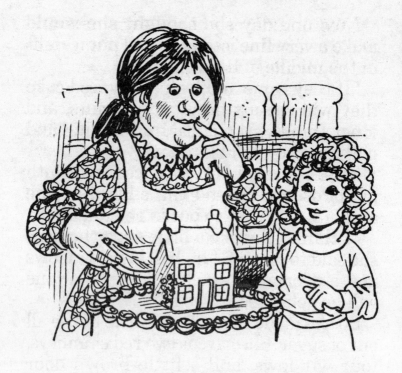

sugar houses? Why don't you go to the Very-Little-Goblins and ask one to live in your sugar house? Then people would come every day to see him opening the chocolate door and looking out of the sugar windows at the pink roses."

Well, Mrs Biscuit thought that was a very good idea. She put on her bonnet and went to where the Very-Little-Goblins lived in their mushroom houses.

"Would one of you like to come and live in a sugar house with pink roses on the walls?" she asked. "It's not like your mushroom houses, up one night and gone the next, so that you have to keep on moving. It stays on my big iced cake for weeks and weeks, and is very beautiful indeed."

The Very-Little-Goblins came out of their mushroom houses and stared at her. "We have heard that you tell stories," said their chief goblin. "We are very truthful

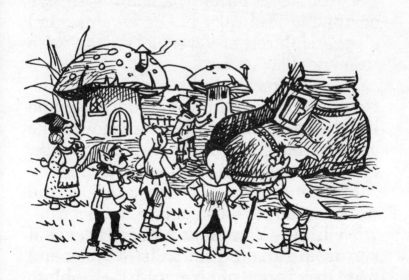

people, you know, and we couldn't live with anyone who didn't tell the truth."

"Of course I tell the truth!" said Mrs Biscuit, crossly. "Why, I've never told a story in my life!"

"Well, that's splendid," said the chief goblin, quite believing her. "I shall be very pleased to let my eldest son come and live in your little sugar house tomorrow."

"Thank you," said Mrs Biscuit, delighted, and she went home.

Soon everyone knew that one of the Very-Little-Goblins was coming to live on the big iced cake in the window, and all the children of Tweedle Village were tremendously excited.

The next day Twinkle, the Very-Little-Goblin, arrived at Mrs Biscuit's shop. She lifted him up on to the iced cake in the window and showed him the sugar house. He was simply delighted with it.

He opened the little chocolate door and went inside. He had brought no furniture with him, so he asked Mrs Biscuit if she would make him a little chocolate bed, two sugar chairs, and a chocolate table. He said he would put up curtains

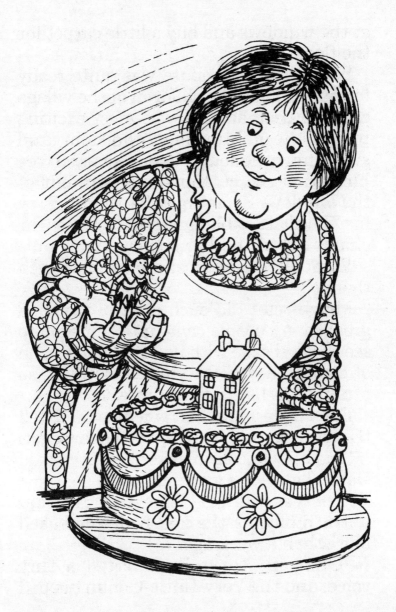

at the windows and buy a little carpet for the floor.

Soon the sugar house was quite ready for him, and all the children of the village came to peep at it. It was most exciting to see the goblin open the door and shake his little mats. It was lovely to see him draw the curtains and lean out of the window. Sometimes he would carry his chocolate table and one of his sugar chairs on to the big sugary space out-side the little house, and have his lunch there.

Mrs Biscuit did such a lot of trade. A great many people came into the shop to see the iced cake with its sugar house, and of course they had to buy something, so Mrs Biscuit began to be quite rich.

For a little while she remembered to tell the truth to people – and then she forgot.

"Is this chocolate cake fresh?" asked Dame Tippy one morning.

"Oh yes, quite!" Mrs Biscuit said untruthfully, for the cake had been baked more than a week ago.

"Oh, you storyteller!" cried a tiny voice, and the Very-Little-Goblin peeped out of the sugar house. "You baked that last week."

"Dear, dear, so I did!" Mrs Biscuit said crossly, very angry to hear the goblin's voice. "Take this one instead, Dame Tippy."

The next day a little girl came in for fresh buns. But Mrs Biscuit quickly took six stale ones from a tray at the back of the shop and popped them into a bag.

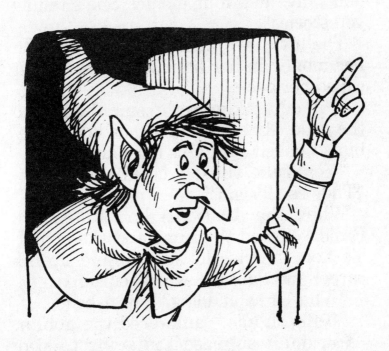

"These are nice and new," she said to the little girl.

"You naughty storyteller! They're as hard as bricks!" cried the little goblin, poking his head out of the window of the sugar house.

"You be quiet! These buns were only baked this morning," said Mrs Biscuit angrily.

"Oooh, the storyteller! Oh, little girl, don't give her your money. She's telling you stories!"

The little girl ran out of the shop with her money in her hand, but Mrs Biscuit called her back.

"I'm only joking with you," she said to the child. "See, here are some lovely new buns I baked early this morning."

"Yes, take those," cried the goblin. "They're all right."

When the little girl had gone, Mrs Biscuit turned to grumble at the goblin. To her surprise he was rolling up his carpet and taking down his curtains.

"What are you doing?" she asked.

"Going home," answered the goblin. "You don't suppose I'm going to stay

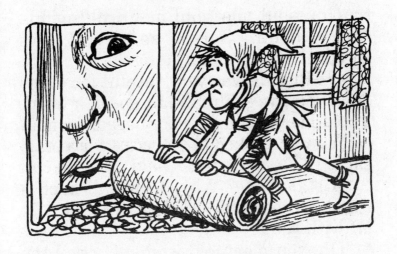

here with a nasty old woman who tells stories, do you? We Very-Little-Goblins hate that!"

"Oh, don't go," begged Mrs Biscuit. "Don't go! Everyone will wonder why you've gone."

"Oh no, they won't, because I shall tell them," said the goblin, tying up his carpet into a roll.

"Please, please, Goblin, stay with me. I'll make you a beautiful little garden seat out of chocolate and ginger if you'll stay," begged Mrs Biscuit. "And I won't tell stories any more, I promise."

"Well, if you do, I'll tell people the

truth," said the goblin, unrolling his carpet again. "So you be careful, Mrs Biscuit."

Mrs Biscuit was very careful for a few days and the goblin didn't speak a word. Then one morning, a poor beggar-woman came in and asked Mrs Biscuit for a stale cake.

"A stale cake? Why, I haven't such a thing in the place!" cried Mrs Biscuit. "Be off with you!"

"Oh, you mean old woman!" cried the

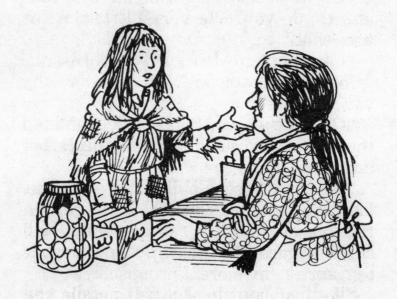

goblin's tiny voice, and he flung open his chocolate front door. "Where are those cakes you baked last Thursday that haven't been sold yet?"

"I've eaten them myself," said Mrs Biscuit in a rage. "Mind your own business!"

"You're a storyteller," said the goblin. "There they are up on that shelf. You give them to the poor beggar-woman this very minute, or I'll go back to Mushroom Town."

Mrs Biscuit dragged the cakes down, put them into a bag and threw them across the counter. The beggar-woman thanked her and went off with them.

Mrs Biscuit didn't care to say anything to the goblin, but she was very angry. He went into his sugar house and slammed the door. He was angry too, to think that anyone could be so mean.

That afternoon a thin little boy crept into the shop and asked for a stale crust. He was dreadfully hungry, and Mrs Biscuit stared at him crossly. Another beggar!

She was just going to say that she had

no stale crusts when she saw the goblin peeping at her out of one of the windows of his sugar house. She hurriedly took down half a stale loaf and gave it to the little boy.

He was so grateful that he took her plump hand and kissed it. It was the first time that Mrs Biscuit had been kissed for years, and dear me, she did like it! She suddenly smiled at the little boy, and felt sorry to see how thin he was. And then she took down a fine new chocolate cake, and gave it to him.

"Oh!" he said in delight. "You kind woman! Is that really for me?"

He went out of the shop singing. Mrs Biscuit looked at the place on her hand where the little boy had kissed it, and a nice warm feeling crept into her heart. It was really rather pleasant to be kind, she thought. She would try it again.

She looked up and saw a crowd of people looking in at her window. And she saw that the goblin was doing a strange, light-hearted little dance round and round the top of the cake, making all the passers-by stare in surprise.

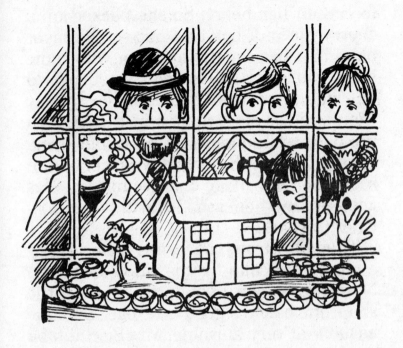

"What are you doing that for?" she asked in astonishment.

"Oh, I'm so pleased to see you do a kind act that I've got to dance!" said the tiny goblin. Everyone watched him, and soon quite a dozen people came in to buy cakes. Mrs Biscuit did a good morning's trade.

The next time someone came begging, Mrs Biscuit decided to be kind and generous again, to get the nice warm feeling in her heart. So she packed up a cherry pie in a box and put some ginger buns in a bag for the old man who came asking for a crust. He was so surprised and delighted that he could hardly say thank you. The little goblin threw open his door and began to sing a loud song all about Mrs Biscuit's kindness, and soon half the village came to hear it. Mrs Biscuit blushed red, and didn't know where to look.

Then Mr Straw, the farmer, came to buy a big ginger cake for his wife's birthday. Now, there were two ginger cakes in the shop, one baked a good time back and one baked that very morning. Mrs Biscuit took up the stale one and popped it into a bag.

"You're sure that's fresh, now?" said Farmer Straw. Mrs Biscuit opened her mouth to say untruthfully that it was, when she stopped.

No, that would be a mean, unkind thing to say, especially when the cake was for Mrs Straw's birthday.

"Er – well, no, this one isn't very fresh," she said. "I'll give you a fresher one, only baked this morning."

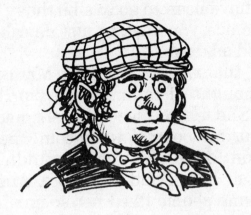

The little goblin, who was peeping out of his window, ready to cry out that she was a storyteller, gave a shout of delight.

"She's a truthful old dame!" he cried. "She's a kind old woman!"

"Dear me," said Farmer Straw, looking round. "That's your little goblin, isn't it? Well, it's nice of you to let me have the fresh cake, Mrs Biscuit, when you've got one that is not quite so fresh. I'm much obliged to you. Perhaps you'll be good enough to come to my wife's birthday party this afternoon?"

"I'd be very pleased to," said Mrs Biscuit, thankful that she hadn't given him the stale cake – for how dreadful it would have been to go to a birthday party and see everyone eating a stale cake she had sold as fresh?

Well, that was the last time Mrs Biscuit ever thought of telling a story or being mean. She felt so nice when she had told the truth or been kind to someone that she soon found she simply couldn't tell a story or be unkind any more. And in a short time people liked her so much that they always bought their cakes and pies from her, and she became rich enough to buy a little cottage and go there to live.

She took the iced cake with her, with the little sugar house on top. She put it on a table in the front window to remind her of the days when she had kept a cake shop – and would you believe it? – that Very-Little-Goblin is still there, shaking his carpet every day and opening his windows to let in the sunshine!

That shows she is still a truthful, kind old dame, and if you ever pass her cottage and see the iced cake in the window, with the little sugar house on top, don't be afraid of knocking at her door and asking if you may see the Very-Little-

Goblin. Mrs Biscuit will be delighted to show you round.

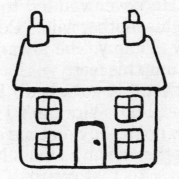

The Boy Who
Wouldn't go to Bed

Timothy was such a naughty boy at
bedtime. He never wanted to go to bed,
and when his mother said, "Put your toys
away now, Timmy," he always began to
cry and stamp his feet.

"I don't want to go to bed!" he shouted.
"Why must I go? Why can't I stay up all
night? I'm not sleepy. Let me stay up!"

And Mother always said, "No, Timmy
dear, you can't stay up. Little boys
must go to bed early. Nobody stays up
all night."

One night Timmy was so very naughty
about going to bed that his mother really
didn't know what to do with him. You
should have heard how bad he was! He
kicked all his bricks round the nursery, he
stamped on his best soldier, he shouted at
his mother, and tried to slap her when she

made him pick up his toys. In the middle of it all, in came Timothy's father to see what was the matter. When he heard Mother's story, he looked very serious.

"Very well, Timmy," he said, "you shall do what you want. We won't bother with you any more this evening. You shall stay up all night if you want to." Stay up all night! Timmy could hardly believe his

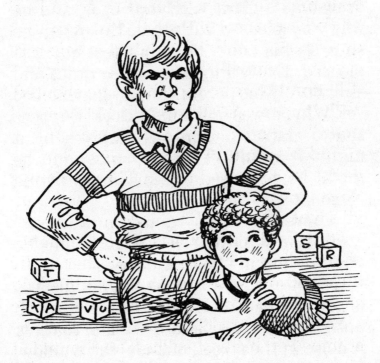

ears! Good! He had got his own way at last. His parents went out of the room and shut the door. Timmy was left alone in the playroom and his parents went downstairs.

He had a lovely time until eight o'clock, building an enormous tower with his bricks. Then until nine o'clock he drew in his drawing-book. The last thing he drew was a giant with four eyes, and he was very pleased with that. But when he shut up his book, he didn't feel quite so pleased. Everything seemed so quiet and still. Surely his parents hadn't gone to bed yet! Why, it was only nine o'clock! Suppose that a giant came into the playroom at night! It wouldn't be very nice, and he might be surprised to see Timmy sitting up so late.

"There aren't any giants nowadays," said Timmy to himself. "What shall I do now? I'll get my book and read."

He got out his big book of animals and began to read it. He liked it very much until he came to a picture of a lion roaring. A noise in the street, outside the window, suddenly made him jump.

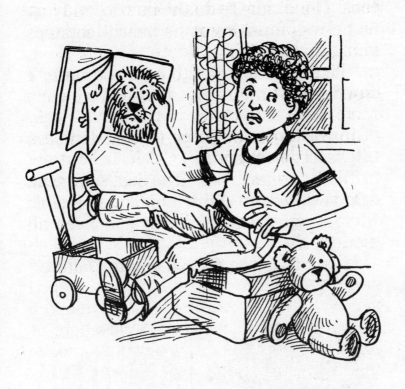

"I quite thought it was a lion for a
moment," said Timmy, shutting up his
book. "It's ten o'clock – I'll get out my big
puzzle and do it on the rug."

He took his box of jigsaw puzzles from
the toy cupboard and emptied the bits on
to the rug. Timmy felt rather cold, so he
sat as near the radiator as he could. It

took a long time to do the puzzle, and just as he was finishing it he heard footsteps going up the stairs.

"That's Jane going to bed," he said. "I wonder if Mummy and Daddy have gone too."

Just then the door opened and Jane, his big sister, looked in.

"Well, Timmy, I'm off to bed," she said. "Do you want to come too, like a sensible little boy, or shall I leave you here all alone?"

"I'm not going to bed tonight, Jane,"

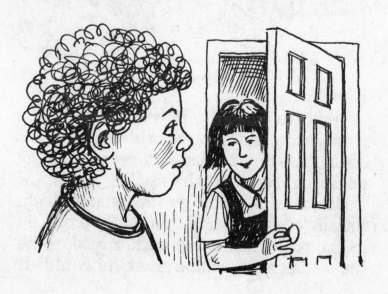

said Timothy. "Mummy said I could stay up all night, and I'm going to."

"Oh, very well," said Jane, and she closed the door and went into her bedroom. Timmy heard her running the water in the bathroom, and then heard the creak of her bed as she got into it. He opened the playroom door and looked out. Everything was dark. There wasn't a light on anywhere.

"The house will soon be asleep too," said Timmy. "I shall be the only one awake!"

He went back to the radiator, which was getting cold now, and sat down to his puzzle again. He put a few pieces of the puzzle into their places, and then suddenly he yawned. His eyes felt as if they had sand in them, and he rubbed them hard. He wasn't going to go to sleep, not he! He was going to stay up all night!

He didn't want to do any more puzzles. He put all the pieces away, and then sat down in his little chair. How quiet the house was! There wasn't a sound to be heard.

Crack! What was that? Timmy sat up straight and listened. *Crack!* There was the noise again. Why, it was the big toy-cupboard making that noise. It sometimes did it in the daytime, but it didn't sound so loud then. It sounded very loud indeed at night.

Then the old wicker-chair in the corner creaked all by itself, and Timmy was very much surprised. Could somebody be sitting down in it? And whatever could that be, scampering over the floor? Ooh, he didn't like it!

Poor Timmy! It was only a little mouse come out to pick up the crumbs on the floor. When it saw Timmy it was frightened – but not nearly so frightened as Timmy was! He didn't know it was only a mouse. He couldn't think what it was!

Then the wind began to blow outside, and it puffed round the window and said "Hoo-hoo-hoo," in a very loud voice. How Timmy jumped with fright!

"Hoo-hoo-hoo," said the wind. "HOO-HOO-HOO!"

"I wish I was in bed," thought Timmy, "I wish I was cuddled down fast asleep under my warm blankets. It's cold in here, and I'm sleepy and frightened – but I daren't go to sleep in case the wind comes right in through the window and shouts in my ear."

He sat curled up in his chair and listened to the wind blowing. A twig tapped on the window and he didn't like that at all. And then suddenly he heard the front door being opened!

"Burglars!" thought poor Timmy, and

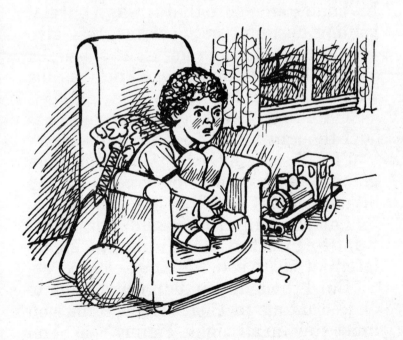

he was so frightened that he couldn't move a finger.

But it wasn't burglars! It was his mother and father coming home late from a party. They hadn't gone to bed, they had been out all the evening!

Mother ran upstairs to see if Timmy was still up, and when she opened the playroom door, what a sleepy, frightened little boy she saw! He was curled up in his chair, quite sure that it was a burglar coming upstairs, and dear me, how glad he was to see his mother!

He ran to her and hugged her as if he would never let her go.

"Oh, I'm so glad it's you!" he said.

"I thought I'd just pop in and see how you felt," said Mother. "Daddy and I are going to bed now, but you want to stay up all night, don't you?"

"Oh no, please, no," said Timmy. "I want to go to bed. I don't like staying up late. Put me to bed, Mummy, please."

"But I thought you didn't like going to bed," said his mother. "Oh, I think you must stay up all night, Timmy dear. You said you wanted to, you know."

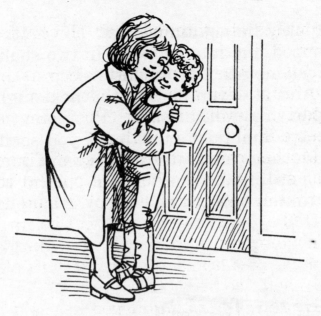

"Well, I don't want to now," said Timmy. "Let me go to bed, Mummy. I promise I'll never, never be naughty about going to bed again, if only you'll put me to bed now."

"Very well," said his mother. "I'll put you to bed – but mind, Timmy, if ever I have any more naughtiness at bedtime, you will certainly stay up all night – and you won't like that at all, will you?"

"No, I shan't," said Timmy, and goodness me, you should have seen how quickly he got undressed! His mother popped him into bed, and in two shakes of a lamb's tail he was fast asleep.

And at seven o'clock the next night, when his mother said, "Put your toys away, Timmy, it's bedtime!" you should have seen him hurry. He wasn't going to miss his bedtime again! No, he was definitely going to bed!

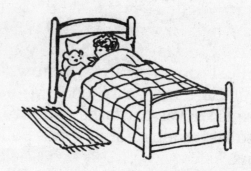

You Bad
Little Dog

John and Fiona took their little dog Wuff down to the sands with them. It was such a lovely beach for little dogs, as well as for children!

There was fine golden sand stretching right down to the very edge of the sea and tiny waves to play in, and warm pools to bathe in. Wuff liked it as much as John and Fiona did.

That morning the children had their spades with them. They meant to build the biggest castle on the beach – bigger even than Tom and Peter and Dick had built the week before. That one was so big that the sea just couldn't knock it all down, but left half of it for the next day.

Wuff wanted to build, too – but as his idea of building was to dig enormous holes and scatter the sand all over the place,

John and Fiona wouldn't let him help.

"No," they said. "You keep away today, Wuff. You're just being a nuisance. As soon as we get a heap built up you scrape a hole in it. That's not building!"

So Wuff went a little way away and sat down sadly to look at the two children building. Soon an old man came and sat down in a deckchair nearby. He opened his newspaper and began to read. He wasn't near the children, and they took no notice of him at all.

But Wuff was quite near him, sitting still, feeling rather bored. He suddenly smelled rather a nice smell. He got up and ambled round and about, sniffing at the sand. Ah – here was the smell!

Someone had left a bit of cake in the sand and Wuff felt that he really must dig it up. So he began to scrape violently with his front paws. Up into the air went great showers of fine sand – and the old man found himself being covered from head to foot.

"Stop it," he growled to Wuff. But Wuff was too happy to hear. He was getting near that bit of cake! Up flew some more

You Bad Little Dog

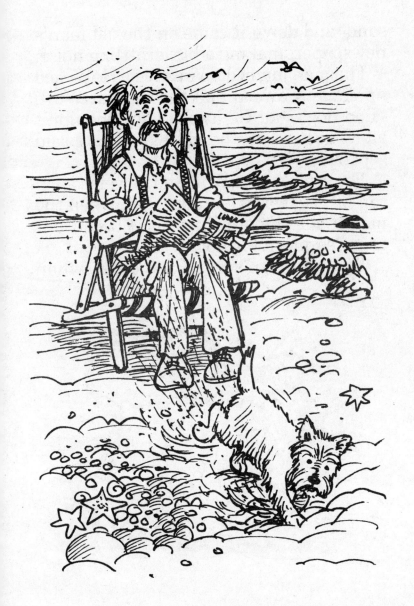

sand, and down it came on the old man's newspaper, making a little rattling noise.

The man jumped up in anger. He picked up some seaweed and threw it at Wuff. "Bad dog, you! Go away! They shouldn't allow dogs on the beach. I've always said so! Grrrrr!"

The seaweed hit Wuff and he yelped and ran off. He was frightened, too, when the man made the growling noise because it sounded like a big dog!

The children were very cross when

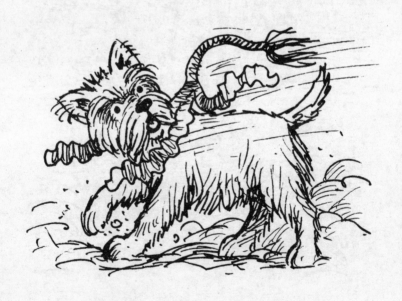

they saw the old man throwing seaweed at Wuff and heard him shouting. "Just because Wuff threw some sand over him by mistake!" said Fiona.

"You take that nasty little dog of yours away from this beach!" shouted the old man. "If he comes near me again he'll be sorry!"

Fiona and John were upset. They left their castle half-finished, and Wuff left the hidden bit of cake, and they all went right to the other end of the beach. They began to build another castle, but it was lunch-time before they had done very much. They were very disappointed.

"Now the sea will be able to sweep away all we've done," said John. "The castle ought to be twice as high if there's to be any left when the tide goes out again."

They went home to lunch, Wuff dancing round their legs. The old man had gone, too. The deckchair was empty and the deckchair-man was just about to pile it with all the others, so that the sea wouldn't take it away when the tide came in.

Next morning the children went down

to the beach again. Wuff went, too. The old man was there in his chair, and John and Fiona decided not to go too near him.

"We really must work hard this morning," said John. "Granny is coming this afternoon and it would be lovely to show her a really magnificent castle, bigger than any on the beach."

"Wuff," said Wuff, quite agreeing.

"You go away till we've finished," said Fiona to Wuff. "Look, take your ball and go over there to play with it. You aren't much good at castles, Wuff."

Wuff took his ball. But it was really very boring to play by himself, and he suddenly remembered the bit of cake he had smelled in the sand the day before. Suppose it was still there? He could perhaps find it this time. He began to run about, sniffing, to see if he could smell it again.

He came near to the old man and stopped. Why, here was the man who growled like a dog and threw seaweed at him! He'd better be careful or he might be hit by another piece of soggy seaweed.

The old man sat quite still. He didn't

speak or move. Wuff sniffed the air. Was he asleep? When people were asleep they didn't shout or throw things. He could look for that bit of cake if the old man was asleep.

He *was* asleep – fast asleep in the warm sun. His newspaper lay on his knee. The wind tugged at it, trying to get it.

Wuff began to scrape in the sand for the bit of cake. A few grains flew into the air and fell on the newspaper on the man's knee. He didn't stir at all. The wind suddenly blew strongly and the newspaper

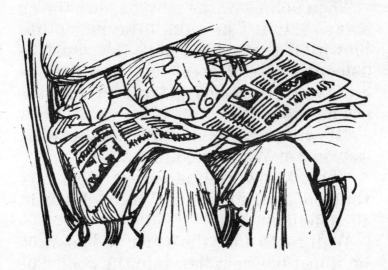

flapped hard. It flapped itself right off the man's knee on to the sand.

Wuff stopped burrowing and looked at it. Soon that newspaper would blow right away. He didn't know why people liked newspapers so much, but he knew they did. This one belonged to the old man. Did he want it? Would he mind if his paper blew right into the sea?

The children suddenly saw Wuff near the old man again. They called to him. "Wuff! Wuff! Come away from there! You know you got into trouble yesterday."

Then John saw the newspaper blowing away. "Look," he said, "the paper has blown off that man's knee. He must be asleep. There it goes! Oh, won't he be cross when he wakes up and finds that the sea has got it!"

"It will serve him right for throwing seaweed at Wuff," said Fiona.

"There goes the paper – almost into that pool," said John. "Wuff – fetch it, then, fetch it, boy!"

Wuff raced after the paper and pounced on it just before it flew into the pool! The old man, awakened by the shouting, sat

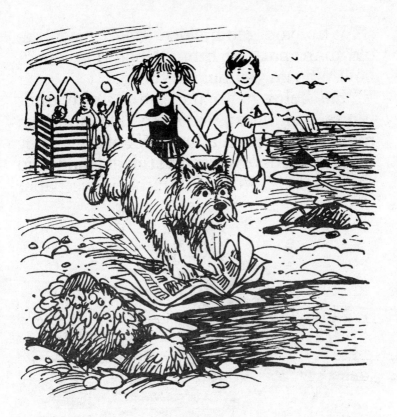

up and looked round to see what the noise was about.

He saw Wuff pouncing on his paper – and then the little black dog turned and ran all the way back to the old man with it and put it down by his feet, just as he did when he ran after a ball and took it back to the children.

"Why, you good, clever dog!" said the old man, patting him. "Good dog, good boy! Who do you belong to?"

"He belongs to us," said John and Fiona, coming up, astonished to find the man making such a fuss of Wuff.

"Well, he's a very clever dog," said the

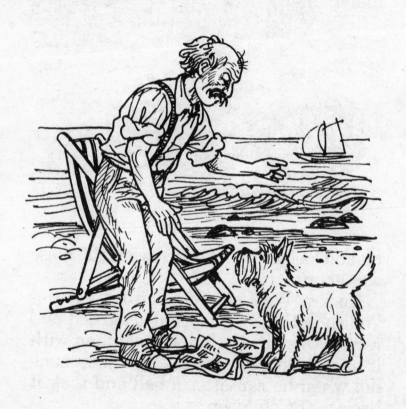

man, folding up his newspaper. "Not a bit like a horrid little dog I saw here yesterday, who threw sand all over me. Oh, he was a dreadful little thing!"

"Wuff!" said Wuff, trying to tell the man that yesterday's dog and today's were exactly the same. But the man didn't understand.

"I must buy a bone for this good dog," said the man. "Does he like bones?"

"Yes. But he likes ice creams even better," said Fiona.

"Well, well – what good taste he has!" said the man, getting up. "Shall we all go and buy ice creams? Come along, then."

They went to the ice cream man and the old man bought four ice creams, one for each of them and one for Wuff too, of course. Then he went down to look at the castle the children were building.

"I'd better help you with this," he said. "I can see you won't finish it if I don't. We'll make it the biggest one ever seen!"

They finished their ice creams, Wuff too, and set to work. My goodness me, how the old man could dig! You should have seen that castle when it was finished. All the children on the beach came to admire it.

"Well, thank you very much indeed for the ice creams and the digging," said John and Fiona.

"I'll help you again tomorrow," said the man, smiling. "Goodbye – and goodbye, little dog. I'm glad you're not like the nasty little dog I shouted at yesterday!"

Off he went. The two children looked at one another. "Well! He may think Wuff is a different dog – but honestly he's a different man, too!" said John. "Who would have guessed he could be so nice?"

It was funny, wasn't it? What a good thing Wuff ran after his paper!

The Enchanted Egg

Now once upon a time Sly-One the gnome did a marvellous piece of magic that nobody had ever done before.

He stirred together in a golden bowl, lit by moonlight, many peculiar things. One of them was the breath of a bat, another was a snippet of lightning, and yet another was an echo he had got from a deep cave.

He didn't quite know what would come of all these strange things and the dozens of others he had mixed together – but he guessed it would be something very powerful indeed.

"Whatever it is, it will bring me greatness and power," thought Sly-One, stirring hard. "I shall be able to do what I like."

Sly-One was not a nice person. He was mean and unkind and sly. Nobody liked him, though most people were afraid of him because he was very cunning. But he did not use his brains for good things, only for bad ones.

He stirred away for two whole hours, and soon the curious mixture in the golden bowl began to turn a colour that Sly-One had never in his life seen before. Then it began to boil! As it boiled, it twittered!

"Very strange indeed," said Sly-One to himself, half scared. "A very curious twitter indeed. It sounds like the twitter of the magic hoolloopolony bird, which hasn't been seen for five hundred years. Surely this magic mixture of mine isn't going to make a hoolloopolony bird! How I wish it was, because if I had that bird I could do anything I liked. It is so magic that it has the power to obey every order I give it. Why, I could be king of the whole world in a day!"

But the mixture didn't make a bird. It twittered for a little while longer, turned another curious colour, and then boiled away to nothing.

Or almost nothing. When Sly-One, disappointed, looked into the bowl, he saw something small lying at the bottom of it. It was a tiny yellow egg, with a red spot at each end.

Sly-One got very excited indeed when he saw it. "It's not a hoolloopolony bird – but it's the egg! My word, it's a hoolloopolony's egg! Now, if only I can get it hatched, I shall have one of those enchanted birds for my very own – a

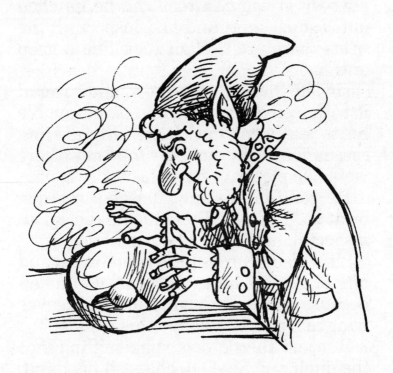

slave that can obey any order I think of making!"

He picked up the egg very gently. It hummed in his fingers and he put it back into the bowl. How was he to get it hatched?

"I'd better find a bird's nest and put it there," thought Sly-One. "A really fine nest, safe and warm and cosy, where this enchanted egg can rest and be hatched out. I must go round and inspect all the nests there are. I shall soon find a good one."

He left the egg in the bowl and covered it with a silver sheet. Then he put on his boots and went out. It was the nesting season for birds, and Sly-One knew there would be plenty of nests to choose from.

He soon found one. It was a robin's, built in a ditch. Sly-One walked up to inspect it, and kneeled down beside it.

"It's made of moss and dead leaves and bits of grass," he said. "It's well-hidden because there are plenty of dead leaves lying all round. Perhaps this will do."

But just then a dog came sniffing into the ditch and Sly-One changed his mind.

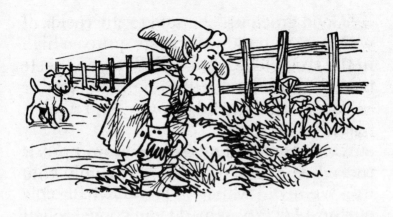

"No, no! It's not a good place for a nest, if dogs can tramp about near it. Why, that dog might easily put his paw on the enchanted egg and smash it, if I put it here!"

So he went off to find another nest. He saw some big ones high up in a tree and he went up to look at them. They were rooks' nests, big and roomy.

"They look safe enough, high up here," thought Sly-One. "Made of good strong twigs too. No dog could tread on these high nests!"

He sat down in one to see what it was like. Just then a big wind blew and the tree rocked the nest violently. Sly-One was frightened. He climbed out quickly.

111

"Good gracious!" he said to the rooks. "I wonder you build your nests quite so high in the trees. The wind will blow your nests to and fro and out will come your eggs!"

"Caw!" said a big rook, scornfully. "Don't you know that when a stormy summer is expected we build lower down and when a calm one comes, we build high up? We always know! No wind will blow our nests down. Why do you come to visit them, Sly-One? You don't lay eggs!"

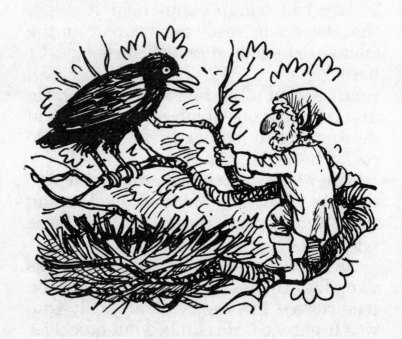

Sly-One didn't answer. He slid down the tree and came to a hole in the trunk. He put his head in and saw a heap of sawdust at the bottom. It was a little owl's nest. Sly-One felt about, and didn't like it.

"Not at all comfortable for an enchanted egg," he thought. "A good idea though for a nest, deep down in a tree-hole. Very, very safe!"

"If you want another kind of hole, ask the kingfisher to show you his," hissed the little owl. "Do you want to hide from your enemies or something, Sly-One? Then the kingfisher's nest is just the place!"

So Sly-One went to the brilliant kingfisher who sat on a low branch over the river and watched for fish. "Where is your nest?" asked Sly-One.

"Down there, in that hole in the bank," said the kingfisher, pointing with his big, strong beak. "Right at the end. You'll see it easily."

Sly-One found the hole and crawled into it. At the end was a peculiar nest, made of old fish-bones arranged together. It smelled horrible.

"I feel sick!" said Sly-One, and crawled

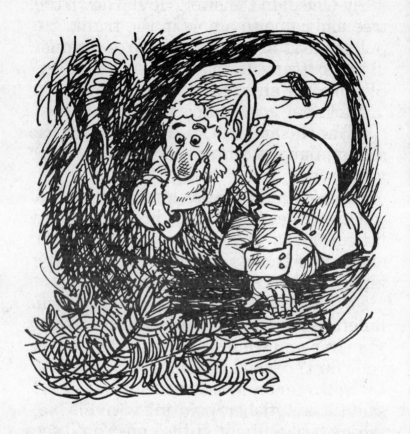

out quickly. "Fancy making a nest of smelly old fish-bones! Certainly I shan't put my precious enchanted egg there!"

He saw the house martins flying in the air above him and he called to them. "Where are your nests? I want to find a nice, cosy, safe one to put something precious in."

"See that house?" said a house martin, flying close to him. "See the eaves there? Well, just underneath we have built our nests. They are made of mud, Sly-One."

"What!" said Sly-One, looking up at the curious mud-nests in amazement. "Are those your nests – those peculiar things made of mud, stuck against the walls of the house? They might fall down at any minute! And fancy living in a mud-nest! No, that won't do, thank you."

"Coo-ooo," said a woodpigeon, flying near. "Would my nest do for you, Sly-One? I don't know what you want it for – but I have a very nice nest indeed."

"What's it made of?" asked Sly-One.

"Oh – just two sticks and a little bit of moss!" said the woodpigeon, and showed Sly-One the tree in which she had built her nest.

"Why, you can see right through it, it's so flimsy!" said Sly-One in horror, thinking that his enchanted egg would certainly fall through the pigeon's nest, and land on the ground below.

Then he went to the lark, but the lark said that she just laid her eggs in a dent in the ground. She showed him her eggs, laid in a horse's hoofmark in a field.

"Ridiculous!" said Sly-One. "Why, anyone might run over those eggs and smash them. A most stupid place for a nest. I want somewhere that nobody could possibly tread in."

"Well," said the lark, offended, "why not go up to the steep cliffs, then, where some of the sea-birds lay their eggs. Look, do you see the great bird there? He's a guillemot. Call him down and ask him to carry you to where he puts his eggs. They are up on the steep cliffs, where nobody can even climb."

Soon Sly-One was being carried on the guillemot's strong wings to the high cliff. There, on a ledge, was a big egg, laid by the guillemot.

"Do you mean to say you just put it there on this ledge?" said Sly-One. "It might fall off at any moment, when the wind blows strongly."

"Oh no it won't," said the guillemot. "Do you see its strange shape? It's made

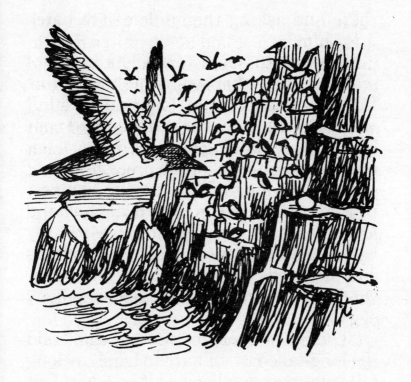

that way, narrow at one end, so that when the wind blows, it just rolls round and round in the same place. It doesn't fall off."

"Oh," said Sly-One. He thought of his enchanted egg. No, that wasn't the right shape to roll round and round. It would certainly roll right off the cliff if the wind blew. It wouldn't be any good putting it there and asking the guillemot to hatch it for him.

He went to see a few nests made of seaweed, that other sea-birds showed him. But they smelled too strong, and he didn't like them. He went back to the wood near his home, wondering and wondering what nest would be best for his precious egg.

He saw a long-tailed tit go to her nest in a bush. He parted the branches and looked at it. It was a most extraordinary ball-shaped little nest, made of hundreds and hundreds of soft feathers! Perhaps it would be just right for the hoolloopolony egg.

"There's no room for another egg," said the long-tailed tit. "I have to bend my long tail right over my head as it is, when I sit in my ball of a nest. When my eleven eggs hatch out, there won't be any room at all!"

Then Sly-One met a big grey bird, with a barred chest. The bird called "Cuckoo!" to him and made him jump.

"Oh, cuckoo, so you're back again," said Sly-One. "Where's your nest?"

"I don't make one," said the cuckoo. "I always choose a good, cosy, safe nest to put my eggs in, belonging to somebody else. I don't bother about building!"

"Well," said Sly-One, "as you're used to finding good nests for your eggs, perhaps you can help me. I want one for an enchanted egg. I want a good safe nest, with a bird who will hatch out my egg and look after the baby bird for me, till it's old enough to come to me and do magic spells."

"Ah, I'm the one to help you then," said the cuckoo at once. "I can pick up eggs in my beak easily. I've just put an egg into a wagtail's nest. Wagtails make good

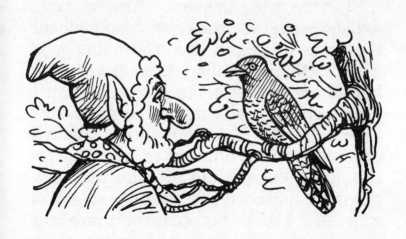

parents. I'll put your enchanted egg there too, if you like."

And that's just what the cuckoo did. Sly-One fetched the little egg from the golden bowl, and the cuckoo took it in her beak and popped it into the wagtail's nest up in the ivy. She showed Sly-One her own egg there too.

"The wagtail had four eggs of her own," she said. "I took one out and dropped it on the ground when I put my own there. I've taken a second one out now to make way for your enchanted egg. The wagtail will sit on all four eggs and keep them warm, mine, yours, and two of her own."

Sly-One was pleased. "Now my egg will be safe," he thought. "How clever the cuckoo is! She's used to finding good nests for her eggs. I ought to have asked her advice at first, instead of wasting my time inspecting all those other nests."

One day Sly-One went to see how his egg was getting on, and to his surprise the cuckoo's egg had already hatched, though it had been laid after the wagtail's eggs. And also to his surprise, there was only one wagtail egg in the nest, besides his own enchanted egg. Sly-One saw the other one lying broken on the ground. He wondered what had happened.

He didn't know the habits of the baby cuckoo. That little bare, black, baby bird didn't like anything in the nest with him. He had actually pitched the wagtail's egg out of the nest! Now he was lying resting, waiting for strength to pitch the other eggs out too!

He did pitch out one egg – the other

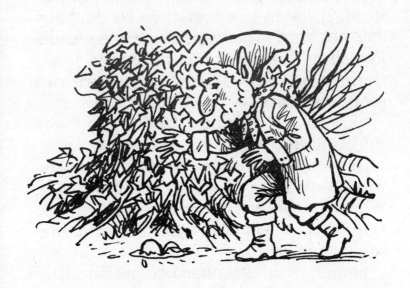

wagtail egg. He waited till the mother wagtail was off the nest for a few minutes, then he set to work. He got the wagtail egg into a little hollow on his back, climbed slowly up the side of the nest – and then over went the little egg to the ground below. Another egg gone. Now there was only the hoolloopolony egg left to deal with. The baby cuckoo sank back, exhausted.

Then the enchanted egg hatched out into a dainty little yellow bird with a red head. It lay in the nest close to the baby cuckoo. When the wagtail came back she looked at the two baby birds and loved them. She didn't know they were not really her own.

"I'll go and fetch grubs for you," she said, and flew off.

As soon as she was gone the baby cuckoo wanted to have the nest all to himself. What was this warm bundle pressing close against him? He didn't like it. In fact he couldn't bear it!

Somehow he managed to get the tiny bird on to his back. Somehow he managed to climb up the side of the nest to the top.

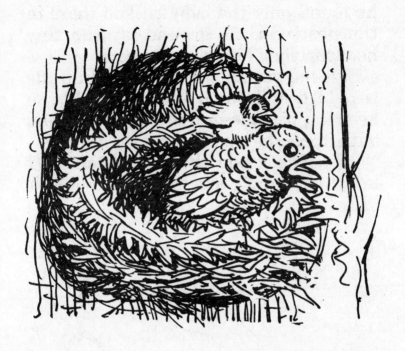

He gave a heave – and over the top of the nest went the baby hoolloopolony bird, right to the ground below.

It twittered there helplessly. The wagtail came back but didn't notice it. She fed the hungry baby cuckoo and thought what a wonderful child he was. She didn't seem to miss the other at all.

When Sly-One came along to see how his wonderful egg was getting on, he found only the baby cuckoo there in the nest! On the ground lay the tiny hoolloopolony bird, almost dead.

Sly-One gave a cry. He picked up the tiny bird and put it into his pocket to keep it warm. He sped to the wise woman with it, and begged her to keep it alive.

"Sly-One," said the wise woman. "I know why you want this bird. When it

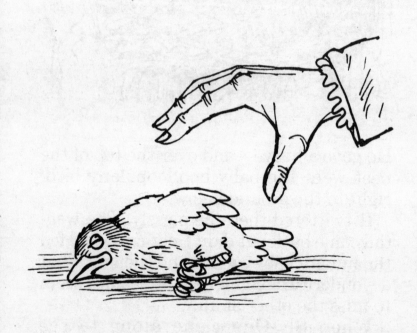

grows, it will be able to do powerful magic for you. Well, Sly-One, you are not a nice person and I am not going to rear up a bird to work for you. It must die!"

Sly-One was very angry. "How was I to know the bad ways of baby cuckoos?" he cried. "The cuckoo is not a good bird. It puts its eggs into other birds' nests and throws out their own eggs. And the baby cuckoo throws them out too, and even throws out the baby birds. They are both bad – but how was I to know?"

"You are not really very clever, Sly-One," said the wise woman, softly. "I could have told you the ways of all birds and animals, though you should know them yourself. I am glad you chose the cuckoo to help you! Now you will never own a hoolloopolony bird, and you will never be king of the world!"

He wasn't of course, and a very good thing too. As for the tiny bird, it did live, though Sly-One didn't know. The wise woman kept it alive, and then set it free. It is full of magic, but no one knows that. It's no good trying to catch it if you see it, because it can't be caught.

Whose nest would you have put the egg into? There are such a lot of different ones to choose from, aren't there?

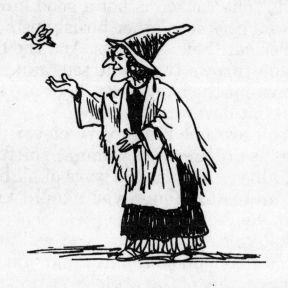

Silly Simon and
the Goat

Simon had had a cold and his ears had ached. He had been very miserable. Now he was better and up again, but he was rather deaf. That was horrid.

"You'll be able to go to school again tomorrow," said his mother. "That will be nice for you. Today you can stay at home and help me."

So Simon helped his mother. He fetched in the washing from the line. He ran to the shop to get some butter, and he took the baby out for a little walk. He really was a great help.

"You have been quite a sensible boy for once," said his mother, pleased. Silly Simon wasn't always sensible. He sometimes did very silly things, and then his mother was cross.

He was pleased. "Well, you always think

I haven't got brains," he said. "But I have, Mum. I'm really a very clever boy."

"Well, I hope you go on being a clever boy for the rest of the day," said his mother. "Now, I'm going upstairs to do some things. Baby is fast asleep."

She went upstairs, and then she remembered that she wanted her old coat to mend. So she called down to Simon.

"Simon! Fetch me the old coat, will you?"

Simon didn't hear her very well. He thought his mother said, "Fetch me the old goat." He was rather surprised, but still, as he was feeling very good and obedient, he set off to fetch the old goat in from the field.

He caught the goat, and led him to the house on a rope. He called up to his mother. "I've got it for you."

"Well, bring it upstairs, and hang it over the banisters," called his mother. Simon felt more astonished than before. It was funny to want the old goat brought into the house, but still stranger to want it upstairs hung over the banisters.

"The goat won't like it!" he called up

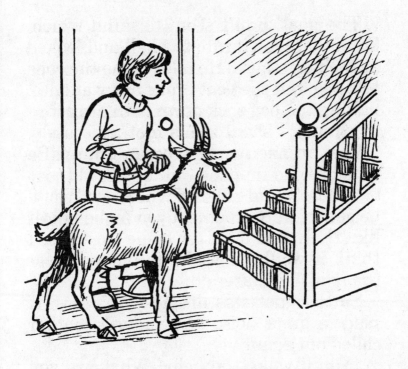

after a bit. But his mother only half-heard what he said.

"Don't be silly!" she said. "It won't hurt the coat. But hang it in the hall, if you'd rather."

"Hang you in the hall?" said Simon to the surprised goat. "Which would you rather, goat? I can hang you in the hall, or take you upstairs and put you over the banisters."

The goat didn't seem to mind which. So Simon took it into the hall and looked at the pegs there. He tried to tie the rope to a peg, but the goat broke away at once, pulling the peg-rack down with a crash.

"Simon!" shouted his mother crossly. "What in the world are you doing? Be quiet."

"There!" said Simon to the goat. "You'll be getting into trouble if you make noises like that. You'd better come upstairs. I think it would be easier to put you over the banisters, after all."

So the goat was dragged upstairs. It made a great noise and Simon's mother called out again.

"You'll wake the baby! What are you making all that noise for?"

"I'm dragging the goat up," panted Simon. "It won't come."

"A coat isn't as heavy as all that," said his mother, crossly. "What a fuss you make to be sure! I hope you're not dragging it on the floor."

Simon at last got the goat to the top of the stairs. He tried to get it across the banisters, but the goat simply wouldn't

Silly Simon and the Goat

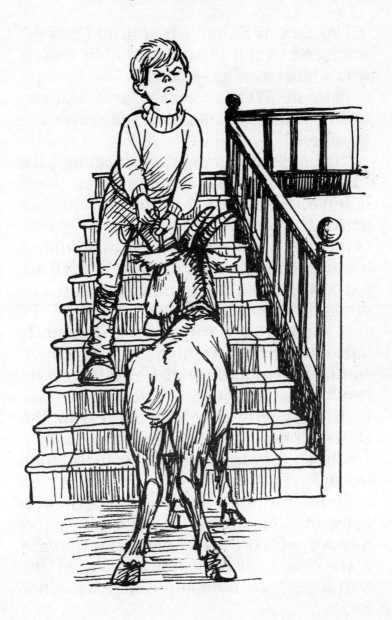

go. As fast as Simon lifted it up one end, it slipped to the ground the other end. It was a most annoying goat.

"Simon! Whatever are you doing out there?" called his mother. "Why can't you be quiet?"

"There!" said Simon to the goat fiercely. "You'll get me into trouble if you don't behave. Now, just you let me put you across the banisters!"

But it was no good. The goat wouldn't be at all helpful. It clattered with its four feet, it slid here and there, and was altogether most obstinate.

It suddenly got very tired of Simon. It backed a little way, put its head down, ran at Simon and caught him full on its head. It butted him hard, and Simon rose in the air with a yell, sailed down the stairs, and landed at the bottom with a crash. He howled loudly. The baby woke up and yelled, too.

Simon's mother flung open the door to glare at Simon – but instead she found herself glaring at the old goat, who glared back, and looked as if he might butt her at any moment. Simon's mother

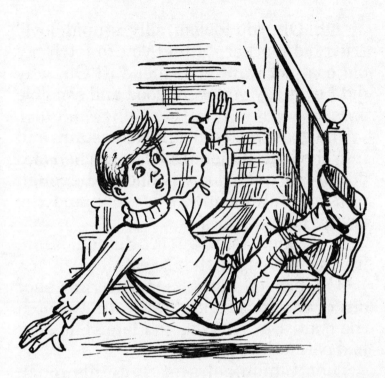

hurriedly stepped back into the room and shut the door.

She called through it. "You bad boy, Simon! How dare you bring that old goat up here? Take him back to the field at once!"

"Well, you told me to bring him here and hang him over the banisters," wailed Simon. "You did, you did!"

"Oh! Oh, you foolish, silly, stupid boy!" cried his mother. "I told you to fetch my old coat – I wanted to mend it! Oh, why did I ever say you were good and sensible today?"

The goat trotted neatly downstairs and into the hall. It went into the kitchen and out of the back door. It had had enough of Simon and Simon's mother and the crying baby.

"It's gone!" said Simon. "But, oh, Mum, it's taken a rug with it to eat!"

"Oh, has it!" cried his mother, and shot out of the room and downstairs to catch the goat. But she was too late. The goat had eaten the rug.

Then Simon got sent up to his room, and he was very upset about it.

"I try to be good and sensible and obedient and this is what I get for it!" he wept. "I'll never try again."

"Well, if you do things like that when you are trying to be good, you'd better stop!" said his mother.

Poor Simon! You wouldn't think anyone would be so silly, would you?

Silly Simon and the Goat

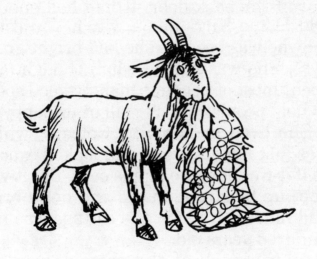

The
Witch's Cat

Old Dame Kirri was a witch. You could tell she was because she had bright green eyes. She was a good witch though, and spent most of her time making good spells to help people who were ill or unhappy.

She lived in Toppling Cottage, which was just like its name and looked exactly as if it was going to topple over. But it was kept up by strong magic and not a brick had fallen, although the cottage was five hundred years old.

At the back of the cottage was the witch's garden. Round it ran a very, very high wall, taller than the tallest man.

"I like a high wall. It keeps people from peeping and prying," said old witch Kirri. "In my garden I grow a lot of strange and powerful herbs. I don't want people to see them and steal them. I won't have people making spells from my magic herbs – they might make bad ones."

The witch had a cat. It was black and big, and had green eyes very like the witch's. Its name was Cinder-Boy.

Cinder-Boy helped the witch with her spells. He was really a remarkably clever cat. He knew how to sit exactly in the middle of a chalk ring without moving, while Kirri the witch danced round and sang spells. He knew how to go out and collect dewdrops in the moonlight. He took a special little silver cup for that, and never spilled a drop. He never drank milk.

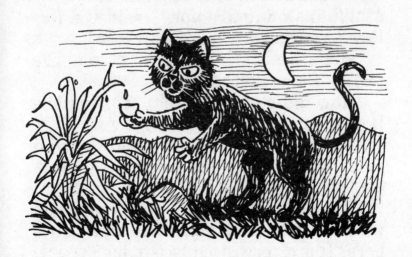

He liked tea, made as strong as the witch made for herself. Sometimes he would sit and sip his tea and purr, and the witch would sip her tea and purr, too. It was funny to see them.

Cinder-Boy loved to sleep in the walled-in garden. He knew all the flowers and herbs which grew there. No weeds were allowed to grow. Cinder-Boy scratched them all up.

But one day he came to a small plant growing at the foot of the wall. It had leaves like a rose-tree. It had pale pink flowers, with a mass of yellow stamens in the middle. It smelled very sweet.

"What flower are you?" said Cinder-Boy. "You smell rather like a rose."

"Well, that's just what I am," said the plant. "I'm a wild rose."

"How did you get here?" said Cinder-Boy, surprised.

"A bird dropped a seed," said the wild rose. "But I don't like being here, black cat."

"My name is Cinder-Boy," said the witch's cat. "Why don't you like being here? It is a very nice place to be."

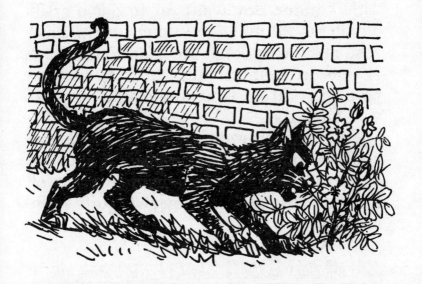

"Well, I feel shut in," said the wild rose. "I'm not very large. If I was taller than the wall I could grow up into the air, and see over the top. I don't like being down here at the bottom, shut in."

"Well, grow tall then," said Cinder-Boy. "I can give you a spell to make your stems nice and long, if you like. Then you can reach up to the top of the wall and look over. There's a nice view there, I can tell you."

"Oh, would you do that?" said the wild rose in delight. "Thank you!"

So Cinder-Boy went off to get a spell which would make the stems of the wild rose grow very long. He soon found one. It was in a small blue bottle, and he poured it into a watering-can. The spell was blue, too.

Then he watered the wild rose with the spell, and it began to work almost at once. In two or three days the stems of the wild rose plant had grown quite high into the air.

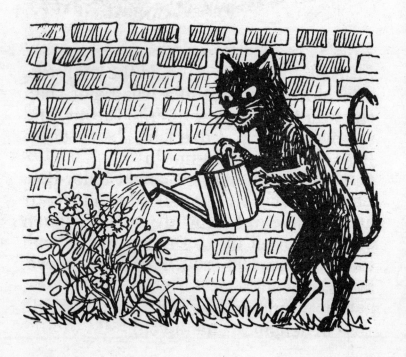

"Go on growing. You will soon be at the top of the wall!" said Cinder-Boy. So the wild rose went on, making its stems longer and longer, hoping to get to the very top of the wall.

But when Cinder-Boy next strolled out into the garden to see how it was getting on, what a shock he had! Every single stem was bent over and lay sprawling over the grass!

"Why, what has happened?" said Cinder-Boy, waving his tail in surprise.

"My stalks grew tall, but they didn't grow strong," said the wild rose, sadly. "Just as I reached the top of the wall, they all flopped over and fell down. They are not strong enough to bear their own weight."

"Well, how do plants with weak stems manage to climb high then?" said Cinder-Boy, puzzled. "Runner beans grow high and they have very weak stems. Sweet-peas grow high, and they have weak stems too. I'll go and see how they do it." So off he went, for the witch grew both in the garden. He soon came back.

"The beans twine their stalks round

poles," he said, "and the sweetpeas grow little green fingers, called tendrils, which catch hold of things, and they pull themselves up high like that. Can't you do that?"

The wild rose couldn't. It didn't know how to. Its stems wouldn't twist themselves, however much it tried to make them do so. And it couldn't grow a tendril at all.

"Well, we must think of another way," said the cat.

"Cinder-Boy, how do you get up to the top of the wall?" asked the wild rose. "You are often up there in the sun. I see you. Well, how do you get to the top?"

"I run up the trees," said Cinder-Boy. "Do you see the young fruit-trees near you? Well, I run up those to the top of the wall. I use my claws to help me. I dig them into the bark of the trees, and hold on with them."

He showed the wild rose his big curved claws. "I can put them in or out as I like," he said. "They are very useful claws."

The wild rose thought they were too. "If I grew claws like that I could easily climb

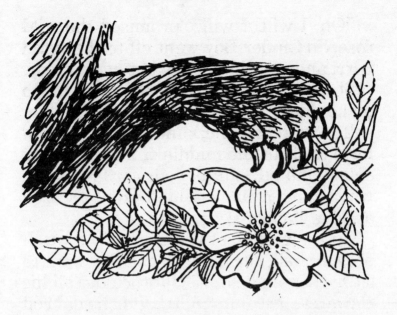

up the fruit-trees, right through them to the top, and then I'd be waving at the top of the wall," it said. "Can't you get me some claws like yours, Cinder-Boy?"

The cat blinked his green eyes and thought hard. "I know what I could do," he said. "I could ask the witch Kirri, my mistress, to make some magic claws that would grow on you. I'll ask her today. In return you must promise to grow her some lovely scarlet rosehips which she can trim her hats and bonnets with in the autumn."

"Oh, I will, I will," promised the wild rose. So Cinder-Boy went off to the witch Kirri and asked her for what he wanted.

She grumbled a little. "It is difficult to make claws," she said. "Very difficult. You will have to help me, Cinder-Boy. You will have to sit in the middle of a blue ring of chalk, and put out all your claws at once, while I sing a magic song. Don't be scared at what happens."

In the middle of the garden the witch drew a chalk ring and Cinder-Boy went to sit in the middle of it. He stuck out all his claws as she commanded and she danced round with her broomstick singing such a magic song that Cinder-Boy felt quite scared. Then a funny thing happened.

His claws fell out on to the ground with a clatter – and they turned red or green as they fell. He looked at his paws and saw new ones growing. Then those fell out, too. How very, very strange!

Soon there was quite a pile of claws on the ground. Then the witch stopped singing and dancing, and rubbed out the ring of chalk.

"You can come out now, Cinder-Boy,"

144

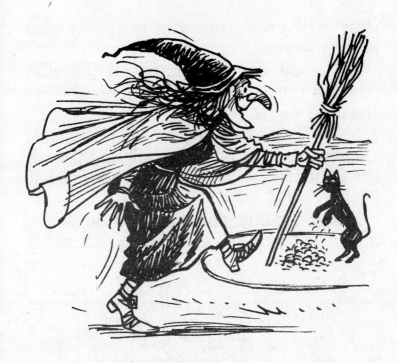

she said. "The magic is finished."

Cinder-Boy collected all the red and green claws. They were strong and curved and sharp. He took them to the bottom of the garden, and came to the wild rose.

"I've got claws for you!" he said. "The witch Kirri did some strong magic. Look, here they are. I'll press each one into your stems, till you have claws all down them. Then I'll say a growing spell, and

145

they will grow into you properly and belong to you."

So Cinder-Boy did that, and the wild rose felt the cat-claws growing firmly into the long stems.

"Now," said Cinder-Boy, in excitement, "now you will be able to climb up through the fruit-tree, wild rose. I will help you at first."

So Cinder-Boy took the wild rose stems, all set with claws, and pushed them up

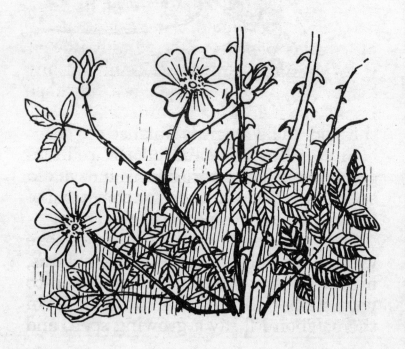

into the little fruit-tree that grew near by. The claws took hold of the bark and held on firmly. Soon all the stems were climbing up high through the little fruit tree, the claws digging themselves into the trunk and the branches.

The wild rose grew higher. It pulled itself up by its new claws. It was soon at the top of the wall! It could see right over it to the big world beyond.

"Now I'm happy!" said the wild rose to Cinder-Boy. "Come and sit up here on the wall beside me. Let us look at the big world together. Oh, Cinder-Boy, it is lovely up here. I am not shut in any longer. Thank you for my claws. I do hope I shall go on growing them now."

It did. And it grew beautiful scarlet berries in the autumn, for witch Kirri's winter bonnets. You should see how pretty they are when she trims them with the rosehips!

Ever since that day the wild roses have grown cats' claws all down their stems, sometimes green and sometimes red or pink. They use them to climb with. Have you seen them? If you haven't, do go and look. It will surprise you to see cats' claws growing out of a plant!

It was a good idea of Cinder-Boy's, wasn't it?

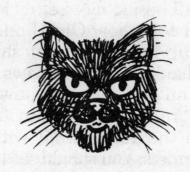

Mr Squiggle

"Cathy, will you stop scribbling over everything?" said her mother. "Look here – you've made squiggles and scribbles on the kitchen wall – and I've found some silly squiggles on the door of the shed outside. Why do you do it?"

"Well, I can't write words properly yet," said Cathy, "and I'm not very good at drawing. So I just do squiggles – like this!"

And will you believe it, she took her pencil and did a squiggle on the nice clean tablecloth!

Her mother took her pencil away from her. "Very well – if you are as silly as all that, you shan't have a pencil!" she said.

But Cathy had got such a habit of scribbling here, there and everywhere that she simply couldn't do without something in her fingers for scribbling. She found a blue crayon and began scribbling on the doorstep with it.

So her mother took that away, too. Then Cathy found a piece of white blackboard chalk, and dear me, the mess she made with that! There were squiggles on the garden gate and scribbles on the garden seat!

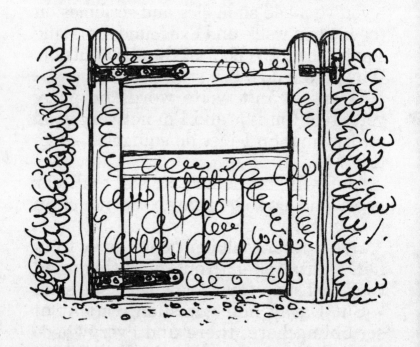

Even her father got angry. "Each time I find a squiggle, I shall smack your fingers," he said. "If *you* can't stop them scribbling, I will!"

"I do hope she won't grow up into one of those dreadful people who sign their names everywhere," said Mother. "I can't think why she does it – she doesn't even write words – it's just squiggles!"

Cathy didn't stop squiggling and scribbling. She got into trouble for it at school, too, because she scribbled all over the wall next to her seat in class.

"One of these days," said Miss Brown, the teacher, to Cathy, "you'll meet Mr Squiggle, who knows the language of squiggles – and, dear me, won't you be surprised at the nonsense you've written! You can't understand it, but he'll be able to!"

Cathy was certain that Miss Brown was joking, and she laughed. But will you believe it, the very next day she did meet Mr Squiggle!

She was going home from school. She had with her a piece of red chalk, and she was simply longing to scribble on something with it. When she came to one of the sheds belonging to Mr Straw, the farmer, she began to scribble all over it in red. It really looked horrid, and quite spoilt the shed.

And then she heard a squeaky voice behind her. "How dare you sign my name like that! I wondered who it was writing my name everywhere – and oh, my goodness, what naughty things you write – and then sign my name to them!"

Cathy turned round in surprise. She saw a thin little man bristling with pencils and pens and crayons. They were in rows of pockets, and he even had a row of red pencils in his hat, and some behind his ears. He looked rather like a brownie, she thought.

"I *don't* sign your name!" said Cathy, indignantly. "I don't even know it!"

"My name is Mr Squiggle," said the thin little man. "And look – here's my name. You've written it three times on this wall!"

He pointed to some funny little squiggles. "See? That's my name – and that, and that. Watch while I sign it and you'll see it's really exactly like my signature."

He scribbled something with one of his pencils – and sure enough it was exactly like the three squiggles Cathy had made.

"Well, I didn't know I was signing your

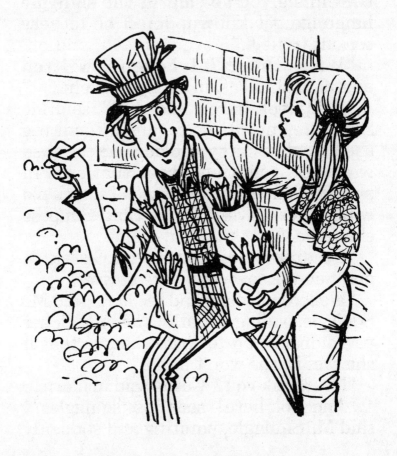

name," said Cathy. "It just looks like a squiggle to me."

"Well, it is. I told you my name was Squiggle, so, of course, it's a squiggle like that when I write it," said Mr Squiggle. "And let me tell you this – if some of the things you've said in the squiggle language get known, you'll be in very serious trouble."

"What things? I haven't written anything at all!" said Cathy in fright.

"Well, look here – see this?" said Mr Squiggle, pointing to a silly-looking squiggle that Cathy had done on the shed wall. "Do you know what that says in squiggle language? It says, 'I'll smack old witch Green-Eyes.' Fancy that! Suppose she came along and read that!"

"I didn't write that," said Cathy. "I don't even know witch Green-Eyes."

"Well, come along and see her," said Mr Squiggle, pulling at Cathy's arm. "Tell her you didn't mean to write that, so that if she sees it, she won't mind."

"No, thank you," Cathy said in alarm.

"And look here – see those squiggles?" said Mr Squiggle, pointing and suddenly

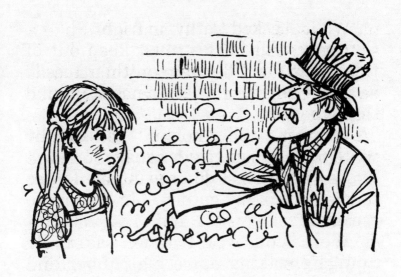

looking very fierce. "You've actually written 'The goblin Long-Nose is always poking his nose into things. It wants pulling.' You're a very rude little girl. I've a good mind to bring Long-Nose here and show him what you've written about him."

"No, don't," said Cathy, almost in tears. "I tell you, I don't know him. Why should I write things about people I don't know?"

"Just part of your silliness, I suppose," said Mr Squiggle "I passed through your garden yesterday and what did I see written on your garden seat?"

"What?" asked Cathy, in fright.

"I saw, 'All fairies must keep out of this garden or I'll stamp on their toes'!" said Mr Squiggle. "That's a nasty, unkind thing to write!"

Cathy was full of horror. "Did I really write that in squiggle language? I didn't know I had. Oh, I don't want the fairies to keep out of my garden. I'm longing to see one."

"Well, you won't now," said Mr Squiggle, taking out a big rubber and beginning to rub out some of Cathy's silly squiggles. "Not one will come near you. You're a rude little girl!"

"I'm *not*! I didn't know what I was writing!" wept Cathy. "Have I said anything else dreadful?"

"Good gracious me, yes," said Mr Squiggle, rubbing out hard. "There was one thing I had to rub out at once, in case you got the Jumping Imps after you. You'd written it on your school playground. You wrote, 'If ever I catch a Jumping Imp I'll slap him and put him in the dustbin.' Fancy being so rude. If I hadn't rubbed that out at once, you'd have had dozens

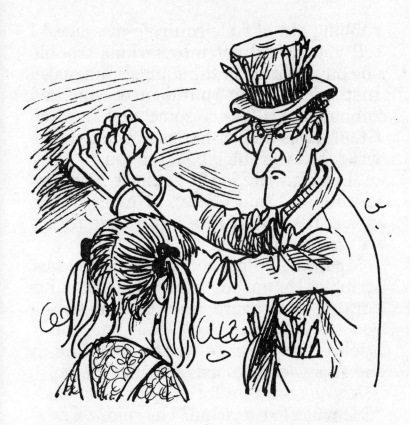

of Jumping Imps giving *you* a few slaps!"

"Was it you who rubbed out what I'd chalked in the playground, then?" said Cathy. "I thought the rain had washed it away."

"I couldn't wait for the rain," said Mr Squiggle. "It had to be rubbed out at once. You give me a dreadful lot of work. All this rubbing out of rude squiggle messages! I tell you, you'll get into serious trouble one day, writing in the squiggle language! Instead of going round after you and rubbing out, I'll fetch someone like witch Green-Eyes and let her read what you've written. Then she'll be after you."

"I won't write in the squiggle language any more," said Cathy. "Never, never, never. It's dreadful to write rude things without meaning to."

Mr Squiggle rubbed out the very last scribble. He put his rubber back into his pocket. "I've heard your mother telling you to stop," he said. "And you don't. Look – I'm going to write something in the squiggle language now – watch me!"

And he wrote a lot of quick scribbles. "See what I've written?" he said. "'Cathy is a rude girl. Give her a smack whenever you go by. Signed, Mr Squiggle'!"

Then, before Cathy could say another word, he raised his hat to her, making all the pencils in it click together, jumped over the hedge and completely disappeared.

Cathy stared at the squiggles he had

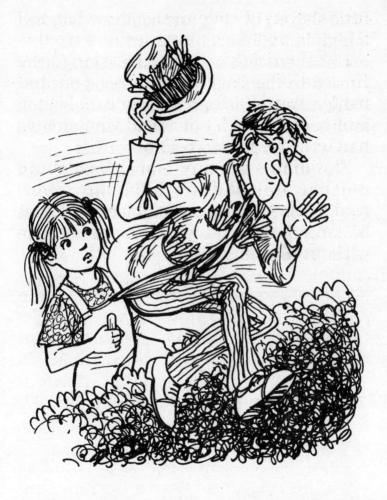

written neatly on the shed wall. Did they really mean what he had said? She didn't want to get sly slaps wherever she went! And then, quite suddenly, she felt a sharp little slap on her leg, and someone laughed a high laugh like a blackbird.

But there was no one to be seen. Cathy turned to the shed wall. She took out her hanky, wetted it in a nearby rain-barrel, and began to rub out what Mr Squiggle had written. No more slaps for her!

She didn't get any more slaps – and neither did she scribble any more squiggles. Are you a scribbler, too? Just be careful you don't write something rude without meaning to!

Clever Old
Green-Eyes

Green-Eyes belonged to Morris. She was a big black cat, with a thick, silky coat, and the greenest eyes you ever saw.

"They are as green as the cucumbers you buy in the summer, Mummy," said Morris. "I do love Green-Eyes. She purrs so loudly, and she loves sitting on my knee. She is the nicest cat in the world."

Morris bought Green-Eyes a lovely Christmas present. It was a cat-basket made of wicker. Morris begged an old cushion from his mother, and an old bit of blanket. Then he picked up Green-Eyes and sat her down in the basket.

"It's yours, Green-Eyes, with my love," said Morris. "Mummy, may I have Green-Eyes's basket in my bedroom, please? Do let me. She is very good, and she won't make my room untidy or smelly at

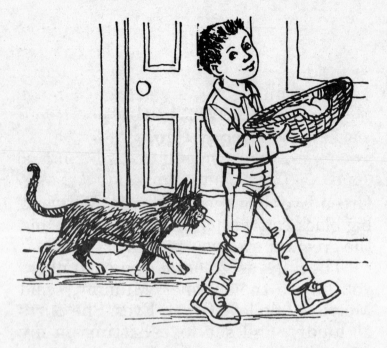

all, I promise you."

Well, Mother didn't very much like a cat sleeping in Morris's room, but certainly Green-Eyes was a very good, quiet cat – so she said yes.

And, in great delight, Morris carried the basket up to his own little bedroom, with Green-Eyes following at his heels.

"There," he said to Green-Eyes, "you can sleep in my bedroom every night now, Green-Eyes – you in your basket and I in my bed. I will always leave the window open a little way so that you can come in and out as you want to. You can easily scramble up the tree outside and come in through the window, if you are not in your basket when I have to go to bed."

Green-Eyes was delighted. She purred loudly. "Thank you, Morris. It is a very lovely basket and I like it very much. You are a kind little boy."

For three or four months Green-Eyes slept in her basket in Morris's bedroom – and then one morning Morris gave such a yell of surprise and delight that his mother came running to see what was the matter.

"Mummy, oh Mummy! Green-Eyes has got four tiny little kittens in her basket! Oh, Mummy, we've got kittens. Isn't it exciting?"

"Very exciting," said Mother. "But Green-Eyes will have to go to the barn now, Morris. I can't have five cats in your bedroom."

"Oh, Mummy – but four of them are only tiny kittens!" said Morris, almost in tears. "Mummy, Green-Eyes is so used to sleeping in my room now – she loves it. Don't make her unhappy by turning her out just when she's got four dear little kittens to look after. They will be safe with me. The rats might get them out in the barn."

"Dear me, Green-Eyes will certainly see that they don't!" said Mother. "She has killed a good many rats in her time. No, Morris dear – she and her kittens must go to the barn. There is plenty of straw there to make her a nice soft bed. She will be very happy there."

"She will miss me so at night," said Morris. "And I shall miss her, too."

But Morris's mother was quite firm about it. Green-Eyes had got to go to the barn with all her kittens, and go she did. Mother picked up the kittens, which squealed loudly. She went downstairs with them and Green-Eyes followed at once.

Mother took the four tiny kittens to the barn. They were all as black as could be, just like Green-Eyes, and one of them had tiny white feet.

Green-Eyes made a bed for them in the straw and lay down. Mother gave her the

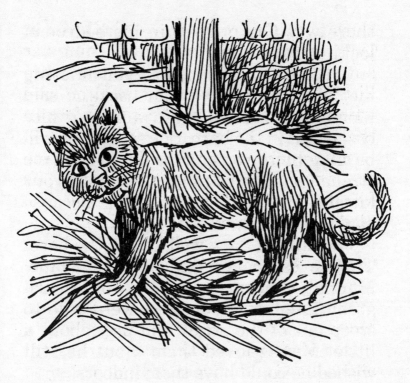

kittens and they nestled up to her, asking her for some milk. Green- Eyes purred loudly.

"There, you see!" said Mother to Morris. "Green-Eyes is quite happy."

But when night-time came and Morris looked at the empty basket, he felt sure that Green-Eyes wasn't at all happy. Then he heard a little soft jump, and there was Green-Eyes in his bedroom, looking up at him.

"Oh, Green-Eyes – are you missing me? Are you missing your basket?" said Morris. "Mummy doesn't want your nice basket out in the barn. She says straw will be all right for you and the kittens. Let me stroke you. There now, go back to your kittens, and don't be miserable because you've been turned out!"

The kittens grew well, out in the barn. Their eyes opened and were very blue. Morris's mother said they would turn green later on. Soon they were able to creep out of the straw and play about a little. Morris loved them – but he still wished he could have them indoors!

One night about four weeks after the kittens had been born, Morris woke with a jump. His window was shut, and something was knocking against it. *Thud, thud, thud*, went the knocking, very soft and slow. He opened the window and Green-Eyes jumped inside, carrying a kitten by the skin at the back of its neck, the way all mother-cats carry their kittens. She dropped it into the basket nearby, gave a tiny mew, and then sprang out of the window and climbed down the tree.

Morris was astonished. "Green-Eyes! What are you doing? Why have you brought your kitten here?"

Soon the cat was back with yet another

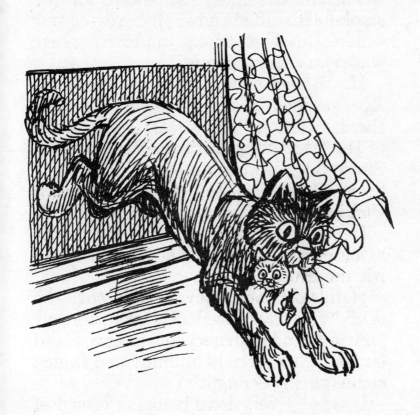

kitten. Morris was more astonished than ever. What could Green-Eyes be doing? Was she tired of the barn? Had she suddenly taken it into her head to bring her kittens to the place that she herself liked so much? It was all very puzzling.

Then Morris smelled something funny – smoke! He sniffed and sniffed. Yes – it was smoke. But what smoke could it be? There was no bonfire burning, he knew that.

He slipped downstairs just as Green-Eyes jumped in at the window with her third kitten in her mouth. He ran out of the back door and went to the barn. Smoke was coming out of it!

"Fire! Fire!" yelled Morris. "Mummy! Daddy! The barn's on fire! Quick, quick!"

He saw Green-Eyes come out of the smoking barn, dragging her last kitten in her mouth.

"Oh, you good, clever little cat!" he said. "You have saved all your kittens by yourself! And perhaps you will have saved our barn, too, if only Mummy and Daddy come quickly enough."

It wasn't very long before a crowd of grown-ups were hosing the smoking barn

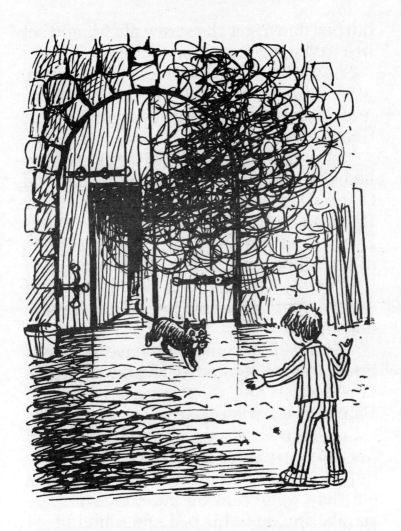

with water. Inside, fast asleep, was an old tramp. He had lit a candle there and fallen asleep without putting it out. It had burned down, set the straw alight, and set fire to the big barn.

Soon the fire was out. The tramp was rubbing his eyes in amazement, and Morris was telling everyone about Green-Eyes.

"She brought her kittens to my bedroom, where her old basket is, and that's what woke me. I went out and saw the barn on fire. Mummy, Daddy, Green-Eyes saved the barn – and saved the life of that old tramp, too!"

They all went back to bed, happy and excited. Mother peeped into Morris's room and smiled.

"Well, well, I suppose I'll have to let you have Green-Eyes and all the kittens there now, Morris. She saved our barn for us, so I must give her a reward!"

So Green-Eyes slept in the basket with her four kittens, and Morris was very happy. But when they were six weeks old they woke him up every morning by clambering on to his bed and nibbling his nose. So, in the end, he had to take them down to the kitchen!

"As soon as they go to their new homes

you can come back to my bedroom and sleep in your basket," he told Green-Eyes. "You'll like that, won't you?"

"Purrrrr-rrr-rrr," said Green-Eyes, and Morris knew what *that* meant.

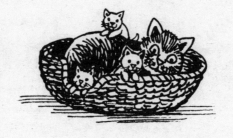

The Two Bad Boys

There were once two bad boys called Tom and Jim. They were not truthful and they were not honest – in fact, they stole apples from outside shops, and once Tom had taken a full milk-bottle from a doorstep!

This was really dreadful. The apples were green and gave them both a pain, and Tom fell with the milk-bottle, broke it, and cut his hand, so they didn't get any good out of their stealing; but how sad their mothers were to know they had children like that!

"Nobody gets happiness out of badness," said Tom's mother, as she bandaged his hand.

Tom didn't believe her – but when he found that the Sunday school party was to be held on Saturday and that he and Jim were not invited, be began to wish he hadn't been so bad!

He grumbled about it to Jim. "There's going to be crackers and balloons and blow-up pigs that squeak, and all kinds of goodies and oranges and sweets and a toy for everybody!" he said. "I wish we were going."

"Well!" said Jim. "What about creeping in before the party begins and taking a few things for ourselves? We could easily do that. We could creep in at a window."

Jim was a very bad boy as you can see. Tom nodded his head. "All right," he said. "We will. Let's go and peep in at the window on Friday and see what sort of toys are there."

So on Friday they peeped in at the window. They saw Mrs Jones and Miss Brown arranging everything ready for the next day. They saw the dishes of sweets put out, the plates of oranges. There were no cakes or buns yet, because they would be made next day. They saw the big balloons being blown up, and watched the balloon-pigs being stood all down the table for the children.

There was a big table for the toys too.

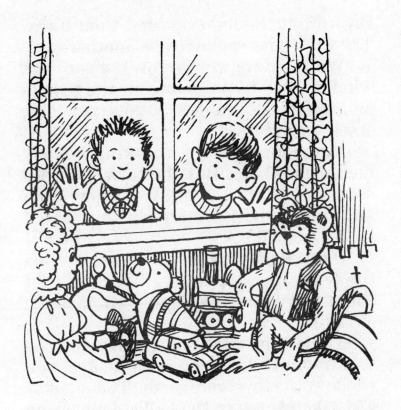

My goodness, what lovely toys! There were
two big humming-tops, a train that could
whistle, a doll that could say "Ma-ma,
Pa-pa", some tiny motor-cars with little
hooters, a bear that growled, a monkey
that squeaked – oh, more toys than Tom
and Jim could count.

They watched until Mrs Jones and Miss

Brown put the light out and went away. Then the boys spoke to one another.

"We'll come tomorrow, when the windows will be opened to air the room – and we'll take oranges, sweets, balloons, crackers and toys!"

They slipped away, thinking nobody had heard them. But the toys had both seen and heard them! They knew Tom and Jim all right! Everybody knew about those two bad boys.

"Did you hear what they said?" cried the bear, in excitement. "We won't let them steal us! We'll give them such a fright!"

So when the next night came, and the two naughty boys crept in at an open window, the toys were ready. The monkey had taken three of the balloon-pigs from the table, and he and the doll and the bear pulled the little corks from the pigs' mouths as soon as the boys came in.

You know what noise a balloon-pig makes when the air goes out of him, don't you? "Eeeeeeeeeeeeeeeeee!" they all said in their mournful voices. "Eeeeeeeeeeeeeee!"

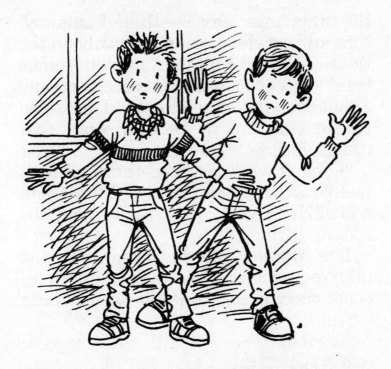

Tom and Jim stood still in fright. Whatever was that? The pigs stopped making a noise and fell over, quite flat. Then the teddy bear pressed himself in the middle.

"Grrrrrrrrr!" he said. "Grrrrrrrrrr!"

"Ooooh!" said Tom and Jim. "Is it a dog growling!"

"Grrrrrrrrr!" said the bear again, quite enjoying himself. Then the monkey and the other toys took the three humming-tops and set them spinning madly on the floor. They all hummed like enormous bees! "Zooooooooooom! Zeeeeeeeeeeeeem! Zooooooooom!" they went. Tom tried to run away and he fell over a mat that caught his foot. *Bang!*

"Ow!" cried Tom. "Something's caught me! What's making that noise? Are we in a beehive? I wish we could see, but the room's all dark!"

The monkey pressed himself in the middle and made loud squeaks. "Eeoo, eeoo, eeoo, eeoo!" Jim fell over Tom in

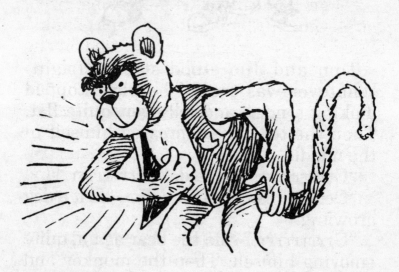

a fright. The monkey nearly laughed out loud!

Then the engine of the train began to whistle. "Pheeeeeeeeeeee!" it went, as loudly as it could. Good gracious, what a fright it gave the two bad boys! They could hardly get up!

"Where's the window? Where's the window?" cried Jim.

Now the talking doll began to call, "Mama, Papa, Mama, Papa!" at the top of her voice, and the monkey and bear pressed the little hooters of the motor-cars at the same time.

"Honk, honk, honk! Honk, Mama, Papa, honk, honk, Mama, honk, Papa, honk!" What a noise! Tom and Jim rushed for the window and tried to climb through – and then the monkey had a bright idea. He took the brooch off his coat and drove the pin into a big balloon hanging near him.

BANG! It went off with such a loud pop that even the toys were startled. Jim and Tom fell to the ground.

"I'm shot!" groaned Tom.

"So am I!" cried Jim. "Somebody's shot us. Didn't you hear the bang!"

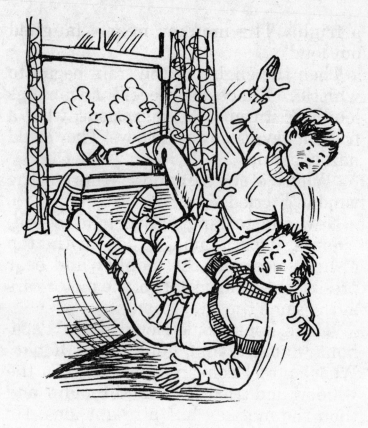

And there they lay groaning, thinking they were shot, till the door opened and in trooped all the children who had been invited to the party! How surprised they were to see Tom and Jim – and you may be sure they guessed at once what those two bad boys had come for!

They shooed them out of the door, they laughed at them – and they banged the door behind them. Tom and Jim began to cry. How they wished they could go and join the happy children in the room, with all the balloons and toys!

"It's our own fault," said Tom, wiping his eyes. "Mum says nobody gets any happiness out of being bad. I'm going to be good for a change. I've had a real fright tonight, and I'm going home to find out where I've been shot!"

Well, he won't find where he's shot, and neither will Jim – but the toys will have done a good deed if they have stopped those two boys from being bad. The monkey still laughs when he remembers all that happened that evening!

Buttons and Bows

"You're lazy, Janie," said her mother. "You're over six years old and you can't tie a bow or do up your buttons properly yet!"

"Well, there's always someone who will do them up for me," said Janie.

"So I suppose you think you need never learn, and you'll grow up to be an old woman who runs round the world asking people to do up her shoes and tie her apron strings for her!" said her mother. "I'm ashamed of you."

"I shall wear shoes without buttons or bows, and I shan't wear an apron when I grow up," said Janie. She just didn't mean to learn things that were a nuisance!

"I'll teach you," said John-from-next-door. He had been to borrow a book, and he had heard all this.

"Thank you, John, that's kind of you,"

said Janie's mother.

But Janie turned away. "No, thank you," she said. "I'm busy just now. I have to practise my skipping."

"You don't have to," called John. "You're just making an excuse!"

Now the next day John went to the woods to find blackberries. Janie saw him going and called, "I'm coming with you. I want some blackberries, too."

"Well, you can come – but you can pick your own blackberries," said John.

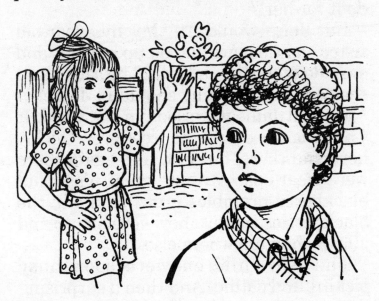

"And if your shoe comes undone you can do it up yourself, and if your hair-ribbon comes untied you can tie that, too. I'm not going to do things for you, lazy little Janie."

"I don't care," said Janie. "I shall get someone else to do them, that's all."

She went off with John. She liked him, although he wouldn't run round after her as the other children often did. "Poor little Janie!" they would say. "She's only little – she can't do this, she can't do that – we'll do it for her!"

But John wouldn't. "My five-year-old sister can tie bows and do up buttons and even do up hooks and eyes," he said. "And she can sew, too. Why shouldn't Janie?"

He and Janie were soon in the wood. It was a big wood, and the trees grew thickly here and there, but now and again there were clear spaces where great masses of blackberry brambles grew. And, oh, the blackberries there! They were bigger and juicier than anywhere else.

The two children were soon busy picking and eating. And then a surprising thing happened.

Something pulled at John's shorts, and a small, high voice spoke a few quick words to him. John looked down, alarmed and surprised.

He was even more surprised when he saw what was pulling at his shorts! It was a small goblin with bright green eyes and big, pointed ears!

"Boy! Listen to me! Can you help me for a minute?" said the goblin's strange, high voice.

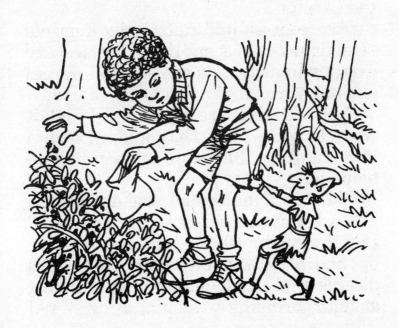

"Good gracious – who are you?" said John. "Hi, Janie, look here – what do you suppose it is? A goblin?"

"Oh!" squealed Janie. "Yes, it must be. Or perhaps a brownie. No, brownies have beards. What are you, little man, and what do you want?"

The goblin went to her, smiling. "I didn't see you," he said, "or I would have asked you to help me! You'd be better than a boy. I'm a goblin, and I'm just off to an important meeting with the King of the Goblins."

"Are you really?" said Janie, amazed. "Goodness me, a goblin – this is very extraordinary. I've never seen a real goblin before."

"You wouldn't see me now if I hadn't wanted you to," said the goblin. "But I'm in a real fix and I had to ask someone to help me."

"What is it you want?" said Janie.

"Just wait a minute and I'll show you," said the goblin. He ran to a nearby bank, opened a little green door there and disappeared. He came out again almost at once, bringing with him a lovely red

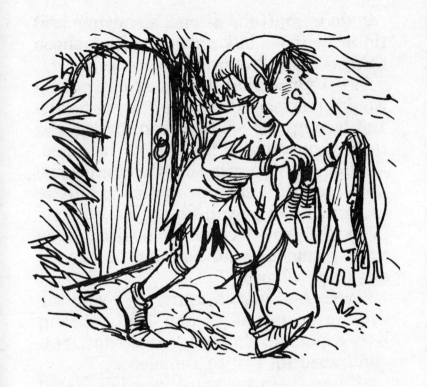

tunic and a pair of pointed shoes with long
green laces.

"Look," he said. "I have to wear these to
go to the meeting. My aunt usually helps
me to dress, because the tunic buttons
all the way up the back and I can't reach
to do the buttons up. And my shoes have
to lace all the way up my legs and tie in
a bow behind my knees. Well, of course I

can do up buttons as well as anyone and tie laces too – but nobody can do those things behind themselves very well."

He stopped and looked at Janie. "So would you please do up the buttons for me and lace up the shoes round my leg and tie the bows behind my knees?" he asked.

Janie shook her head. "Good gracious, no. I couldn't do up buttons as little as that. I can't even do up big buttons properly. And I couldn't possibly lace those things up your legs and tie bows. I don't know how to."

"Well! And you're a girl, too!" said the goblin, in disgust. "I don't believe you. Every girl can do things like that. You don't want to! You're a spoilsport!"

"I'll do them for you if you like," said John. "Put on your tunic and the shoes and I'll do my best to do them up."

The goblin put on his tunic and his shoes, and then stood with his back to John. John had quite a job to do up all the buttons! There were sixty-two of them, very small indeed, but he managed all right.

Then he looped the laces round the

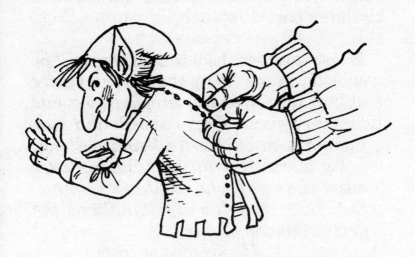

goblin's legs and tied them into neat bows at the back of his knees.

"There you are," he said. "All done! You look very nice!"

"Thank you very much indeed!" said the goblin, and he ran off in delight. "I'll send you a reward some time!"

"Well, I'm glad I couldn't do up buttons or tie bows," said Janie, when he had gone. "I would have hated to do up so many."

But she didn't feel like that when she saw how the goblin rewarded

John. He sent him an invitation to his birthday party!

Please do come, he wrote. *There will be everything you like best to eat, and there will be a present-tree growing presents for every guest. You just wish and pick your present off the tree! And will you bring a friend with you? But not that nasty little girl who wouldn't help me. Somebody nice. It's at midnight on the next full-moon night.*

Happy wishes from
Humpy the Goblin

"Oh, take me, take me, John, please, please do!" begged Janie when John showed her the letter. But John shook his head.

"Of course I can't, Janie. You must have seemed very horrid to him. He really couldn't believe that a little girl couldn't do such simple things. You'd better begin learning straight away, in case you miss some other treat!"

So Janie is busy learning to do up buttons and tie bows and do up hooks and eyes as well – just in case! I hope you'll teach your small brothers and sisters what to do with buttons and bows – you just never know when things will come in useful, do you?

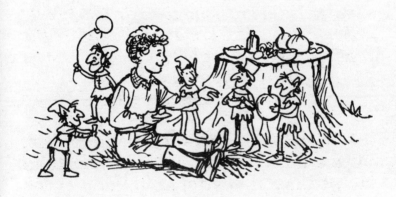

SELECTED PLAYS
OF
GEORGE MOORE
AND
EDWARD MARTYN

Chosen, with an introduction by

David B.Eakin and Michael Case

1995
COLIN SMYTHE
Gerrards Cross, Bucks.

THE CATHOLIC UNIVERSITY
OF AMERICA PRESS
Washington D.C.

This collection first published in 1995 by Colin Smythe Limited,
Gerrards Cross, Buckinghamshire

British Library Cataloguing in Publication Data

A catalogue record for this book is available from the British Library

ISBN 0-86140-144-1
ISBN0-86140-145-X pbk

First published in North America in 1995 by
The Catholic University of America Press, Washington, D.C.

Library of Congress Cataloging-in-Publication Data

Moore, George. 1852-1933.
[Plays. Selections]
Selected plays of George Moore and Edward Martyn/chosen, with an
introduction by David B. Eakin and Michael Case.
p. cm. – (Irish drama selections, ISSN 0260-7962: 8)
Includes bibliographical references.
ISBN 0-8132-0822-X (cl) – ISBN 0-8132-0823-8 (pa)
1. English drama – Irish authors. 2. Ireland – Drama.
I. Martyn, Edward, 1859-1923. Plays. Selections.
II. Eakin, David B.   III. Case, Michael.   IV. Title.   V. Series
PR8865. M66. 1995
822'.8 – dc20   94-22021 CIP

Produced in Great Britain

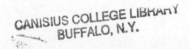

Contents

Introduction

Neither George Moore nor Edward Martyn was a playwright by profession. Moore was a novelist by vocation, a sinner by way of avocation. Martyn seemed to make a vocation out of saintliness, for certainly his other pursuits were so evenly distributed that none of them stands out as being a primary calling. A man of considerable wealth, he was sole heir to a large tenant estate, centred around the ancient family mansion Tulira, in the west Ireland county of Galway. Moore's ancestral home was in the neighbouring county of Mayo. The two were in fact distant cousins and, for a time, close friends, bound together by what Yeats called their 'mutual contempt'. Despite the centrifugal nature of their friendship and despite the secondary nature of their interest in playwriting, they pooled and concentrated their talents in making important contributions at a critical juncture of the Irish literary renaissance.

George Moore's interest in the revival of Irish literature and culture did not begin until he was well into middle age. He had moved to London as early as 1869 at the age of seventeen and did not reestablish residence in Ireland until he was forty-nine. After coming of age in 1873, Moore left for France, believing that Paris was the indisputable home of Art. He spent most of the 1870s in Paris, at first trying his hand at painting but, frustrated by his lack of talent, he quickly turned to literature. Although *The Strike at Arlingford*, produced in 1893, is the first of Moore's plays in the present volume, it was by no means his first venture with the theatre. In fact, Moore's first printed book was a comedy of manners called *Worldliness* (c.1874). No copies of the play have survived, and very little is known about it other than what Moore says in his autobiographical *Confessions of a Young Man* (1888). In all probability the play was privately printed for purposes of interesting prospective theatre managers in London. In *Confessions* Moore says he took his play to London but, having failed to interest a manager, he shook the dust from his sandals and returned to France. He had completed his three-act comedy 'after a month's study' of the Restoration playwrights and concedes that 'it was, of course, very bad'.[1]

vii

Moore's interest in drama had been ignited by Bernard Lopez, a fellow resident at the Hôtel de Russie in Paris and a French playwright whose prolific output included many collaborations with such eminent dramatists of the previous generation as Scribe, Gautier, Dumas *père*, and Gèrard de Nerval. After the failure of *Worldliness*, as well as a small volume of poetry called *Flowers of Passion* in 1878, Moore once again went to Lopez and this time suggested a collaboration. The result was a five-act verse tragedy entitled *Martin Luther*, published in London in 1879 but never produced. In later years Moore had very little regard for this early effort and never considered its reissue in any of the collected editions of his works. Clearly he hoped that the play's religious subject and the authors' fifty pages of preliminary matter attacking the English theatre of the 1870s would cause a mild commotion in the London press. Neither the play nor the prefatory matter, consisting of eighteen contrived letters between the collaborators, generated any excitement in the London literary world, yet the authors can be credited with an early articulation of the flaws of the sentimental drama which dominated the London stage in the 1870s. The play itself is made almost unreadable by the poor quality of verse and by the wooden characterization of the principal characters.

In the 1880s and early 1890s, now established in London, Moore turned his attention to the novel, producing two of his more successful works, *A Mummer's Wife* (1885) and the novel for which he is most known, *Esther Waters* (1894). *A Mummer's Wife* is based in part on Moore's experiences with a theatre troupe with whom he travelled briefly, probably some time in 1883, in Hanley and other nearby factory towns. During the 1880s Moore occupied his spare time with several collaborations on minor dramatic productions, and he began to make a name for himself as a drama critic in articles and letters contributed to numerous periodicals, some of which were collected in his *Impressions and Opinions* (1891), an anthology which received generally favourable reviews. As in the preface to *Martin Luther*, Moore continued to voice his dissatisfaction with native English drama. He loudly impugned 'the soul-wearying conventionalities of the modern stage'.[2] Moore's views were generally in accordance with those already heralded by William Archer, the most eminent of the more liberal critics, but Moore's sometimes brash words nonetheless reached a wide audience and helped pave the way for J.T. Grein's Independent Theatre. The goal of this Theatre was to make serious literary drama, both continental and native, regularly available to English playgoers. Moore's service to the Independent Theatre, besides writing *The Strike at Arlingford*, was essentially twofold: first, through his journalistic

efforts he publicized the idea of free theatre; second, in various capacities he helped produce the theatre's crucial early offerings.

The production of *The Strike at Arlingford*, in London on 21 February 1893, was the immediate result of a wager by George R.Sims, a conservative critic who challenged the Theatre to produce a play written by Moore. Well aware of the Theatre's impoverished state, Moore quickly agreed and set about revising a five-act version of the play which he had written some years earlier but which had never been produced. The production was received in the following days with very mixed critical reaction. All the critics concurred that the play had been poorly acted and that the political and economic themes had been treated inaccurately. Many reviewers complained about the lengthy political discussions of capital and labour which bog down the action of the play. A number of critics, however, found the play an admirable and literary attempt to revive English drama. William Archer gave the play its most glowing praise, calling it 'a play with an excellent motive, worked out with an occasional uncertainty of touch, but on the whole very ably – and ruined, defaced, massacred by the most unfortunate acting conceivable'.[3]

Later in 1893 when Moore published the play, he prefaced it with a short note emphasizing that the labour dispute was far less important than 'the development of a moral idea'.[4] Moore was obviously trying to rebut the unanimous critical opinion that the political issues had been mishandled. Thus he wanted to emphasize the moral conflict between private sensibility and public duty in the protagonist, John Reid. In the *Pall Mall Gazette* Moore tried to explain that he wanted 'to depict a weak man in a position too strong for him – a kind of modern Hamlet, so to speak, whose mind and resolution were overborne by circumstance'.[5] In the play Reid, a poet and socialist, finds himself caught between two extremes, represented by the militant socialist Ellen Sands, his fiancée, and Lady Anne Travers, owner of the coal mines and the woman Reid had loved some ten years earlier. The moral dilemma for Reid is double-edged. He is not long in realizing that Anne is the only woman he ever truly loved, in large part because his aesthetic sensibilities are in tune with her aristocratic tastes; yet his political conscience eschews the economic inequities perpetuated by her class. The dilemma is brought to its climax when Reid must decide whether to withhold an anonymous cheque for the strikers' subsistence fund. The effect of this moral quandary on the play's action is minimal, however, for Reid is easily persuaded by Anne to withhold the cheque. He does acknowledge to himself that had it not been for his love for Anne he would have held to his socialist convictions, but this self-

knowledge has no positive value: the unruly colliers, having discovered his deception, pursue Reid to Anne's house; Anne herself makes a hasty retreat to Italy; and Reid is left despondent and trapped, his only escape a bottle of strychnine. Truly overborne by circumstances, deprived of his political convictions, and forsaken in love, Reid is the Hamlet who accomplishes absolutely nothing.

After the production of *The Strike at Arlingford* in 1893 and the success of *Esther Waters* in 1894, most of Moore's time was spent on his novels and short stories. Until the end of the decade, when Martyn coaxed him to lend his helping hand to the Irish Literary Theatre, Moore only twice dabbled in playwriting, both times in collaboration with Mrs Pearl Craigie, a popular novelist then publishing under the pseudonym John Oliver Hobbes with Moore's publisher, T. Fisher Unwin. The two apparently met in the winter of 1893 and were soon working on *The Fool's Hour*, a comedy of manners that was never produced, though one act of it was published in the first volume of *The Yellow Book* (April 1894). Shortly afterwards, Moore and Craigie collaborated on *Journeys End in Lovers Meeting*, a 'proverb in one act' which was first produced at Daly's Theatre on 5 June 1894. This play, another comedy of manners, was mildly successful, but professional and personal discord between Moore and Craigie soon precluded any further collaboration for the time being.[6]

The years that saw Moore's desultory development in the world of letters were for Martyn largely devoted to an eclectic education that produced a cultural refinement of rare breadth. His father, who boasted an aristocratic pedigree dating back to the reign of Henry II, had died in 1860, leaving the devoutly Catholic mother to conduct the child's education. For a while she raised Edward austerely at Tulira, but later they moved to Dublin and finally in 1870 to London, where he attended Beaumont College, a Jesuit school, for seven years. From 1877 to 1879 he attended Christ Church, Oxford, but left without taking a degree. His early education was capped by a grand tour of the Continent, conducted by Moore. During the 1880s Martyn resided at Tulira, assuming management of the estate. From this point on he began to exhibit a curious alloy of cultural taste. On the one hand he nurtured a strong appreciation for the aesthetic, or at least avant garde, in art. For instance, he collected impressionistic painting, made pilgrimages to Germany for Wagner festivals, and understood Ibsen better than most critics of his day. However, this strong tendency to sensual aestheticism was dominated by a yet stronger ascetic impulse, which surfaced in dutiful submission to Catholic ecclesiastical authority. The ascetic aspect of his personality – the visionary idealist who finds

naught but vanity in the fallen world – is reflected in his first literary work. *Morgante the Lesser* (1890) is a wide-ranging prose satire which mocks materialistic outlooks on life, using the caustic manner of Swift and Rabelais.

Martyn's career as dramatist commenced in the late 1890s. His *Heather Field*, produced in May 1899, proved the major success of the Irish Literary Theatre's first season. Thereafter his plays declined steadily in quality, though almost all are preservable for historical reasons. Some are precocious attempts to apply Ibsenian technique to Irish subject matter. Others veer in the opposite direction and become thinly disguised burlesques targeted at his flamboyant literary colleagues. Despite his later failures, however, his initial accomplishments, that is, his many contributions to the Irish Literary Theatre, were sufficiently notable to ensure him an honoured place in the history of Irish letters.

The story began in 1897 when Yeats, Martyn and Lady Gregory decided to form a theatre whose special mission was to provide a platform for the work of serious native dramatists. By showcasing the country's best talent, such a theatre would further the cause of Irish cultural independence. Martyn guaranteed the first year's expenses. His *Heather Field* and Yeats's *Countess Cathleen* were chosen for the all-important opening programme. Lady Gregory did most of the organizing work. The trio of founders had a timely idea and the enthusiasm to activate it. They had the financial backing and they had two formidable plays to present. What they conspicuously did not have, however, was a technical knowledge of stage company management. The rehearsals of both plays, conducted in London during the early part of 1899, were going very badly when Martyn thought of his cousin Moore, who did have the needed experience, whose notoriety would provide useful advertisement for the venture, and who was in fact Irish by birth. At first Moore hesitated to accept the invitation to join the cause, but once the commitment was made he threw his energies wholeheartedly into the task. By late spring 1899, both plays were ready for performance, thanks to Moore, but then an eleventh-hour crisis nearly caused the suspension of Yeats's play: Martyn threatened to withdraw financial support after a censorious priest detected supposedly anti-clerical passages in the play. Disaster was averted when Yeats produced two priests who found no offense in the questioned passages. With Martyn appeased, the curtain rose for the fledgling Irish Literary Theatre. Amid much agitation, an outcome of the religious controversy, *The Countess Cathleen* premiered successfully in Dublin on 8 May 1899. *The Heather Field* opened the following night, immediately eclipsing Yeats's play in popularity. It was to be Martyn's only enduring theatrical triumph, creating sufficient interest to justify brief revivals in England, Germany, and the United States.[7]

The Heather Field possesses a thematic strain held in common by virtually all Martyn's non-satiric plays, namely the opposition between idealistic and realistic approaches to life. Carden Tyrrell, with his dreams of turning wasteland into productive farmland, clearly embodies the idealistic point of view. His practical-minded wife, the realist, opposes the reclamation project. These points of view are extreme, however: Tyrrell's dream is obsessive and futile; the wife's common sense deteriorates into a warped materialism when she schemes to have her husband institutionalized. The more humane centre is occupied by Barry Ussher, who rues Tyrrell's self destructive expenditure but sympathizes with the nobility of the man's vision, 'our ideal of beauty that for ever haunts and eludes us through life'. Unfortunately, in the profit-and-loss world the uncompromising ideal is destined to elude us ultimately: hence Tyrrell retreats into madness. In this spectrum of attitudes Ussher's seems the most reasonable, but one suspects that Martyn identified himself more closely with the tragic Tyrrell who, for instance, shared his creator's taste for the music of Palestrina. The discrepancy between the reader's identification with Ussher and the author's apparent identification with Tyrrell creates a powerful dramatic tension in the play's subtext and serves to enhance its inherent ambiguity, the sense that the choice between idealistic and realistic courses of action is seldom clearly defined but rather based upon a complex mixture of temperament, motive, and circumstance. This ambiguity is embodied symbolically by the heather field, whose presence, at once threatening and beautiful, is felt in every scene. At times its commonness, its choking weediness, seems more akin to the wife's narrow prosaic view of life. At other times its untamed beauty is emphasized, and then the field suggests Tyrrell and his quest for the ideal. The natural world, it would appear, integrates the material and the spiritual, whereas such perfection is impossible for man.

Maeve, a highly lyrical piece, shares its predecessor's theme of frustrated idealism. Its protagonist, Maeve O'Heynes, is plighted to a wealthy Englishman, but she prefers to dream herself into the romantic past, where a legendary Celtic warrior courts her. Like Tyrrell, she seeks a drastic refuge when the world of fact closes in on her. *Maeve*, along with Alice Milligan's *The Last of Fianna*, opened the Irish Literary Theatre's second season on 19 February 1900. Andrew Malone has claimed that *Maeve* was the best received of the three plays the

Theatre offered that year. The general impression seems to be, however, that its enthusiastic reception was based less upon its many artistic merits than upon its incidental political implications. Reputedly the opening night audience cheered when Peg Inerny, Maeve's mysterious counsellor, proudly declares, 'You think I am only an old woman; but I tell you that Erin can never be subdued'.[8]

Originally Martyn's full-length play *The Tale of a Town* was scheduled to have top billing in the second season, but after reading the manuscript the others deemed it inappropriate for a serious, literary theatre. Yeats pronounced it 'crude throughout, childish in parts, a play to make our movement and ourselves ridiculous'. When Moore reluctantly concurred, Martyn, after a brief internal struggle, gave them the play unconditionally, to do with as they would for the good of the Theatre. Yeats and Moore were surprised, but they accepted the magnanimous offer to rework the play. In the course of events responsibility for the revision devolved upon Moore.

So it came to pass that *The Tale of a Town* became *The Bending of the Bough*, joining the programme for the Theatre's second season. It premiered the night following *Maeve*, on 20 February 1900, and played five times that week, one more than originally scheduled. Audiences, noting the play's political implications, responded favourably, and contemporary reviews also gave generous appreciations.[9]

Moore asked Martyn to cosign the new play, but the latter refused, claiming that the revisions expunged the spirit of the original, an objection for which he had some justification. It is true that the construction remains essentially the same, and that even many lines of dialogue are left verbatim, but Moore's version provided a crucial element that Martyn's conspicuously lacks – compelling dramatic conflict. The central dilemma in both plays, as also in *The Strike at Arlingford*, puts in opposition political and romantic choices. The protagonist must choose between political activism and romantic attachment, between his noble desire to do public service and his equally noble longing for the private happiness of domestic fulfilment. This matrix, with appropriate ambiguity added by shading character motivation, gives the playwright an effective vehicle with which to explore a prime condition of the human predicament, the difficulty of moral choice. The problem with Martyn's original is that the protagonist's dilemma lacks force. The love story is pallid because Millicent Fell is an ineffectual *belle dame*; her virtues are so negligible that one wonders how Jasper Dean became attached to her in the first place, much less why he chose to marry her and not follow Kirwan. However, Dean's temptation to follow the political path does not seem compelling either, because Kirwan is depicted more as a grumbling malcontent than a galvanizing national leader. These deficiencies are corrected in *The Bending of the Bough*. Millicent becomes provocative and appealing; Kirwan becomes a man of vision and action, one capable of exacting commitment from his disciples; the difficulty of Jasper's choice thus becomes much more consequential, much more agonizing. Since the three principal characters are given flesh and blood, most readers would agree that *The Bending of the Bough* is the better play. We have included both plays in the present volume, the first time they have been published together.

In defense of *The Tale of a Town*, it should be said that dramatic conflict was not Martyn's chief concern. The earlier two plays had already proven that Martyn at his best did have the ability to create a fairly interesting battle of minds and wills. With *The Tale of a Town* he was quite purposefully striking out into a radically different type of play, for it is a fast-paced, caustic satire, slashing out at several aspects of Irish life. Its principal aim was to ridicule folly in the Juvenalian manner. Naturally the British received much of Martyn's wrath but, like Swift, he did not whitewash the sins of his own people. Particularly he targeted the petty jealousies and the opportunism that divided local political leaders and made concerted resistance to British dominance impossible. Also targeted was the tendency of the Irish upper classes to ape the most snobbish aspects of British social fashion. At times the satire becomes so unrestrained that it breaks into the realm of burlesque: Dean tosses Foley down the stairs for flirting with his fiancée; Alderman Cassidy gets drunk despite his wife's constant vigilance; an Irish charwoman, representative of the fickle masses, ties a Union Jack to her broomhandle. It is not surprising that Yeats objected to such high jinks, yet neither is it surprising that Martyn, who grew increasingly nationalistic in his later years, thought the play's topicality would ignite Irish theatregoers. Unfortunately, by the time Martyn did get the play produced, in October 1905, the proper ripeness of moment had passed, and it excited little interest. His embarrassing defeat in the matter, despite the relative success of *Maeve*, caused him to withdraw from active participation in the Theatre after the second season and, consequently, from the mainstream of the Irish dramatic revival.[10]

Moore's final contribution to the Irish Literary Theatre was *Diarmuid and Grania*, a collaboration with Yeats, which launched the third season on 21 October 1901 at Dublin's Gaiety Theatre. It proved popular with audiences but objectionable to critics, who thought the authors took immoderate liberties in their handling of the ancient Celtic myth upon which the play was built. In particular, they thought the legend's heroic grandeur had been excessively modernized, deflated into a tawdry tale of romantic intrigue. Apparently the strain of collaboration also put pressure on the unstable relationship already existing between two such independent personalities, because a perceptible estrangement occurred. For this and other reasons, Moore's association with the Irish dramatic revival ended after the 1901 season. When Yeats and Lady Gregory reorganized the Theatre, they did not ask Moore to participate in their new venture, and he joined Martyn on the sidelines. Though excluded from the scene in subsequent years, both Martyn and Moore did unquestionably great service to the cause of Irish drama. Their efforts on behalf of the Irish Literary Theatre helped make it a success, and from that solid foundation rose its more acclaimed and enduring successor, the Abbey Theatre.

When Moore was excluded from the new Theatre, he did not by any means decide to abort his mission in Ireland. In fact, he remained in Dublin until 1911, gathering material for his three-volume account of his Irish sojourn (*Hail and Farewell!*) and writing his book of Irish short stories (*The Untilled Field*) as well as *The Lake*, a short novel about the moral qualms of an Irish priest. This same time also saw Moore working sporadically on the idea that would, after major rewritings, find its final form in *The Passing of the Essenes*, the last of his plays included in the present volume.

Moore's interest in the subject of *The Passing of the Essenes* began some time between 1898 and 1910 and ended with the production of *Essenes* in 1930, just three years before his death. The central idea of the play is a chance meeting in an Essene monastery between the Apostle Paul and a non-divine Jesus who had survived the crucifixion some twenty years earlier. Moore claims he became interested in the subject largely because of a belated initial reading of the Bible, given to him in 1898 by an old friend,[11] and because of his talks with John Eglinton of the National Library of Ireland, who acquainted Moore with current continental scholarship positing the view that Jesus had not died on the cross but had merely fallen into a 'cataleptic swoon'. What particularly interested Moore was not new or fashionable Biblical exegesis but the figure of Paul as a man of faith confronted with spiritual contradictions. Indeed, the anguish of the religion-haunted man (or woman) permeates many of Moore's works from the beginning of his career.

Despite Moore's fascination with the core idea of this new subject, he did not readily find a satisfactory way to execute the idea. In fact, he worked on the idea in six separate pieces of writing, all remarkably different. Space limitations do not permit a detailing of these differences, but a brief note on the various forms will prove indicative both of Moore's obsession with this idea and his lifelong adherence to Gautier's dictum that the correction of form is virtue. He first drafted a short narrative entitled 'The Apostle' for publication in *The English Review* in 1910. In the following year he published a scenario with the same title in dramatic form. Clearly Moore was not satisfied with either of these two writings, and it is probable that he published them only to protect his interest in the novelty of the subject matter until he had time to work out the proper format. Several years later he thus worked the material into a novel which he called *The Brook Kerith* (1916). Certainly the novel was one with which Moore was pleased, but he still hoped to find the appropriate dramatic form. His next venture with the subject was apparently a scenario called 'The Brook Kerith: A Spiritual Drama in Four Acts and Seven Scenes'. The exact date of this unpublished scenario is not known, but it was some time between the publication of the novel in 1916 and the publication of a full-length play entitled *The Apostle* (published in 1923 but never produced). The final version with its wholly new title, *The Passing of the Essenes*, was published seven years later in 1930. The play also premiered on 1 October 1930 at the Arts Theatre and almost without exception was favorably reviewed.

The subject of *The Coming of Gabrielle* (1920) occupied Moore for nearly as long as *The Passing of the Essenes*. His work on the play began in 1904 when, after a ten-year silence, Pearl Craigie suggested they once again pool their talents. The two collaborators soon quarrelled, however, and it was nine years later, seven years after Craigie's death, before Moore took up the play again, publishing it as *Elizabeth Cooper* in 1913. Much of his interest in this play, in both of its published forms, arose from personal circumstances. The plot, theme, and titular character are based on his correspondence with an Austrian countess he never met. The correspondence apparently began in late 1903 when this countess, using the assumed name of Gabrielle von Hoenstadt, wrote Moore an admiring and provocative letter. He quickly responded and exhorted her to be as forthright as possible, assuring her that no one would ever see her letters. In fact, Moore was disingenuous not only in that he afterwards considered publishing the letters but also in that much of the dialogue in the play is taken directly from them.[12] Though Moore never met 'Gabrielle', he did have the opportunity, and he was long intrigued with the idea of a famous, middle-aged author meeting a younger flirtatious admirer. It is this idea that Moore executes in his play, relying heavily on his earlier experiences with the Restoration comedy of manners. In effect, the play in its various forms is Moore's attempt to work out in literature what he could not, or would not, in life.

Two other plays by Moore that we also do not include are *Esther Waters: A Play* and *The Making of an Immortal*. The former, produced in London in 1911, is an adaptation of Moore's most famous novel (1894), a realistic account of a servant girl's struggle to keep and raise her illegitimate son over a twenty-year period of economic and emotional setbacks. The latter, produced in London in 1928, is a lightweight one-act piece capitalizing on the Shakespeare-Bacon controversy, Moore humorously taking the view that Bacon wrote *Richard II* and pawned it off on Shakespeare only after Queen Elizabeth took offense. Neither of the plays is representative of Moore's major interests at the times they were written. The dramatization of *Esther Waters* clearly harks back to Moore's long-abandoned interest in the realistic and naturalistic fiction of the 1880's and 1890's. In part, it can be surmised that Moore was hoping to profit again by his most commercially successful novel, but it is equally true that a successful adaptation would have boosted his ego, for none of his plays had been a long-running success. Evidently, even after the play was panned by the critics, Moore did not give up hope, for a decade later he started work with Barrett H.Clark on a new dramatic version, a project that was, however, abandoned.[13] *The Making of an Immortal* sprang from a superficial and intermittent interest in the plays of Francis Bacon, and Moore agreed to put his idea in dramatic form only when J.R.Wells of the Bowling Green Press expressed interest in producing a deluxe edition.

Martyn's later plays return to themes and techniques employed in the first three. *An Enchanted Sea*, produced in April 1904, is a short lyrical play conceived along the same lines as *Maeve*. It depicts the fatal fascination the sea has over the mind of a young Irish aristocrat, Lord Mask. To him the ever beckoning sea represents a seductive realm of beauty, a magical beauty uniquely Celtic. *Grangecolman*, produced in January 1912, returns to an Ibsenian drama of ideas. Like *The Heather Field*, it presents a domestic tragedy. The protagonist, Catherine Devlin, a highly educated doctor with frustrated feminist ambitions, finds suicide the only solution for her problems. *The Privilege of Place*, produced in November 1915, exposes political corruption in the same satiric manner as *The Tale of a Town*. It is based upon a sketch, published in *The Leader*, 26 July 1902, which features a venal public official named Steppingstone Feathernest.

Two of the later plays are interesting for their mischievous satirical portraits of Moore and Yeats. In *Romulus and Remus*, published in 1907 but never acted until nine years later, Moore (Romulus) and Yeats

(Remus) are apprentice hairdressers. Remus is followed about by an infatuated, fawning shopwoman, intended for Lady Gregory. His claim that he is no mere man but rather an 'ethereal spirit' introduces a scene apparently adapted from an actual incident witnessed by Martyn, wherein Yeats reclined on a sofa in trance, pretending to be in mystical communication with some legendary Celtic hero, while Lady Gregory fed him chocolates with a pair of long silver tongs.[14]

The Dream Physician, produced in November 1914, takes further swipes at Yeats's spiritualism. As the character Beau Brummell he suddenly discerns 'oracular virtues' in a common washbowl stand, which he takes to be a type of ancient tripod, then conducts a ridiculous seance replete with hysterical medium and prophecies chanted to a banjo accompaniment. The play also levels heavy artillery at Moore (George Augustus Moon) whose unflattering portrait of Martyn had recently appeared in *Ave*. Martyn retaliates by lampooning Moore's half-affected pose as literary and social lion; Moon, for instance, brags about fighting duels in Paris then cowers after a loud knocking at the door. When Moon claims to be a modern day Swift, another character retorts, 'While Swift was a terror to his enemies, you have only succeeded in being a terror to your friends'.

Martyn used *The Dream Physician* to inaugurate the Irish Theatre (1914-1920), a little theatre group he established to combat the Abbey's then almost exclusive restriction to the peasant play. By contrast, the Irish Theatre would open its doors to nonpeasant plays written by Irish writers, plays in Gaelic, and Continental drama. All programmes except the first were staged at a small theatre (100 seats) in Hardwicke Street in north Dublin. Players were drawn from a pool composed of experienced amateurs, aspiring students, and professionals looking for the challenge of a different type of role. They performed without remuneration. Although the Hardwicke venture could not compete for popularity with the powerful Abbey, it did make available the alternative artistic theatre Martyn thought was vital to a broadly-based literary renaissance. It also paved the way for the Dublin Drama League, formed by Lennox Robinson in 1918, a more successful organization which had aims similar to those of Martyn's company. Over a third of the Irish Theatre's productions were Continental works, rarely seen plays in that corner of the world, by the likes of Chekhov, Ibsen, Strindberg and Maeterlinck. True to its manifesto, the Theatre also presented several non-peasant plays, satires and intellectual dramas, written by Irish authors. Most of these were first productions. In fact, in 1917 Martyn went so far as to offer a prize to the native writer who submitted the best intellectual drama of nonpeasant life. Besides

The Dream Physician, among his own works to be performed by the Irish Theatre were *The Privilege of Place* (1915), *Romulus and Remus* (1916), revivals of *The Heather Field* (1916) and *Grangecolman* (1917), and his very last play, *Regina Eyre* (1919).[15]

None of Martyn's later plays quite rise to the quality of *The Heather Field*. He was hampered by too many constricting impulses to be a consistently effective dramatist. Weak dialogue and wooden characterization were compounded by an entrenched misogyny, which prevented portrayal of rounded female personalities, and by an almost fastidious submission to Catholic dogma, which tended to limit his aesthetic freedom. In his attitudes toward women and toward religion Martyn stands in diametric contrast to Moore, who was both amorous and irreverent. By temperament Martyn was essentially unsociable, at times even monastic in his austerity. Though he was more cosmopolitan in his artistic tastes than many of his countrymen, his unsociability militated against a broad understanding of human nature.

Ultimately, however, it was an anomalous opposite impulse towards activism that fragmented his creative powers. During the later years he devoted his energies to an incredible number of activities, including reformation of Church decoration and Church music, service in political organizations, and contributions to polemical journalism. The Church was his first love, reformation of the ecclesiastical arts his primary mission. For instance, in 1902 he donated a large sum to establish a Palestrina Society for the performance of plain chant, and later he worked hard to guarantee that a new cathedral rising at Loughrea would display nothing less than excellence in native sculpture, wood carving and stained glass. A full description of his contributions to the advancement of Irish art would fill many pages. Martyn's second love – and a close second at that – was political activism. In the latter half of his life his politics became progressively more nationalistic, evinced by a term (1904-08) as president of the Sinn Fein organization. His activities ranged from stirring minor agitations, such as protesting the visit of Edward VII to Ireland in 1903, to supporting the most important movements, such as the Gaelic League's effort to promote use of the Irish language. Given the breadth of his involvement, he must be considered a significant force in Ireland's endeavour to forge a truly independent cultural identity.[16]

Martyn died in 1923 and Moore ten years later in 1933. For Martyn, an early and perhaps premature dismissal by his colleagues in the theatre prompted him to turn his attention to other areas. For Moore, drama never commanded the sustained attention that his longer prose works did, though clearly he had hoped from the very beginning of his

INTRODUCTION

career for a major success in the theatre. While the plays of neither will challenge the best of Synge or O'Casey or Yeats, both Moore and Martyn are slowly being afforded a secure place in the history of Irish drama.

NOTES

1 *Confessions of a Young Man*, ed. Susan Dick (Montreal and London: McGill-Queen's Univ.Press, 1972), pp.66-67.
2 Moore's words in a letter to the *St.James's Gazette*, 19 July 1890.
3 'The Theatre', *Saturday Review* (London), 75 (25 February 1893), 208.
4 (London: Walter Scott, 1893).
5 *Pall Mall Gazette*, 21 February 1893.
6 Craigie went so far as to publish *Journeys End in Lovers Meeting* in her *Tales About Temperaments* (1902) without anywhere acknowledging Moore as the co-author, even though his name had appeared in the playbills at the time the play was produced and in the reviews.
7 A convenient source for excerpts from contemporary reviews is Robert Hogan and James Kilroy, *The Irish Literary Theatre 1899-1901* (Dublin: Dolmen Press, 1975).
8 For more recent interpretations of *The Heather Field* and *Maeve*, refer to the following: Sister Marie Therese Courtney, *Edward Martyn and the Irish Theatre* (New York, Vantage Press, 1956); Jan Setterquist, *Ibsen and the Beginnings of Anglo-Irish Drama* (New York: Gordian Press, 1974); and Wayne Hall, 'Edward Martyn (1859-1923): Politics and Drama of Ice,' *Eire-Ireland*, 15:ii (1980), 113-22; Katharine Worth, 'Ibsen and the Irish Theatre', *Theatre Research International*, Spring 1990, Vol. 15, pp. 20-28.
9 The *Irish Daily Times*, for instance, entitled its review 'George Moore's Brilliant Play'. English reviewers were less enthusiastic, but they may have been put off by the play's anti-British sentiment.
10 Courtney and Setterquist are among the very few recent critics who prefer Martyn's version to Moore's. The fullest discussion of improvements made by Moore is given by Una Ellis-Fermor, *The Irish Dramatic Movement* (London: Methuen, 1939), pp.125-32. William J.Feeney, in the introduction to his edition of *Bending of the Bough*, Irish Drama Series, Vol.III (Chicago: DePaul Univ.Press, 1969, pp.1-21) also explores differences between the two versions, and he adds helpful background information about the contemporary political situation in Ireland. In a September 1900 letter to Moore, recorded in the second volume of Lady Gregory's *Journals* (Gerrards Cross: Colin Smythe, and New York: Oxford University Press, 1988, pp. 542-44), Martyn describes both *The Tale of a Town* and *The Bending of the Bough* as 'unfitting' for the Irish Literary Theatre. This illuminating letter also gives Martyn's reasons for leaving the Theatre – partly because he had been 'snubbed' by the other founders and partly because he had given more than his fair share of financial support to the venture.
11 See his 'A Prefatory Letter on Reading the Bible for the First Time', printed in the Feb.1911 issue of *The English Review* and included as the introduction to *The Apostle* (London: Maunsel, 1911).

xx

12 'Gabrielle's' letters to Moore are preserved in the typescript Moore apparently had made (now housed at the Humanities Research Center, The University of Texas at Austin). There are twelve known letters by Moore to 'Gabrielle', all located in the National Library of Ireland. Moore's letters to 'Gabrielle', as well as hers to him, have been published in *George Moore's Correspondence with the Mysterious Countess*, by David B. Eakin and Robert Langenfeld (University of Victoria English Literary Studies, 1984).

13 See Barrett H.Clark, 'George Moore at Work', *American Mercury*, 4 (Feb.1925), 202-9; later absorbed in 'George Moore: At Home in Paris', *Intimate Portraits* (New York: Dramatists Play Service 1951), pp.57-153. Clark's article is based in part on letters from Moore to him, in Yale University Library, which also houses typescripts of two versions of the dramatization.

14 The incident is reported in Courtney, p.127.

15 For information about the Irish Theatre see William J.Feeney's introduction to *Edward Martyn's Irish Theatre*, Lost Plays of the Irish Renaissance, vol.2 (Newark, Delaware: Proscenium Press, 1980). The collection includes *Romulus and Remus*. It should be noted that slightly earlier in his career Martyn had helped establish another little theatre group, The Theatre of Ireland (1906-1912), which shared many of the goals of the Irish Theatre. For excerpts from and commentary on *Regina Eyre*, which survives only in the form of an acting script, see Stephen P.Ryan, 'Edward Martyn's Last Play', *Studies* (Summer 1958), 192-99.

16 The standard biography on Martyn is Denis Gwynn, *Edward Martyn and the Irish Revival* (London: Cape, 1930); interesting supplementary material, including a supposed eyewitness account of Martyn and Moore's last meeting, can be found in Philip Rooney, 'The Turret Room', *The Capuchin Annual* (1962), pp.71-80. There are two excellent studies of the relationship between and the accomplishments of the literary cousins: F.S.L.Lyon, 'George Moore and Edward Martyn', *Hermathena* (Spring 1964), 9-32; Ann Saddlemyer, 'All Art is a Collaboration? George Moore and Edward Martyn' in *The World of W.B.Yeats*, rev.edn., eds. Robin Skelton and Ann Saddlemyer (Seattle: University of Washington Press, 1967), pp.169-88.

THE STRIKE AT ARLINGFORD

PLAY IN THREE ACTS
BY
GEORGE MOORE

NOTE

In my own conception of my play the labour dispute is an externality to which I attach little importance. What I applied myself to in the composition of 'The Strike at Arlingford' was the development of a moral idea. I leave the play itself to explain this idea.

G.M.

CHARACTERS.

JOHN REID
BARON STEINBACH
FRED HAMER
LADY ANNE TRAVERS
ELLEN SANDS
FOX, } *Miners*
SIMON,
FOOTMAN

ACT I

SCENE – *Drawing-room at* LADY ANNE TRAVERS'. *Bow window opening on lawn at back right. Door back, window left, door right. Writing-table, couch, arm-chairs, rich furniture. When the curtain rises the door at back, middle of stage, is opened by the* FOOTMAN.
MR. HAMER *is shown in.*

FOOTMAN. I will give her ladyship your card. *(The door is closed,* HAMER *looks round, and having assured himself that he is not observed, opens a note-book and begins taking notes of the contents of the room.* BARON STEINBACH *appears at window opening on to lawn. After watching* HAMER *a moment he enters;* HAMER *turns to him with some slight embarrassment.)*

HAMER. I come from the *Durham Mercury*. Here is my card.

STEINBACH *(reads).* 'Mr Fred Hamer, representative of the *Durham Mercury*'. *(Speaks)* You want to see Lady Anne?

HAMER. I should like to. I've come from Durham for the purpose of writing some descriptive articles on the state of the town during the strike of colliers. I hope that Lady Anne will be kind enough to grant me an interview.

STEINBACH. In any case you intend a descriptive article on her drawing-room.

HAMER. I'm afraid you caught me in the act – just a memorandum of the room. This is her drawing-room, the room she lives in, I suppose? (HAMER *looks at* STEINBACH, *wondering who he is.* STEINBACH *speaks with lofty superiority, and yet without vulgarity.)*

STEINBACH. This is Lady Anne's drawing-room. But I do not think that she will be able to grant you an interview. Lady Anne, you see, has only just returned from abroad. She has a great deal of business to attend to, and I hardly think that the present time is a convenient one. She has not yet got over the fatigue of the journey.

HAMER. She has been, I believe, about a week in Arlingford?

STEINBACH *(looking at him sharply, and answering sharply).* Yes, about a week.

HAMER. I presume that these labour troubles had something to do with her ladyship's sudden return?

3

STEINBACH. I am afraid I cannot answer you. However, I may tell you that it is not likely that Lady Anne will be able to spare the time for an interview this morning. I have come to speak to her on business. I tell you this, for I know that you newspaper people are very hard worked, and that your time is not your own.

HAMER. Thank you. But – I have sent in my card, stating my business, and if Lady Anne is as busy as you say, she will probably make an appointment. I am in no hurry. (*Sits down and takes up book. Annoyed, the* BARON *walks towards the window; he turns, and seeing that* HAMER *does not intend to leave, he crosses left, stops, reads the card, pauses, and then speaks.*)

STEINBACH. I see you come from Durham, Mr Hamer.

HAMER (*lays down the book, and looks up quite pleased at the interruption.*) How are things in your neighbourhood? Any signs of fresh labour troubles?

HAMER. The miners are, I think, waiting to see how things will turn out in Arlingford.

STEINBACH. Very likely; and if the battle is lost here, we may expect strikes all over the North of England. (HAMER *looks at him curiously, wondering who is this grand and somewhat authoritative individual.*) Wattsbury ought to have taught trades unionism a lesson; it received a severe defeat there.

HAMER. It did indeed. But the men would have won all along the line if it had not been for the energy and decision of Baron Steinbach. He is the most determined foe that trades unionism has. He sees that the concessions which the men ask in the name of Justice are stepping-stones to the utter destruction of capital.

STEINBACH. Don't you think he is right?

HAMER. Unquestionably, from his point of view.

STEINBACH (*in a more conciliatory tone*). Were you at Wattsbury?

HAMER. Yes, I interviewed the strike leaders and as many of the directors as I could. I was most anxious to get an interview with Baron Steinbach, but he was always engaged. An interview with him would have been most interesting. He is a man of ideas, and could express his views regarding the necessity of capital.

STEINBACH (*laughing*). Your flattering remarks make it impossible for me to leave you any longer in doubt as to whom you are talking to – I am Baron Steinbach.

HAMER (*jumping up and somewhat overcome*). Oh, indeed, I am sure I had no idea – I am pleased to have had the honour of meeting you.

STEINBACH (*bows*). I read your interviews, and must confess that they were singularly free from prejudice. You have the talent of conveying an interesting and truthful reflection of life.

HAMER (*delighted*). I am glad you liked my articles. I was just saying that I tried to get an interview with you during the Wattsbury strike, but you were always engaged.

STEINBACH. Did it occur to you that perhaps I did not want to be interviewed?

HAMER (*laughing*). Perhaps it did. But are you sure you're not mistaken? The strike leaders are always anxious to express their views.

STEINBACH. The position of the socialist leaders and the capitalists regarding publicity is quite different. They have everything, we have nothing to gain by the publication of our views. In my opinion the battle on our side should be conducted in silence. (*Perceiving that* HAMER *is listening intently he stops short.*) But I see that you are interviewing me.

HAMER. I wish you would develop that idea. You were saying that the battle on your side should be conducted in silence.

STEINBACH. If I were to develop that idea I should be acting contrary to the principles I profess.

HAMER. But while we are waiting for Lady Anne it would be most interesting if –

STEINBACH (*laughing*). I see you are a born journalist – the effective article is your principle.

HAMER. My principle and my interest.

STEINBACH (*laughing*). Even if I wished to express my views I'm afraid this is no time to do so. I have come to Arlingford to see my friend Lady Anne Travers.

HAMER. I hope you have come with some project of settlement. But you are against all compromise; you would force the miners to accede to your terms. But perhaps Lady Anne may incline towards the principle that labour disputes should be settled by arbitration.

STEINBACH. If ever I desire to express my views on capital and labour I shall be glad to entrust their transmission to your intelligence; in the meantime, do not try to interview me against my will.

HAMER. You will excuse my hoping that Lady Anne will see no harm –

STEINBACH. I think that all expressions of opinion at the present moment would be injudicious.

HAMER. I will not presume to argue that point with you, Baron Steinbach. But may I ask you if you think that Lady Anne will keep us waiting much longer?

STEINBACH. I have already told you, Mr Hamer, that I believe Lady Anne is still suffering from the fatigues of her journey – that I have come to talk with her on important business..

HAMER. If I were in your house, Baron Steinbach, I should at once retire, but as I am in Lady Anne Travers's, perhaps you will excuse me if I wait until Lady Anne herself decides if she can see me. (*The door on the right opens and* LADY ANNE *enters.*)

LADY ANNE. Oh, how do you do, my dear Baron? How good of you to come! Who is –

HAMER. I come from the *Durham Mercury*. You have my card in your hand, Lady Anne.

STEINBACH. I have told Mr Hamer that I do not think it is advisable that you should express any opinion regarding the strike.

LADY ANNE. You see, Mr Hamer, I only arrived a few days ago from abroad. I have been little in Arlingford since my husband's death; besides, I have exceedingly important business to discuss with Baron Steinbach. You must excuse me.

HAMER. I was about to explain to Baron Steinbach when you entered that the object of this visit was not merely to interview you regarding the strike – I easily divine what your views are – but to ask you if I may be present at one o'clock, when you receive the deputation.

STEINBACH (*to* LADY ANNE). Have you consented to receive another deputation?

LADY ANNE. I could hardly refuse. Do you think I was wrong?

STEINBACH. I don't think much good will come of re-opening the question. You intend to stand by your first offer and to grant nothing further?

LADY ANNE. I can make no further concession, that is certain. But I do not think it would look well to refuse to receive the deputation.

STEINBACH. Perhaps not.

HAMER. The account I shall furnish will be impartial; you know that, Baron Steinbach. But should you refuse to allow me to report the proceedings, John Reid or his *fiancée*, Ellen Sands, will send in a report, and you know what a one-sided version that will be.

STEINBACH (*stops to think*). Yes, it is as you say; I prefer your report to theirs, and I have no objection to offer. Lady Anne, will you allow Mr Hamer to accompany the deputation?

LADY ANNE. I shall be very glad if you will consent to be present.

HAMER. Thank you. At one o'clock then. You have just come back from the south, Lady Anne? This is the room you live in. That cabinet is Chippendale?

LADY ANNE. No, old Italian.

HAMER. I should like to have the impressions gathered on your journey, but when you are less busy. Your drawing-room looks on a garden. You are fond of gardening, I suppose? One of these days, before you leave, Lady Anne, you will favour me, I hope, with your views and your impressions; and, perhaps, Baron Steinbach, I shall be able to persuade you to favour me with your views regarding the necessity of capital? Most interesting, I'm sure.

STEINBACH. We'll talk about that later on.

HAMER. I hope so. (*Exit.* BARON STEINBACH *returns from the door.* LADY ANNE *advances to meet him, her hand extended.*)

STEINBACH. It is such a pleasure to see you again, Anne.

LADY ANNE. (*with an almost imperceptible moving away from him*). And I am so glad to see you. I wrote to you, because I believe you to be my friend.

STEINBACH. You have no better friend. When I received your letter, I called for the Bradshaw, and I told my servant to pack my portmanteau at once. Then I threw myself into an arm-chair and read your letter over and over again.

LADY ANNE. There was not much to read.

STEINBACH. No; your letters are always the same curt little epistles...A little statement in a fine, delicate handwriting. (*Taking her hand.*) Your hand is your handwriting – that decisive little writing with its very distinctive slope. (*She withdraws her hand.*) It was a great pleasure to receive your letter, and in the train I watched the hedge-rows, thinking that with every one I was some yards nearer to you.

LADY ANNE. It was very good of you. You are very good to me. I want you to be my friend.

STEINBACH. If I were not your friend, do you think that I would have left important business and come to you at an hour's notice? I didn't wait for the express. I came by the slow train, because it arrived here ten minutes sooner.

LADY ANNE. You've arrived none too soon. Things are in a frightful way here. I don't know what will become of me! What would you advise?

STEINBACH. We've all the afternoon to talk business. I want to tell you that I think you as charming as ever.

LADY ANNE. If you wouldn't make love to me.

STEINBACH. Have I not a right?

LADY ANNE. I'd sooner have you as a friend.

STEINBACH. You didn't always think like that, Anne.

LADY ANNE. I always told you that I was a cold woman, and I'm in too great trouble now to think about love. (STEINBACH *looks at her doubtfully.*) I know you don't believe me; men never will

7

believe. (*A pause.*)

STEINBACH. I never could make out whether you liked me, or what you intended.

LADY ANNE. I always liked you, my dear Baron, but –

STEINBACH. My dear Anne, let us be frank with one another; you've treated me very badly.

LADY ANNE. Have I?

STEINBACH. Think of it. We met at a dinner-party about two years ago, and it has been going on ever since.

LADY ANNE. You took me down to dinner.

STEINBACH. And we were friends before we got to the dining-room; and next day you wrote asking me to lunch, and you began your letter 'My dear Baron'.

LADY ANNE. I didn't mean anything by that. I told you in the drawing-room that very night that you were mistaken in me.

STEINBACH. It wasn't so much that I was mistaken as that I was unlucky. It was not to be; I felt from the first I was not going to be your lover. One always knows.

LADY ANNE. How strange men are! Is that what a man thinks when he is introduced to a woman – am I or am I not going to be her lover?

STEINBACH. Only when one is in love. I thought you the most fascinating woman I had seen for a long time. You seemed to like me, yet I only once thought that my instinct had deceived me.

LADY ANNE. When was that?

STEINBACH. The first time I lunched alone with you. I was standing on the hearth-rug smoking a cigarette, thinking how I should tell you that I loved you. You must have guessed my embarrassment, for you got up and walked so close to me that I quite naturally took you in my arms.

LADY ANNE. It was then that you thought that you were mistaken.

STEINBACH. Yes, and the mistake was pardonable, for with your head lying on my shoulder, you told me you were going out of town, and it was arranged that I was to meet you.

LADY ANNE. What could I do? My friends wrote to say they were going to send for me to the station.

STEINBACH. You put me off till the summer, till you went abroad to take the waters at Carlsbad or Contrexville, I forget which. The day was arranged for your departure, but I knew that something would happen to prevent it, and something did happen.

LADY ANNE. It was not my fault. You know it wasn't.

STEINBACH. Apparently not. You told me the whole circumstances three months after.

LADY ANNE. I could not have acted otherwise than I did. But when I asked you to come to the Riviera you couldn't leave London. That was not my fault!

STEINBACH. Nor mine; it was the moment of the Baring crisis, and for a fortnight I did not know that I should have a thousand left to go on with. When I wrote to you later on, you sent a telegram telling me not to come.

LADY ANNE. I had friends staying with me. There always did seem to be some hitch. And now I am like you were in the Baring crisis; in a week's time I may not have a thousand pounds to my name. How can you expect me to think of love at such a time? (*Rises and crosses.*)

STEINBACH. Tell me exactly what your position is.

LADY ANNE. I cannot go into details.

STEINBACH. I don't want the details. I'll get them from the books; just the main facts. (*Lights a cigarette*).

LADY ANNE. As far as I understand, the dispute resolves itself to this: The men want a rise of twenty per cent all round. There are other demands, the abolition of what they call 'Billy Fairplay'. It has something to do with getting rid of the refuse.

STEINBACH. I know. Have the men had an increase before?

LADY ANNE. Yes; last year an increase of five per cent was demanded on account of an anticipated advance in the price of coal.

STEINBACH. You conceded the rise in wages and the advance in coal did not come off?

LADY ANNE. Exactly.

STEINBACH. So the money in the mine, out of which you all get your living, is five per cent poorer than last year?

LADY ANNE. I suppose so. (*Sits R. table.*) They contribute nothing towards the working expenses, and now they want another rise of twenty per cent. If the mine belonged to the miners, it could not be worked on such a scale of wages.

STEINBACH (*walking to and fro*). I should think not indeed. It is impossible to work a mine on the co-operative principle. At the end of six months they would have to reduce the scale of wages; in a year they would be in bankruptcy, and the mine in ruins.

LADY ANNE. My manager tells me that we could not grant this twenty per cent and work the mine at a profit. Even if it were possible, nothing would be left for me. I cannot afford to grant more than five per cent.

STEINBACH. I would not have you raise their wages one per cent, nor grant any concession whatsoever. Admit the principle of

9

concession, and bit by bit they will wring our property from us. Our interests are common, and if we were half as united in our actions as these fellows we should very soon trample out the labour movement. (*Sits.*) When did the men leave work?

LADY ANNE. Three weeks ago.

STEINBACH. Do you think they are well supplied with funds?

LADY ANNE. I think not. A week ago they would have accepted our terms.

STEINBACH. A mistake, a fatal mistake, to offer any terms. If *I* had my way, the declaration of every strike should be accompanied with a declaration of a reduction of wages. They accept our terms, or we lose the battle sooner or later.

LADY ANNE. It is easy for you to speak like that; your capital is unlimited, mine is not, and if the pumps were to be stopped, and the water got the upper hand, the mine might never be got back into working order.

STEINBACH. There is always non-unionist labour to be had if you offer the price.

LADY ANNE. They say that there is hardly any non-unionist labour; besides, my resources are limited.

STEINBACH. The other mine-owners should help you.

LADY ANNE. They are afraid the strike will spread.

STEINBACH. Personal selfishness will prove our ruin in the end. That's the weak point in our armour. And you tell me they refused your offer of five per cent. Why was that?

LADY ANNE. The great labour leader, John Reid, came down here to conduct the strike, and it was owing to his influence that the men resolved to accept no abatement on their original demands.

STEINBACH. I know him; we met at Wattsbury. He is a poet as well as a socialist leader; a curious combination, socialism and poetry. I see no connection between hob-nails and sonnets, bull-pups and -

LADY ANNE (*rises*). His poems are not in the least like that. Here is his last volume (*Takes book from table.*) *Nostalgia*; charming title, isn't it? and there are charming things in it.

STEINBACH. It is strange that, notwithstanding all your trouble, you should be able to find time to interest yourself in poetry. This taste in poetry is quite new in you. (LADY ANNE *continues reading.* STEINBACH *watches.*) One would think you were personally interested in the author.

LADY ANNE (*laying the book down*). I'm afraid that that is just it. You see, we are old friends.

STEINBACH. What *do* you mean, Anne?

LADY ANNE. Yes, old friends, though we have not seen each other for

10

ten years. Ten years ago he was my father's secretary – he was eighteen and I was seventeen.

STEINBACH. Oh, I see, a boy and girl flirtation.

LADY ANNE. Yes, I suppose it was that. We used to stand on the terrace and look at the sun setting. He wrote verses which he used to send me. It was a pretty romance while it lasted. (*Sits on sofa.*)

STEINBACH. And how was it broken off?

LADY ANNE. When I was eighteen. I understood that I could not marry my father's secretary.

STEINBACH. And John Reid was dismissed, and he told you that you had broken his heart.

LADY ANNE. John Reid was not Lord Elwin's servant. He was just as much a gentleman as my father.

STEINBACH. Ah! that explains a good deal in John Reid. He used to puzzle me; I could see that his plebeian airs were more or less an affectation. I understand it all now.

LADY ANNE. And do you think better of him?

STEINBACH. No, indeed, I should have liked him better as a working-man fighting the battle of his class. So he is a mere parcel of renunciations, a frantic egotism –

LADY ANNE. Egotism! But he surrenders all things for an idea.

STEINBACH. Renunciations are often but the efforts of the feeble to realise themselves. So he is no more than a convert. I have little taste for conversions of any kind. You know, my dear Anne –

LADY ANNE. I believe it is disagreeable to you that any one should even try to be good.

STEINBACH. Ah! trying to be good! But I see that you can only think of your old lover. Tell me about him. He said that you had broken his heart.

LADY ANNE. He did say that his heart was broken.

STEINBACH. And in the following year you married Sir Francis Travers. Five years ago he died leaving you a rich widow, and your old lover heads a strike of your miners, little thinking that Lady Anne Travers is the Anne that he loved. You were a lovely girl; how much you must have meant to him!

LADY ANNE. Yes, he did love me, perhaps as no one else ever did.

STEINBACH. A most romantic situation; and the young man comes here suspecting nothing?

LADY ANNE. He suspected nothing the day before yesterday.

STEINBACH. Then you have written to him?

LADY ANNE. No; I went to see him.

STEINBACH. Where? At his lodgings?

LADY ANNE. No. At the committee rooms.

STEINBACH. And you saw him?

LADY ANNE. No, I didn't see him. He was not there.

STEINBACH. But you do not care for him?

LADY ANNE. Care for him? No; but I should like to see him again.

STEINBACH. So that, through his influence, you might settle this dispute to your advantage?

LADY ANNE. That is all. (*Rises.*)

STEINBACH. Did you meet any one at the committee rooms?

LADY ANNE. Yes; his sweetheart, Ellen Sands. They are engaged to be married. I can't congratulate him on his choice – a most unformed young person. I have heard since that she is a school-mistress turned socialist; the girl who believes she has a mission, and would hang on to a man for its accomplishment.

STEINBACH. I know the type. The feeble who are in earnest.

LADY ANNE. I cannot think what he sees in her.

STEINBACH. Did you leave any message for him?

LADY ANNE. I wrote a note, but fearing she might see it, I tore it up, and left some flowers I had with me.

STEINBACH. How like a woman! You knew that leaving the flowers would cause Ellen Sands extreme annoyance.

LADY ANNE. I did not care whether I annoyed her. It was a bunch of heliotrope, and he always associated that perfume with me. He will think and think. She will describe me over and over again, and then suddenly he will remember. I don't think I have changed very much.

STEINBACH. It is a pity in a way, for if he knew nothing at all about it, what would his consternation not have been on finding himself face to face with you!

LADY ANNE. I daresay he will be sufficiently troubled as it is.

STEINBACH. You forget that rejected love turns to hate.

LADY ANNE. Do you mean that you are going to hate me? You know, Edward, that it was not my fault. Something went wrong from the first; as you said, we weren't lucky. Why cannot you be my friend? (*Sits.*)

STEINBACH. I'm too much a man of the world to quarrel with a woman because she won't love me. But I understand the whole matter now. When you found that the strike leader was your old lover, you went straight to him, but finding him engaged to be married, you telegraphed to me. Most womanly and most modern.

LADY ANNE (*rises*). How horrible and cynical you are: you like to misinterpret. I wrote to you because I thought you were my friend.

STEINBACH. Don't let us talk any more about friendship – you make the

12

world odious to me. There are two reasons why I should help you. First, because you are a pretty woman; second, because it is my interest to defeat these socialists whenever I can; on triumphing over you they triumph over me. If you consent to put your affair entirely in my hands, I will do the best I can for you.

LADY ANNE. Will you? And will you stop and receive this deputation?

STEINBACH. On conditions that you do not concede anything above your first offer of five per cent.

LADY ANNE. Very well; and now let us talk of other things. What have you been doing all this long while? Who have you been making love to?

STEINBACH. To no one. You're the only woman who interests me. (*Enter* FOOTMAN.)

FOOTMAN. The deputation is waiting, my lady.

LADY ANNE. (*to* BARON STEINBACH). Shall we receive it here?

STEINBACH. Why not?

LADY ANNE. Show them up. (*Exit* FOOTMAN). Do you think you'll be able to get them to accept my offer?

STEINBACH. I think so. These strike leaders are beginning to feel afraid of me.

FOOTMAN. The deputation, my lady. (*Enter* JOHN REID, HAMER, ELLEN SANDS, *and six Miners. The Miners are impressed by their surroundings.* LADY ANNE *signs to the deputation to sit; some do, some do not.* STEINBACH *accosts the men.*)

STEINBACH. So you're out on strike, it appears. (ELLEN *advances.* STEINBACH *interrupts her.*) Well, I shall be pleased to talk over things with you. (*Rolls up his chair, and settles himself comfortably.*) Well, what have you to say to me?

ELLEN SANDS. It is with Lady Anne Travers –

STEINBACH. Lady Anne has placed her business in my hands.

ELLEN. There is no reason whatever, then –

STEINBACH. Oh yes, there is. We have met before, Miss Sands – in the Wattsbury strike, which ended so disastrously for the men. You did not expect to see me here. (*Turning from* ELLEN *to the men.*) Now, you look like quiet, industrious fellows. I daresay you were pulled out against your will; you had nothing to do with getting up this strike, and would have been glad to have accepted Lady Anne's handsome offer of five per cent?

ELLEN. If you think that you are mistaken. It is not the idle and indifferent, it is the real workman that rises against you, and says, 'Since you condemn me to starvation, I prefer to be at liberty, and not to die of hunger whilst I am filling your pockets'.

13

STEINBACH. This is personal animosity, the result of your defeat at Wattsbury. I am not of opinion that these men should suffer to gratify your vanity.

ELLEN. We have not come here to listen to your jibes. John, won't you speak?

REID. Perhaps, Ellen; but from the tone that Baron Steinbach is taking, I doubt if it is worth our while to enter into discussion with him.

ELLEN. That is my opinion. I never saw any good come of discussion. We are strong enough in Arlingford to dictate our own terms.

STEINBACH. You were of the same opinion at Wattsbury. However, as the men are here, they shall have the facts of the case – they shall know what they are doing. If they then please to sacrifice themselves, they can. You would like to know the facts?

FOX. Yes, yes; let's 'ear what e's to say.

STEINBACH. Now, men, I have gone into the calculation, and am prepared to prove what I say, step by step, to any one you may select. At present I will merely state the results. You have had recently a rise of five per cent in wages, which was conceded to you as a rise in prices was anticipated. The rise in prices did not come, and in consequence that rise in wages simply diminished the value of the mine, the property from whose success comes your only chance of livelihood. And in these circumstances you demand a further increase in the rate of wages to the extent of twenty per cent; that, if granted, would again diminish the value of the mine to less than nothing. To work it under such conditions would cost five thousand a year more than it would pay. I can give you the figures for it.

ELLEN. We know that argument, and dispute it no more. We say:- You have convinced us beyond the shadow of a doubt that you cannot give us twenty per cent. We say we don't doubt your word; we say we don't doubt your figures; and then we say, nevertheless, we want our twenty per cent, and somehow the capitalists manage in the end to concede it.

STEINBACH. This is mere violence. I appeal to you men that if your leaders' demand was granted the mine would have to be worked at a loss of five thousand a year for your benefit, and I ask you if you think it likely that we shall do this?

MINERS. Not likely, not likely. (REID *steps forward as if to speak.* LADY ANNE *rises.*)

LADY ANNE. Excuse me a moment. I should like to say a word. Three generations ago no one dreamed there was coal here. The land was waste. My husband's grandfather was a great mineralogist; he found

14

in the soil the signs that told his practised eye that coal lay hidden far beneath it. He had saved a little money by the hard labour of half a lifetime, and with that – all he had – he bought the land we stand on . . . His son, and subsequently my husband, devoted their lives to the mine, and by dint of patience, courage and self-denial they forced it at length to yield a profit. You did not do this; it was not your brains; – it was not your money that created this property.

ELLEN. The sophistries of all capitalists; there is nothing of value in the world save the labour of man.

LADY ANNE. And now to matters that concern you as much as they concern me, for our fortunes are inextricably bound together. Remember, before you decide, that the thing once done cannot be undone. If the furnaces are once stopped, I am ruined, and so are you. The mine will be closed, and your chance of changing your minds will be gone then. In place of some fancied benefit, you will have brought this upon yourselves, that you, your wives, and children, will have to go among strangers and beg of them for that work that you will have made it impossible for me to give you here. (*Goes up to Miners.*)

A MINER. I say, boys, what do you think of it?

ELLEN. Steady men. Take time.

FOX. I'd be main sorry to see the mine closed. I've worked there from a lad – my father and uncle was killed in it.

SIMON. Say, master, what about Billy Fairplay? Will you say the dross shall be paid for?

STEINBACH. Our offer is the same as before. Five per cent rise, or if you like better, three per cent rise and twopence a ton for the dross.

FOX. That's good enough for us; what do ye say, lads? (*Applause, and murmurs of acquiescence among the Miners.*)

ELLEN. John, John! (*They come down together.*) They are all falling away from us. Speak as you did the other day in the market-place.

REID. I never approved of this deputation, Ellen. Such a question as this is not to be discussed in Lady Anne's drawing-room.

ELLEN. There's no better place. (*She turns to the Miners.*) It is here they should tell her the story of their wrongs; of the despair of their wives, of the hungry complaining of their little ones. It is here that they should ask her if she wishes to destroy them utterly. (LADY ANNE *has been talking to the Miners, who are overcome by her condescension; she listens with a look of contempt to* ELLEN'S *speech.*) There is a word to be said, and if you speak it you'll be listened to.

REID (*with the air of a man who has come to a sudden decision*). Lady

Anne, I must remind you that a deputation can only be addressed through its responsible spokesman.

LADY ANNE. Do you dictate to me my behaviour in my own house?

REID. No; but I am responsible for these men. (*He pushes back the men to whom* LADY ANNE *has been speaking.*) I speak for them; and I say that though they are overwhelmed by your consideration in noticing their existence after years of neglect, that though for the moment they are confused by the laws of arithmetic, yet they are not cowards, but men. They come out of your mine because their burden was too heavy to be borne! They will not take it on their shoulders again unless you can lighten it.

LADY ANNE. But it is my wish to do so. I was telling them that their property and mine were linked together.

REID. Words without meaning. (*Murmurs.*) We have a distinct demand; do you grant that?

LADY ANNE. It is unreasonable. It would ruin me.

REID. So it has been said. Then this concession of five per cent is the only one?

STEINBACH. Five per cent, or three per cent and twopence for the refuse.

REID. We cannot accept that.

A MINER. Why not?

ELLEN. Mr Reid will tell you. John, speak as you did the other day! Explain – tell them how this lady's wealth is the result of their labour.

REID. You want to know why you should refuse her ladyship's offer. Because you've taken it into your heads that you intend to live like men and not like beasts. But you're told that if you do not live like beasts, that this lady will be ruined. Look round you, mates; this is a nice place to be ruined in. Never were you in such a place before; feast your eyes upon it, and feel the tread of the carpet under your feet, and breathe the soft scented air. All your homes taken together would not suffice to purchase this room. And the rings on the fingers of that delicate lady are worth more than you can earn in a year of labour. Look at Baron Steinbach and look at yourselves! Look at her, and think of your sisters and wives! She has told you what her husband, her husband's father, and her husband's grandfather did for the mine; but she has not said a word about what your fathers and your grandfathers did for it. From her ancestors she inherited the right to live in idleness, but yours could only bequeath to you the right to labour for her benefit. You've taken up arms against this injustice; you're fighting not only for yourselves, but for your wives and children. You're fighting to give them decent meals and decent

16

homes, and when we've led you within sight of victory, you hesitate
... Have you brought me here to tell her that you'd starve like brutes
rather than she should want for anything? I want to know. Now
which is it going to be?

FOX. Say, Master John, but thee do speak fine; let's 'ave a word about
the strike fund. We cannot see the bairns starve afore our eyes.

REID. This morning's post brought us help and promise of help. The
money is all right.

SIMON. If Mr Reid says the money is right, I'm for the strike.

REID. Will you hold out now, lads?

A MINER. Of course we will; give us yer 'and.

ANOTHER MINER. Hurrah, boys!

MINERS. Never fear, sir; we'll hold out. Hurrah for the strike, boys!
(*Cheers.*) (*Exeunt Miners.*)

LADY ANNE. This is disgraceful. (*To* ELLEN.) Will you persuade your
friend to make a bear-garden of some other place than my drawing-
room?

ELLEN. The men have done no harm to your drawing-room; a few cheers
won't hurt your furniture.

STEINBACH. Then the strike is to go on at all costs.

ELLEN. Certainly. Come, John, you've done excellently well; come.

REID. I will follow you in a moment. I have a word to say to Baron
Steinbach. (*Exit* ELLEN.)

STEINBACH. You are mistaken, Mr Reid. I have nothing to say to you.

REID. Is Lady Anne determined that this battle should be fought out to
the end? (*Catching* LADY ANNE'S *eye.*) I am sorry if the violence
of my words has prejudiced you against the men; I was never in
favour of the deputation.

LADY ANNE. You mistook my drawing-room for a tavern. (*Pauses.*)
Your manner was once more courteous. Have you forgotten?
Perhaps you do not know –

REID. I have not forgotten. I wish you to understand that personal
motives do not count with me in this matter; circumstances forced
me to go further than I intended; but when I meet my comrades in
council, your interest shall not unduly suffer. (HAMER *comes down
the stage and advances towards* STEINBACH, *who is standing near*
LADY ANNE.)

HAMER. Excuse me, Baron Steinbach. You could not state your case to
ignorant men. Now the advantage of the press is –

LADY ANNE (*eagerly*). I should not like any incorrect statement to get
into the papers, Baron; you will oblige me if you give Mr Hamer all
necessary information. (STEINBACH *and* HAMER *go up stage.*) So

you have not forgotten me? There is no need to ask, for you would not have attacked me as you did if you had forgotten – that we were once friends.

REID. I would not have you think that. It was to disabuse your mind of such thought that I stayed to explain – to excuse, if you will, some excesses of language, and to assure you that I shall act with absolute impartiality towards you.

LADY ANNE. But do you think that you can hold the balance as fairly as you propose to? Can you guard your heart so that nothing, no trifle, no bitter remembrance, shall fall into the scale against me? We are not strangers; do you think it is possible to play at being strangers?

REID. That I cannot say; we can only endeavour to be just.

LADY ANNE. I know there are many with you who hardly desire a settlement of this dispute, who at heart believe that the destruction of my property is the best that could happen. Ellen Sands, the young lady you are engaged to marry, is of this way of thinking, or very nearly.

REID. I must leave Ellen to answer for herself.

LADY ANNE. But you would not wish the strike to continue if I could prove by my books that it would be impossible to raise the men's wages twenty per cent and still work the mine at a profit?

REID. No, I should not. But capitalists are not in the habit of submitting their books to strangers – to their enemies.

LADY ANNE (*gently*). We were once friends. I should not mind submitting the books of the mine to you. When will you come and inspect them? Will you come tomorrow?

REID. I can do nothing without consulting my colleagues. But they will raise no objection – it would be impossible to object.

LADY ANNE. Then you will come tomorrow?

REID. Tomorrow? I have to speak at several places tomorrow. But I could be here by four in the afternoon, if that will suit you.

LADY ANNE. That will do very well.

FOOTMAN. Luncheon is ready, my lady.

LADY ANNE. You will stop to lunch, I hope?

REID. That, I regret, is quite impossible.

LADY ANNE. Surely –

REID. You must excuse me. (*He takes his hat and moves towards the door.*) Good day, Lady Anne.

LADY ANNE. Are you going to the committee rooms?

REID. Yes.

LADY ANNE. Then your shortest way will be through the garden. I will show you the way. (REID *hesitates;* STEINBACH *and* HAMER *watch*

18

him. He follows LADY ANNE *through the window.*)

HAMER. Lady Anne seems of a very forgiving disposition. If one had not been present at the deputation one would think they were old friends.

STEINBACH. They are old friends. He was her father's secretary ten years ago. It is said that she broke his heart –

HAMER. What a remarkable story! It is quite dramatic ... I don't suppose Lady Anne would mind my writing an article about it. (*Pause.*) The facts are well known, I suppose?

STEINBACH (*going towards the door*). Such a matter could not be discussed in a public print.

HAMER. But really –

STEINBACH (*opening the door*). No, Mr Hamer, I cannot minister to journalistic curiosity. (*Exit* HAMER. STEINBACH *goes towards the window.*)

CURTAIN.

ACT II

SCENE – *The same as before,* LADY ANNE'S *drawing-room.* LADY
ANNE *discovered.* STEINBACH *enters, right.*

LADY ANNE. You have finished with the books?

STEINBACH. Yes.

LADY ANNE. And they prove all we said?

STEINBACH. Yes, and something more.

LADY ANNE. Then surely I did right in wanting John Reid to inspect the
books; once convinced of the impossibility of the miners'
demands, he will surely not persevere in any adventure that must
end in our mutual ruin – my ruin and their ruin.

STEINBACH. He will understand that this is so; the testimony of the
books is convincing. But I fail to see how the mere opening of Mr
Reid's eyes will alter things.

LADY ANNE. Then you don't believe in Mr Reid's honesty?

STEINBACH. On the contrary, I believe him to be an honest man and a
clever man! But that is not sufficient. I had an opportunity of
studying him the other day.

LADY ANNE. What do you mean?

STEINBACH. I may be wrong, but this is what I think! You take Reid for
a force! I take him for an eloquent interpreter of a force. Let us
suppose that an examination of the books convinces him of the folly
of the men's demands, and that forthwith he goes into the market-
place and says – 'My poor fellows, I was mistaken, and my advice
to you now is to go back to work'.

LADY ANNE. You think they will not take his advice? But yesterday you
saw that he had only to raise his voice and the men followed like
sheep.

STEINBACH. He was then appealing to their brutish instincts; telling
them that their homes were not so comfortable as your drawing-
room. Besides, you have forgotten Ellen Sands.

LADY ANNE. You think that it will be impossible to convince her?

STEINBACH. Her beliefs are not swayed by facts and figures; they are
well entrenched in pure theory, and are practically inaccessible to
argument.

LADY ANNE. Then you think that John Reid's examination of the books will come to nothing?

STEINBACH. Something comes of everything, but what? Briefly, I do not think that this inspection of the books will prove as easy a solution of your difficulties as you imagine.

LADY ANNE. But I did not propose this inspection of books until you had failed.

STEINBACH. Failed! A little vulgar rhetoric answered by a few idiotic cheers; a few caps thrown into the air. Had I had my way, those caps and cheers would have been instantly answered by a withdrawal of your offer of five per cent. But instead, you threw yourself on the man's mercy; you capitulated without terms – you invited him here. This policy may prove successful. He loved you when you were a girl; you come with all the added charms of womanhood. He may lose his head; you may twist him round your finger, but the step is a perilous one.

LADY ANNE. Why perilous for me?

STEINBACH. Supposing your names were scandalously connected together – your name and the name of a socialist leader! Think of it; all help from your family would be at an end. Your father, Lord Elwin, who might assist you –

LADY ANNE. But you'll tell no one of our boy and girl flirtation – that silly love-story which I told you of.

STEINBACH. When you took Reid through the garden, that newspaper fellow – Hamer is his name, I think – and I were standing by the window – you passed out before us.

LADY ANNE. But you told him nothing!

STEINBACH. I had to say something. I told him that Reid had been your father's secretary. It seemed the least compromising thing I could say.

LADY ANNE. I wish you hadn't done this!

STEINBACH. I had to say something.

LADY ANNE. It was wrong of me; I didn't think of what I was doing. If it becomes known it will irritate that girl Ellen Sands still further against me. If I fail it will be through her. She'll prove my stumbling-block.

STEINBACH. Then woman proves woman's stumbling-block as well as man's.

LADY ANNE. Oh! Edward, let me be! This is no time for epigrams – ruin hangs like a sword above me. The overseers are working fifteen hours a day. Only this morning I heard that they will not be able to bear the strain much longer; the mine will be flooded, and I shall be

21

ruined! Oh! it is cruel! Why was I selected? Why do they attack a woman? Why do they choose the weakest?

STEINBACH. The weakest is Nature's instinctive selection. It is the weakest that goes to the wall first. (*Seeing there are tears in* LADY ANNE'S *eyes, his manner softens.*) But why does the weak refuse association with the strong? Dearest Anne, you know that my fortune as well as my heart is at your disposal. (*Takes her in his arms and kisses her.*)

LADY ANNE. Money, my dear Baron, has never influenced my choice. We may be worldly and not as good as we might be, but for our sakes we must keep ourselves free from that taint. I told you yesterday that I was in too great trouble to think of love or lovers. After the battle, who knows? During the battle I want you to be my friend.

STEINBACH. Well, let it be so. I'll be your friend, and if chance should favour me I shall deem myself the most fortunate of men.

LADY ANNE. Is this a compact?

STEINBACH. Yes; and I should be satisfied if I thought, if I were sure, you didn't care for this socialist chief.

LADY ANNE. I in love with John Reid! How absurd!

STEINBACH. It does seem absurd, but I half fancied that this socialist chief -this man you had loved long ago, who comes up to you from an unknown world, halo of poetry about him – had inspired in you some sort of fantastic caprice, some sort of capricious interest.

LADY ANNE (*absent-mindedly*) No, I'm not in love with John Reid; that is all over and done with. He hates me. If you were to ask him, he would describe me as a cruel, heartless woman. I did treat him cruelly, I know I did; but it was not all my fault. He's now going to marry Ellen Sands. Oh, no, I'm not in love with him. That is quite an absurd idea.

STEINBACH. Sweetheart, swear that you do not love him.

LADY ANNE. I do not care for him.

STEINBACH. Then you'll love me. You once did – you will again. (*Putting his arms round her.* LADY ANNE *moves away.*)

LADY ANNE. Hush, someone's coming. (*The door opens and servant announces that* JOHN REID *is downstairs.*)

FOOTMAN. Mr John Reid wishes to see your ladyship. Is your ladyship at home?

STEINBACH. My advice is not to receive him.

LADY ANNE. I cannot do that. What excuse can I give?

STEINBACH. Excuse! The usual excuse – a sick headache.

LADY ANNE. He wouldn't believe it. It would only incense him still further against me. I must see him. (*To Servant.*) Show Mr Reid up. (*Exit Servant.*) Believe me that I do this only in the hope of obtaining a settlement of this dispute.

STEINBACH. In the hope of alienating him from his party?

LADY ANNE. Yes; that is my only reason. I shall expect you this evening to dinner, and will tell you all about it. (STEINBACH *looks at her doubtfully.* REID *enters. The men bow to each other.*)

REID. (*a suspicion of shyness*). I'm afraid I'm disturbing you. You're engaged, I see.

LADY ANNE. Not at all; Baron Steinbach was just leaving. He's been good enough to put my books in order. He has explained them to me so that I can explain them to you.

STEINBACH. Your books are excellently well kept; they can be read at a glance. But perhaps a lady and a poet will not read them as easily as a financier.

REID. I've had some practice with accounts, and unless they're very difficult indeed, I shall be able to understand them. Poets are not such impracticable beings as financiers imagine.

LADY ANNE. Mr Reid's poetry is as well known to the world as his socialism. The world prefers his poetry.

REID. One half the world.

STEINBACH. A strange alliance, poetry and socialism; and yet I don't know, in the modern world mysticism finds expression in socialism and science.

REID. Mysticism! So we seem to you like mystics, a recrudescence of the Middle Ages. And you wonder if we really believe that the future will differ from the present.

STEINBACH. I certainly wonder that an intelligence like yours should never doubt the possibility of man's regeneration.

REID. You believe man to be utterly base.

STEINBACH. The mass of mankind, certainly.

REID. A cruel creed, an ignoble creed. I could not live if I did not hold to some hope of earthly salvation.

STEINBACH. I wonder if your speech comes from conviction, or if it is a mere habit of eloquence. There is one question that I put to men like you. If the capitalists were abolished tomorrow, tell me what you would do with the incorrigibly idle; those who would say, 'We will not work, we prefer to beg,' and wander the world over.

REID. Not long ago I met an old couple on a country road. They had worked forty years in the factory; they could work no more, and were on their way to the Poor-house; yet Baron Steinbach wonders why the poor are not more industrious.

23

STEINBACH. In every system there must be failures.

REID. You think that the successes of the system should reconcile us to its failures?

STEINBACH. There is neither present nor past system; it is human passion that blocks your way. But argument is useless. Lady Anne, the accounts are in the library.

LADY ANNE. I shall expect you to dinner at eight, Baron.

STEINBACH. I'm not leaving. I have some letters to write. I shall find what I want in the morning-room. (*Exit*.)

REID. A strange man. He seems to take pleasure in the knowledge that evil exists.

LADY ANNE. He's a man without illusions.

REID. Has he taught you to think like him?

LADY ANNE. No; I always try to look on the pleasant side. (LADY ANNE *shows signs of emotion, her handkerchief is in her hand.*)

REID. You seem troubled, Lady Anne. Perhaps you're not feeling well, and would like to postpone the examination of accounts?

LADY ANNE. No, I'm well enough. Even so, I should not allow health to interfere, however distraught I may feel.

REID. Distraught!

LADY ANNE. The difficulty of knowing what to do, how to act. Whatever course I take, it seems to be the wrong one.

REID. I think you have acted wisely in submitting to an inspection of your books. For after all it is but a question of facts and figures. I may say that when I reported your decision the majority of the committee was impressed in your favour.

LADY ANNE. But if the books vindicate my position, do you guarantee that the men return to work at once?

REID. I shall certainly advise that the strike be discontinued.

LADY ANNE. Perhaps that advice will be opposed.

REID. Maybe; but the extreme views do not carry a majority of votes.

LADY ANNE. You're alluding to Ellen Sands.

REID. Miss Sands, I admit, holds extreme views; but so does your friend Baron Steinbach. Ellen Sands and Baron Steinbach represent the poles of the social question. Both are for war to the knife.

LADY ANNE. Baron Steinbach anticipates Miss Sands' opposition, and says that this inspection of the books will only end in useless publication of my affairs. (*Pause*.) On certain conditions he would help me with all his wealth to fight the demands of the miners, and with his money I could not fail to force them to accept the terms I was pleased to impose.

REID. And you have declined his aid?

LADY ANNE. I hesitated to accept his offer. (*Pause.*) I do not wish to crush these poor people utterly. I do not believe them to be dissatisfied with their condition; they are merely ill-advised. Nor do I believe that the advice that they follow is altogether disinterested.

REID. Lady Anne!

LADY ANNE. I do not wish to accuse either you or your associates of dishonesty, but did you not tell me just now that Ellen Sands was opposed to an inspection of my books? In other words, was opposed to any amicable settlement of this dispute. Ellen Sands hates me.

REID. No; she merely hates the class to which you belong.

LADY ANNE. Does she know, have you told her, that we were once – well – shall I say sweethearts?

REID. I have told her nothing. She knows nothing for certain. The flowers you left for me seemed to rouse some suspicion in her mind. But it has passed away.

LADY ANNE. Did the perfume tell you who had left the flowers for you?

REID. Not at first. I could not remember where I had met that perfume. It seemed to recall a far-off time, a dead past; but when I tried to define what it did recall, the illusion vanished. Ellen's description of you did not help me. It was when my thoughts were occupied with other things that the haunting odour seemed on the point of whispering its secret. I put the flowers away, but the soft, insinuating odour pursued me, held me sleepless ... Suddenly I cried out – 'It is she!'

LADY ANNE. I remember the day you left Torrington Park. I saw you walk across the park in the rain; you had told me that I had broken your heart.

REID. I did not speak false. You were a cruel, heartless girl, as you are now a cruel heartless woman.

LADY ANNE (*dashes the tears aside*). I am sorry you think so badly of me, but it can't be helped ... I did treat you cruelly, I know.

REID. But have we not other things to discuss?

LADY ANNE. No; this matter demands settlement before all others. How was I circumstanced at the time? Have you forgotten that I was no more than a child, hardly seventeen, when you first told me that you loved me? I was true to my love until –

REID. Until you realised that you could not marry your father's secretary.

LADY ANNE. Have it so, then. Why did I seek to convince you? What is it to me how vile you think me. Still it seems to me strange that, after all these years, so clever a man should not be able to see that I was helpless in the hands of my relatives. What was my will

25

against their will?

REID. You made no effort to resist them. You were determined on a rich marriage.

LADY ANNE. If I had married you, you would be tired of me by now. We should have been married ten years. All the romance would be faded.

REID. You think so. Is that the lesson that life has taught you?

LADY ANNE. You think, then, that you wouldn't have grown tired of me? You used to say so. I still keep the verses you wrote to me. Do you remember the corner of the terrace where the sun set behind the hills? Looking down that valley, we thought that we saw our lives from end to end.

REID. That illusive valley.

LADY ANNE. I like the poem. It is one of the prettiest in your book. You see I have marked it.

REID. Oh, then you have read my poems?

LADY ANNE. Yes, I bought the volume when it first came out. I little thought I should meet John Reid again and in such circumstances.

REID. Or little cared. I remember one evening, we were walking together on the terrace, we had said that we loved one another. The conversation had fallen; I was thinking of our future, and without a word of warning you said, 'But this will never be'. Next time we met I noticed that your manner was wholly changed, and when your coldness forced me to ask you if you wished me to forget you, to go away, you answered, 'I think it would be as well if you did'.

LADY ANNE. It is as I thought. You remember only what was disagreeable in me. You cannot find excuse in childish ignorance. However, you have forgotten me. How could it be otherwise? What we're talking of is ten years ago.

REID. Why do we speak of these things? (*Stops and looks at her.*) I have done nothing but reproach you. I really don't know why. I've come here on a purely business matter. Why do we not confine ourselves to it?

LADY ANNE. Perhaps it would be better if we did. The accounts are in the library. I'll take you there at once. (*She goes towards the door. Looking round.*) But how pale you're looking, and all this time I've not asked you to sit down . . . You're looking ill.

REID. It is nothing. I'm only a little tired. I've been speaking in the Merton district. I'd then to attend a committee meeting. I was detained longer than I expected, and had to run most of the way here.

LADY ANNE. I should have noticed your tired face before. Sit down –

26

rest yourself.

REID. I'll sit down for a few minutes – if you're not pressed for time?

LADY ANNE. I've nothing to do ... But I must be careful what I talk to you about. You do not wish to speak of the past – let us speak of the present. You've made your way in the world since we last saw each other. I should like to hear how you won your success. You must have worked very hard. You must have suffered; for you'd very little, only your younger child's portion.

REID. I was poor then, I'm poor now – now, because my work leaves so little time for earning money. I suppose it was hard at first, but I went through no melodramatic struggle for existence. I could always make money with my pen.

LADY ANNE. I am glad of that. Then why –

REID. Did I become a socialist? Oh, it was not because I could not 'get on'.

LADY ANNE. There must have been a reason.

REID. Oh yes, there was a reason.

LADY ANNE. Perhaps I shall not be able to understand your reasons? I know nothing of political economy.

REID. My reason was a very simple one – so simple that I can hardly call it a reason at all – a mere human sentiment. I felt I was leading a selfish life. I grew aware of the misery around me. When I came home in the morning in evening clothes and white cravat I did not dare to look the poor vagrants in the face – the poor wretches who had just risen from the cold stones and walked shivering onwards in front of the policeman.

LADY ANNE. I remember one summer morning I dropped my fan as I was getting out of the carriage. One of those poor creatures picked it up and handed it to me. It was horrible.

REID. I came to think more and more about the poverty and the misery that three parts of the world live in – of the injustice of what we call civilisation, and gradually –

LADY ANNE. So it was not Ellen Sands who drew you into socialism?

REID. No; I've only known her about a year. But it was her enthusiasm that strengthened me in my convictions; I might say gave me convictions, for before I met her I only felt that things were wrong in the world. I did not know that they could be remedied.

LADY ANNE. And now you're going to marry her; and henceforth you'll live among the people. You're going to take the final step. I wonder if you'll be happy?

REID. I shall be happy as another. Who is happy? Are you happy?

LADY ANNE. I often think I'm not. I often hate my life, and wonder what

27

is the use of all this hurry after mere amusement. But I never had any one to encourage me to think, to help me to think. (*Pause.*) I like to listen to you. It seems quite natural to think as you do. It is interesting to think of things. (*Enter* BARON STEINBACH.)

STEINBACH. Oh, I thought you were in the library examining the books.

REID. Lady Anne has been good enough to take an interest in my book. It is, I'm afraid, too easy to tempt a poet into talking of his verses.

LADY ANNE. I'm quite ready.

REID. But it seems a shame, Lady Anne, to fatigue you with dry account-books. If Baron Steinbach has finished his letters –

LADY ANNE. The accounts will not fatigue me. Besides, this will be an opportunity to obtain an insight into my affairs, which I have neglected. It is I who should speak to you of fatigue. You're really looking very tired and pale.

STEINBACH. I wonder when Mr Reid will tire of work for those who understand nothing of his aims and aspirations, whose ideas are limited to their pint-pots!

REID. Lady Anne, time presses. If you wish me to go into the matter of these accounts, I must do so at once. If the books are in order it will not take us long to get at the results.

LADY ANNE. This is the way to the library. (*Exeunt, right.*)

STEINBACH. I wonder what the effect of this meeting will be – accounts and conversations about poetry. (*Paces the stage.*) Poetry! (*Stops before table, takes up* REID'S *poems, sits down, and turns over the leaves.* FOOTMAN *opens the door; shows in* MR HAMER.)

HAMER. I apologise, Baron Steinbach. I do hope I am not wasting your valuable time. But I thought you might favour me with your views on the capitalistic question before I leave Arlingford.

STEINBACH. My dear Mr Hamer, what can I have to say on a subject so utterly worn out with controversy?

HAMER. For the original mind no subject is worn out.

STEINBACH. You're too complimentary. However, if you'll put some questions, I'll try to answer them.

HAMER. You visited Lady Anne's mine this morning; you were impressed by its gloom, its danger ... Let me remind you that human beings are born for life-long labour in its subterranean night ... How different their fate from yours! In a few weeks you'll be back in your palace on the beautiful Italian coast. I want to ask you if you think such inequality just?

STEINBACH. Of course it is not just. Look into Nature, examine her intentions, and you'll find injustice at the root of every one. What can be more unjust than that one brother should never know a day's illness, and the other brother should never known a day's health? Why do some come into the world criminals, crazed with passion from which they cannot escape, and which lead them by certain steps to the gallows?

HAMER. The socialists know very well that there will always be healthy and unhealthy, stupid and intelligent, but they think that –

STEINBACH. That some day they'll be neither rich nor poor? But poverty and riches are merely the consequence of health and disease, stupidity and intelligence.

HAMER. If it were not legal for the individual to accumulate capital there would be neither rich nor poor.

STEINBACH. But it is nature and not man that is the inexorable tyrant. (*Getting up, holding on to and leaning over the rail of his chair.*) You want me to tell you what I think of the capitalistic system. The capitalistic system is founded on thrift, on industry, and on forethought – three things which the world has agreed to call virtues. It is also founded on the lust of possession, on the pleasure of gambling, and the craving for personal superiority – three things which the world has agreed to call vices. Do you think that a system, founded on six instincts inherited from the beginning of time, can be overthrown?

HAMER. Then you think that our present form of civilisation will endure for ever – that we have reached the highest attainable point?

STEINBACH. New combinations will arise, but nothing will be altered. There have been a thousand reformers and not a single reformation. The misery of man is incurable.

HAMER. Do you go so far as to say that life subsists on misery and vice as much as on happiness and virtue?

STEINBACH. Surely. Misery and vice are antecedent to capital; they exist because Nature believes them essential in her design.

HAMER (*writing, and speaking to himself*). Man cannot live by virtue alone.

STEINBACH. Precisely; man cannot live by virtue alone. Nature and the socialist are at variance on this point, and Nature does not allow any one to contradict her. Socialism would take from life all it has of adventure and excitement; it would reduce the world to the colourless void of monastic life. It would go further than the more ferocious ascetic has yet gone; it would take from life even the excitement of religion! In the socialist monastery gambling for places in Paradise would not be allowed. (*Turning to* HAMER). Have you got that?

HAMER. One moment. (*He finishes writing and looks up.*) But would

29

you deny progress altogether? Surely the world is not as ignorant as it was? Education –

STEINBACH. Education! What has it done? You've taught men to read, but what do they read? Are the books written today, when everyone knows how to read, better than those that were written two thousand years ago, when few knew how to read? You have established schools for instruction in the art of painting and sculpture. Are your painting and sculpture as good as the painting and sculpture done before the world had begun to indulge in dreams of educational advantages?

HAMER. You must admit that there is at least one improvement in modern over ancient life – the abolition of slavery.

STEINBACH. The argument of the socialists is that the factory is the most ferocious form of slavery that the world has ever known. And I'm not sure that they are not right.

HAMER (*getting up and closing his note-book*). There are two more questions I should like to ask you, Baron Steinbach. You're said to be one of the richest men in the world. The other day I saw it stated that your fortune exceeded ten millions.

STEINBACH. Ten millions! When a man is known to be rich he's credited with ten – a thousand times his real wealth. But let the amount be waived. What do you want to ask me?

HAMER. I want to ask you if money is happiness?

STEINBACH (*walking up the stage*). Oh, no. Happiness is another thing. Money, of course, means a great deal, otherwise we should not take the trouble we do to acquire it. But happiness is found not in money, but in work.

HAMER. My last question.

STEINBACH. Ask it.

HAMER. Admitting your contention that all are at liberty to acquire capital, and that capital is acquired by the intelligent and the industrious, do you not think that it is unjust that a man should be allowed to leave his money to children who have not worked for it, and are perhaps neither intelligent nor industrious?

STEINBACH (*coming down the stage*). Are you married?

HAMER. No, not yet.

STEINBACH. When you are, and have children, believe me you'll not question the law of inheritance.

HAMER. I understand. The family is the rock on which socialism goes to pieces. Thank you very much, Baron Steinbach. Your views, I'm sure, will be read with great interest. I will send you a copy of the paper. I suppose that this address will find you. But that reminds me:

you remember the interesting details you were kind enough to supply me with regarding the romantic attachment of Lady Anne and John Reid in early life?

STEINBACH. I hope you've not referred to that in your paper.

HAMER. Well, you remember I asked you if the facts were known?

STEINBACH. I said that the story was not one that could be discussed in a public print. It will injure Reid's position.

HAMER. It may do that; but you see, it was a really interesting item of news, and things are so dull at present. I think you'll find that I've treated the subject delicately. I do hope Lady Anne will not be annoyed.

STEINBACH. She certainly will be annoyed. I'm afraid you cannot come here again.

HAMER. I'm sure I should be sorry to think that – but it's too late now. (*Preparing to go.*)

STEINBACH. Has your article appeared?

HAMER. No, but I'm afraid it is too late to withdraw it. It will probably go into tomorrow's or Wednesday's paper. I'll send it to you, and I hope you'll tell Lady Anne that –

STEINBACH. I'll tell her what you say – that things were dull. But I doubt if she'll be able to see the matter in that light.

HAMER. Thank you for your very interesting views – most interesting, I'm sure. Thank you again, and good morning. (*Exit.*)

STEINBACH. (*returning from the door*). I thought that he would not be able to resist the temptation. I think that his article will bring this ridiculous flirtation to an end. (*Goes to door at back. As he lays his hand on the handle, enter* LADY ANNE *and* REID.)

STEINBACH. Ah, so you've finished with the books. I hope they've convinced you –

REID. Of the impracticability of our demands? Quite.

STEINBACH. I'm glad of that. It says much for your open-mindedness.

LADY ANNE. Mr Reid will advise the discontinuation of the strike?

REID. I shall report the result of my examination of your books – the figures speak for themselves.

STEINBACH. This is a serious refutation of your ideas. (*Enter* FOOTMAN).

FOOTMAN (*approaching* BARON STEINBACH). Mr Hamer has come back, sir, and wishes to know if he can have a word with you.

LADY ANNE. Will you see him in the morning-room, Baron Steinbach? Mr Reid and –

REID. But my business is quite finished. Pray do not let me –

LADY ANNE. Mr Reid, I hope you are not going yet. We've still –

STEINBACH. Will you excuse me? One has never quite done with an interviewer. I'll see you later on, Lady Anne. (*Exit.*)

REID. I see that Baron Steinbach is an intimate friend of yours.

LADY ANNE. I've known him a long while, and when all this trouble came I wrote asking him to help me. He came at once.

REID. Was it love of you or hatred of us that brought him to Arlingford, I wonder?

LADY ANNE. It is difficult to say why men do things. But you see that I preferred to accept your help to his.

REID. I daresay he advised you against me – against this course. I remember you told me he did.

LADY ANNE. He doubts your power to assist me. He says you'll be opposed; he thinks you'll not be able to overcome this opposition.

REID. What opposition? That of that thick-headed fellow the secretary of the committee, and a few fanatics? He's mistaken. I've a hold over the men that they haven't. Ellen knows them all; they're her friends, she visits them in their homes; but when it comes to a pinch it is I whom they obey.

LADY ANNE. I wonder how that is? You're so different – you haven't a thought, not a sympathy in common.

REID. I beg your pardon. At heart I was always of the people. They care little for poetry, it is true. But their sturdy fighting manhood is common ground where hearts – and fists too! – may meet. The other day I took off my coat and gave a fellow a hiding. You should have heard them cheer me. My popularity is ten times what it was. I can do what I like with them.

LADY ANNE. You gave the fellow a thrashing? Tell me about it.

REID. It was about the right to trade away the stores that had been obtained with the tickets – something about the tickets, something about drink. They must accept your last offer. Let me see, the percentage is – I've forgotten. My memory's gone. (*Sinks into a chair.*)

LADY ANNE. Oh, what is this? (*Supports his head with her arm.*) He's fainted; he's seriously ill. (*Runs for scent, wets her pocket handkerchief, and bathes his face. He begins to revive.*) He has only fainted. John, speak to me. Are you better? Lie still. No, no. Let me bathe your temples.

REID. What is it – Anne, Anne! it is you? Tell me what has happened. (*Pause.*) I fainted, didn't I? (*He closes his eyes.*)

LADY ANNE. He's fainted again.

REID. No, I haven't. But my head is swimming. I was saying something to you. What did I say? Did I tell you that –

LADY ANNE. You said nothing.

REID. Ah! that perfume, how it brings back the past! I was writing all last night, and I ate nothing – I had no time. I have overdone it; that's all.

LADY ANNE. You mustn't talk. Rest –

REID. I'm better now. (*Makes an effort to rise.*)

LADY ANNE. Let me help you. (*She helps him to rise.*)

REID (*leaning against the table*). Fainting like a girl. I'm ashamed of myself. I shall be all right when I get into the air. Goodbye, Lady Anne. You'll excuse me.

LADY ANNE. But you're not going yet. Wait until you're better.

REID. May I have a glass of water?

LADY ANNE. I'll ring for one. (*Rings. The* FOOTMAN *enters. To* FOOTMAN.) Bring a glass of water at once – quickly. (*Exit* FOOTMAN). Let me order you some lunch; you're starving!

REID. A glass of water will be sufficient. It is only a little faintness. I shall be all right presently. (*Enter* FOOTMAN *with water.* REID *drinks. Exit* FOOTMAN. REID *prepares to go.*)

LADY ANNE. You must take more care of yourself; your health will break down if you don't. I suppose we've said everything. But you'll find time to come and see me again. I'm not the superficial woman you take me for. I want to hear your ideas. When will you come and see me?

REID. There would be no reason for my coming here again. You forget how different are our positions. Besides, the turn that events have taken will leave little spare time on my hands. I must now consider the best way of getting the men back to work.

LADY ANNE. But you must not think that it was for that I invited you here.

REID. Surely.

LADY ANNE. You think there was no other reason?

REID. Perhaps you felt some sort of interest in seeing me again.

LADY ANNE. Indeed I did. I asked you here because I want you to forgive me. (*Giving him her hands.*)

REID. I wish we had met in other circumstances.

LADY ANNE. Circumstances do not control those who care for each other.

REID. Care for each other!

LADY ANNE. When you fainted just now I learnt from your own lips that you loved me. You do love me; you cannot deny it.

REID. Alas! I've never loved anyone but you. It is too late now.

LADY ANNE. It is never too late. I, too, have a confession to make. I have

33

not forgotten you. I never loved anyone but you.

REID. Ah, I heard you say the same words long ago, and I learnt what your love was worth.

LADY ANNE. I am not situated as I was then.

REID. Nor was I situated then as I am now.

LADY ANNE. Do you doubt my love? Why should I tell you so if it were not true?

REID. Why indeed!

LADY ANNE. It is your duty to tell the men to return to work. Only revenge could prevent you from doing so, and you do not want revenge, do you?

REID. Anne, it is too late; my troth is pledged to another.

LADY ANNE. To whom? You do not love that thread-paper girl with theories instead of blood in her veins?

REID. Not as I once loved you.

LADY ANNE. Nor even as you love me now. (*She draws herself against him like a cat.*) Kiss me! (*He kisses her and breaks away from her. He stands looking into space; she sits down, right. Pause.*)

REID. You want me to betray her as once you betrayed me. To cause her the same suffering. This can only end in shame and ruin. (*With sudden determination.*) I will go at once. (*Exit.*)

LADY ANNE. Gone, gone! I shall never see him again. She'll never let him come here again. (*Throws herself on the sofa.*) Ah, I could have loved that man. (*Getting up.*) I must, I will...I shall see him again. I will write to him. (*Goes to writing-table. Two minutes should elapse between* REID'S *exit and his entrance. The door opens;* REID *enters, a letter in his hand.*) Ah, so you've come back. What has brought you back? Something has happened. Bad news is written in your face.

REID. The worst of news. Irrevocable disaster!

LADY ANNE. What do you mean? Tell me.

REID. As I was leaving, this letter was put into my hand. (*Reading.*) 'Sir, – Knowing the situation to be critical in Arlingford, I send you a cheque for £2000. It is necessary that labour should win this battle. Arlingford is the key to the situation in the North. – A friend of labour'. A friend of labour? Ah, a cruel friend! (*Clenching letter.*) Ah! it is you who have destroyed us.

LADY ANNE. But you'll tell the miners that the books prove that their demands are impossible, that to continue the strike must end in the ruin of my property – of their property. You will appeal to their reason.

REID. With this money in my hand it were idle to advise them to return

34

to work.

LADY ANNE. Then I'm ruined, utterly ruined! (*They sit down,* REID *in a chair next the table,* LADY ANNE *in a chair down the stage on the right.*) When the money is gone, when they would return to work, the property which cost the labour of three generations to create will have disappeared; the mine will be a swamp.

REID. Yes, a vast property lost to a little drunkenness! What a derision! (*Getting up, and going to* LADY ANNE.) But cannot you get money from your relations sufficient to keep the mine in working order?

LADY ANNE. My relations cannot help me; no-one can help me now, except Baron Steinbach.

REID. Baron Steinbach! (LADY ANNE *looks at him. Recollecting himself.*) Baron Steinbach, our bitterest foe; he would crush us with his millions! He would resist until he forced the poor folk to accept his terms; God knows what they'd be! The alternative is a terrible one, but I do not understand why you have not already accepted his help.

LADY ANNE. Let us say because I do not wish to crush these poor people utterly; give me credit for some good intention.

REID (*taking her hands*). Is this really true, Anne?

LADY ANNE. Yes, it is quite true. There is one way out of this terrible situation. No-one knows of the arrival of that cheque; say nothing about it, and advise the men to return to work.

REID. Detain this cheque, and advise the men to return to work! You do not realise what you are asking!

LADY ANNE. Yes, I do. Detain that cheque a few days – a few hours may be sufficient. Tell them to go back to work; save them, and save me!

REID. 'To do a great right to do a little wrong'. But is my wrong little, however noble my purpose. One cannot foresee the end of such an act. Oh, God! my responsibility is greater than I can bear!

LADY ANNE. Save them from Steinbach! Save me!

REID. I'll save you both! (*To himself.*) And will bear the punishment even if it falls upon me from both sides.

LADY ANNE. You do this for me, for me who did you such wrong? How can I thank you, how can I recompense you? Say that you forgive me the past!

REID. Let me not think that it is for you I do this.

LADY ANNE. Why should it not be for me?

REID. Were it so, it would be a shameful act.

LADY ANNE. Shameful to save the woman you once loved from ruin.

REID. Ah, if it should become known that I once loved you, no other explanation except love of you will be believed.

LADY ANNE. Then you hesitate – you're afraid?
REID. No, I am not afraid. I'll do this. But we must not meet again. (*He gets up to go.* LADY ANNE *stands between him and the door.*)
LADY ANNE. We must not meet again.

CURTAIN.

ACT III

SCENE. – *The same as before.* LADY ANNE'S *drawing-room. As the curtain rises,* LADY ANNE *is seating herself on the sofa.* REID *is standing by her.*

LADY ANNE. At last we're alone. The worst of servants is that one can't speak before them, unless one speaks in French. You don't, do you? Come and sit down. (*Enter* FOOTMAN *with coffee and liqueurs.* REID *takes chair.*) Oh, here's the coffee. (*To* FOOTMAN.) You can put it on that table. I will serve it. (FOOTMAN *draws over the wicker table, and places coffee upon it. Exit* FOOTMAN. LADY ANNE *puts her hands on* REID'S *shoulders and looks at him.*) I cannot imagine how you could have ever thought of marrying a woman who wasn't a lady.

REID. Why introduce a subject that you know must be painful to me? Let us not speak of Ellen.

LADY ANNE. I'm jealous of her, of the influence she has had over you. You never could have lived among common people. Admit that you're glad to find yourself in a drawing room again.

REID. Among the refinements of life! I never regretted these things, I only regretted you. (*Enter* FOOTMAN; *offers liqueurs.*) None, thank you.

LADY ANNE. What, no liqueur; not even a glass of Chartreuse? What an ascetic you've become! (*Exit* FOOTMAN.) At last we're alone. How nice it is to have you here! Tell me how you managed to get away.

REID. It was difficult. I had to avoid exciting any suspicion.

LADY ANNE. You're sure you weren't followed?

REID. Quite.

LADY ANNE. Tell me how you managed to deceive them. I love the excitement, the intrigue; it is half the charm.

REID. I told them I was going for a long walk in the country. I walked for a couple of miles, until I made sure I wasn't followed, and then I took a short cut across the fields, and entered the town by the other side. That is all. And you, how did you manage to get rid of Baron Steinbach?

LADY ANNE. Oh, that's rather a good story. I wrote him a nice letter,

37

inviting him to tea. I slipped a tea-gown over my dress, and with the help of some violet powder got myself up to look like an invalid. He found me lying on the sofa, a bottle of smelling salts in my hand, hardly able to speak. I gave him a cup of tea, and told him I was going to spend the evening in my room. Wasn't that ingenious?

REID. It seems so strange that you should take this trouble for me, and after all these years.

LADY ANNE. Why is it strange? I'll not have you look at your muddy boots. I like your loose necktie and your rough clothes; you're far nicer like that. A west-end tailor could only make you look like any other young man. No, I don't think a west-end tailor could make you look like that.

REID. It is the novelty of my roughness that attracts, and when the spice of the novelty is worn off you'll grow tired of me, as you did before.

LADY ANNE. Now don't begin to analyse, or you'll spoil everything.

REID. I analyse nothing. I only know that I am yours, that you can do what you will with me. I am no longer John Reid – I am your lover.

LADY ANNE. And you don't desire any longer to address miners at the street corner, to urge them to destroy everything beautiful in the world? You're content to sit here by me, to be my lover?

REID. I forget all but you. I look on your face, I watch the colour of your eyes, I hold you in my arms.

LADY ANNE. And when you go away from here do you forget me?

REID. Then I'm really yours...words, looks, everything is remembered. I lose myself in memories of you. There never was a more complete abandonment of self.

LADY ANNE. I don't think your love is a selfish love. I must prove worthy of it.

REID. Anne, if you'd only been true to me! Ah, how I loved you! Do you remember those beautiful summer evenings by the river-side? How young we were then! Life had not had its way with us. Do you remember the oak wood and the tree on which I carved your name?

LADY ANNE. I remember everything, John. When I read your poems all that past came back to me; the book used to fall on my knees, and I wondered if we were to meet, if you'd care for me.

REID. But when you heard that I headed the strike on your mine, you hated me.

LADY ANNE. No; I only thought of seeing you again. But you hated me when you came into this room at the head of the deputation. I was madly anxious to find some excuse to speak with you alone. When I caught your eye and you came down to speak to me –

REID. You knew that you would succeed in winning me back.

LADY ANNE. I hoped that we might be friends. I felt that I must speak to you of the old days, that was all. And you, when did you begin to love me?

REID. I hardly know. It was like the giddiness that takes a man on a cliff's edge. I knew that if I looked I should throw myself into the void. And I looked –

LADY ANNE (*freeing herself from his embrace*). How despondent and philosophical you are! You take life very sadly. (*Showing her fan.*) Look at these lovers, how gay and delightful they are! What do you think of my fan? This is an heirloom, a real old Pompadour fan, one of Watteau's designs. Ah! that is a century I should have liked to live in.

REID. Anne, listen. I've come to tell you –

LADY ANNE. You've come to tell me that you love me. I won't hear anything else. Look at my fan, see the ladies and gallants how they're grouped under the colonnade. That little woman in the brown dress, isn't she sweet? And the little gallant at her feet, he's nice too. He doesn't believe much in what he's saying; it's just part of the entertainment.

REID. But, Anne, do you hate deep feeling? Must all love be light?

LADY ANNE. I really don't know. You find fault with all my conversation. You argue everything.

REID. Forgive me, Anne ... In other circumstances you would find me different.

LADY ANNE (*extending her hand to him*). Forgive me. Go and get your poems, they are on that table; read to me. (*He fetches book and reads.*)

REID. One night Temptation came to me
    And woke me with her passing hair,
    And led me captive by the sea,
    Adown the cliffs to the sea's lair.
    The rank grass rustled sharply, stirred
    By puffing winds that gasped and died,
    And through the sundered rocks was heard
    The hollow bellow of the tide.

    She sate me on a narrow ledge,
    And watched me till I could not bear
    Her eyes green spell. Upon the edge
    Of life she held me; in despair
    I took my soul from out my heart
    And let it go for good or ill –

39

For why restrain what would depart;
This soul was weary of my will.

Do you know the poem of which that is the two first stanzas?

LADY ANNE. Yes; it is called 'The Ballad of a Lost Soul'. The soul wanders over the skies unable to choose among the many stars, until at last Venus rises, and then the soul is caught within the attraction of Venus.

REID. It is strange that I should have opened this book at that poem. You do not perceive the allegory.

LADY ANNE. I suppose you mean that I tempted you from honour and duty? Very well, go to Ellen Sands. I'm not accustomed to these hesitations; nor do I think much of those who never know their own minds, or even on what side they're fighting.

REID (*getting up*). Anne, I beg of you to be patient with me. It is not my fault if, on entering this room, I cannot efface from my mind what I have seen during the day.

LADY ANNE. Tomorrow the men will surrender; they cannot hold out much longer.

REID. Perhaps; but this morning their sullen determined faces frightened me. I made every appeal, and failed to move them.

LADY ANNE. How do you account for this obstinacy? Last week you had only to speak for them to obey.

REID. Now Ellen Sands and others are against me. Besides, that article in the *Durham Mercury* telling of our early love-story has done much to undermine my influence. This morning there was talk of promised assistance and unaccountable delay in the transmission of money.

LADY ANNE. Ah! that newspaper article. The letters I have received. It seems that at Torrington Park you're looked upon as my acknowledged lover. I, too, have made sacrifices, but I'm not so eloquent about them as you.

REID. Anne, my position is a terrible one.

LADY ANNE. Are you afraid?

REID. You mean personal fear? I'm not afraid. But my guilt burns in my heart. Let me give them their money.

LADY ANNE. To achieve my ruin your friend would see the men die by inches.

REID. Anne, you do not know the abject suffering of the town, and all within a few yards of you. Let me show you. (*He leads her to window, left.*) Look into the street. Those men are starving. That man, how miserable he seems – his slouching, hungry gait! And those children who follow their mother. She has no bread to give them. A little lath and plaster between this elegant boudoir and miserable garrets. Anne, have mercy!

LADY ANNE. The night is chill, and I cannot remain by this window. (*She wraps herself in her scarf, and they come down the stage and sit at table.*)

REID. Little children in empty rooms crying for bread. The thought is unbearable. The next time the clock strikes I may be a murderer. Anne, Anne! (*Throws himself on his knees.*) Let me beg mercy of you. I beg mercy of you.

LADY ANNE. What am I to say? The situation is a terrible one, I know. (*Buries her face in her hands.*) I am not the cruel, heartless woman you think me. I wouldn't walk over a fly on the ground if I could help it. But what am I to do? Did you not say yourself, that to surrender this money would bring ruin on the miners?

REID. Yes. (*Getting up.*) That is the tragedy of the whole thing, the horror of the situation. But in my heart I know, Anne, that I would not have detained that cheque if I had not loved you.

LADY ANNE. Then you regret?

REID. That I love you? I might as well regret that I breathe, that I was born. My fear is to lose you. Then I should have realised nothing.

LADY ANNE. Perhaps we ought never to have met. I have ruined you. What will be the end of all this?

REID. Let us go away from here; let the cheque be acknowledged. We are not answerable for the catastrophe the miners bring upon themselves. I'll work for you. I cannot give you back your lost wealth, but I can give you a competence. I beseech you, Anne, do this for me; if not for their sake, for the sake of my love. I want to love you, to love you always.

LADY ANNE. You want me to fly with you, to leave everything. (REID *takes her hands.*) It would be nice to go far away, to some beautiful country – far from this trouble. I think we could love one another.

REID. I have often dreamed such a love-story. Is it possible that my dream will be realised?

LADY ANNE. Ah! if I could leave everything for you! Society, friends, riches – but can I? You forget what all this means to me.

REID. I have abandoned all things for you. Honour and truth, and that pity for humanity which was once so dear to me.

LADY ANNE. We cannot abandon the life we were brought up in. You tried to, but you've come back to it.

REID. Anne, your fortune is in desperate peril. You're no longer sure that Baron Steinbach will help you. What will you do if you find yourself utterly ruined?

41

LADY ANNE. You mean if I were left worth nothing, and had to think of – I don't say of earning my bread, but being very poor – two or three hundred a year.

REID. If you loved me you would not hesitate.

LADY ANNE. I do love you, but this is folly. I cannot even think of myself as a poor woman – it is impossible. I should commit suicide.

REID. Suicide!

LADY ANNE. Why not? I'm not afraid of death. It is so easy to die. (*Going to cabinet.*) Last year a favourite dog of mine had to be destroyed. (*Shows a small bottle.*) A few of these white grains, and the poor brute leaped up in the air and fell stone dead.

REID. And if tomorrow you found yourself ruined you would – you shall not. (*He snatches the bottle.*)

LADY ANNE. Give me that, you've no right to – (*The* FOOTMAN *enters.*)

FOOTMAN. Miss Sands is downstairs, your ladyship. She wants to see Mr Reid.

LADY ANNE (*to* REID). I must say that you're not here.

REID. Is not that piling falsehood upon falsehood?

LADY ANNE. Very well, go to her. But before you go, do not forget that you've to make a restitution to me. Give me what you took from me just now.

REID. Let him say that I'm not here.

LADY ANNE (*to* FOOTMAN). Tell Miss Sands that Mr Reid is not here, that he left an hour ago. (*Exit* FOOTMAN.) How did they discover you were here? You must have been followed.

REID. What can she have come for? If news of the cheque has reached them I'm lost.

LADY ANNE. But you'll admit nothing, for my sake, to save me.

REID. Anne, this is ruin. The detention of the cheque must be discovered. You asked for a few hours' delay – nearly a week has passed.

LADY ANNE. Tomorrow the men will surrender.

REID. Children are starving, Anne. You've not seen their haggard faces. Anne, let that cheque be acknowledged – let us go away together.

LADY ANNE. What folly, what folly this is! (*Enter* FOOTMAN.)

FOOTMAN. Miss Sands says she knows Mr Reid is here, and refuses to leave until she has seen him.

LADY ANNE. I dare not have her turned out. (*To* REID). Dare I trust you with her; are you sure that she'll not win you from me?

REID. No-one can win me from you.

LADY ANNE. But she'll speak to you of honour, duty!

REID. You're my only duty.

LADY ANNE. (*to* FOOTMAN). Show Miss Sands up. (*Exit* FOOTMAN). What can she have come for?

REID. She may have come to question – (*Enter* ELLEN SANDS.)

ELLEN. I apologise, Lady Anne, for my intrusion ... You'll readily believe that it is as disagreeable for me to come as for you to receive me. (LADY ANNE *affects occupation with some wool-work.*)

LADY ANNE. Won't you sit down, Miss Sands?

ELLEN. I'm an intruder. Only the most important business could have brought me here, therefore there's no reason why I should sit down.

LADY ANNE. As you like, Miss Sands. I didn't wish you to seem as if you'd come after a situation, that's all. Your business is important, and you see the hour is late.

ELLEN. And yet Mr Reid is here.

LADY ANNE. Mr Reid and I are old friends, as I believe you're aware. He's been dining here ... You see I continue to answer your questions.

ELLEN. Dining here! – one of the few houses where there has been dinner tonight. The town is starving. Ah, the poor little children crying for bread – wild work may happen before morning.

REID. This morning I besought the men to relinquish the hopeless struggle, but you and others opposed my advice. You insisted that the books of capitalists could not be trusted, that to go back to work unless every demand was acceded to was to go back to slavery. Therefore I say, Ellen, let the guilt be upon your head – the suffering endured and the acts it may bring about.

ELLEN. I do not hesitate to accept the responsibility. The fate of unborn generations is involved in the struggle. The men must triumph.

REID. Triumph! Then you really call into question the evidence of the books.

ELLEN. This tale has been disproved a hundred times. All that concerns capital is false and corrupt. Capital must be destroyed.

LADY ANNE. Of course, Miss Sands; but may I ask if it was only that I might hear your views on this all-absorbing question that you forced your way into my house?

ELLEN. No, Lady Anne, it was not. Matters have arrived at a crisis, and we do not know on what side – can I still say our leader, is fighting.

LADY ANNE. Indeed. It seems to me that Mr Reid has very clearly defined his position.

ELLEN. Have you gone over to the other side?

REID. If to state the truth is to go over to the other side, I have done so.

LADY ANNE. Are you satisfied, Miss Sands?

ELLEN. I fully understand! I do not contest Mr Reid's right to change his opinions, but before every dissolution of partnership there is a general settling. There are certain matters on which I must speak to Mr Reid alone.

LADY ANNE. Miss Sands, you're presuming on the tolerance I extend to you – let me remind you that there are limits. But perhaps this is a matter that Mr Reid will settle for himself.

REID (*to* LADY ANNE). I cannot refuse to discuss whatever matters Miss Sands may desire to discuss with me. You'll excuse me, Lady Anne. (LADY ANNE *bows coldly*.) Ellen, I'm at your service. (*To* LADY ANNE.) It is not possible for me to do otherwise. I'll return in a few minutes. (ELLEN *has moved towards the door.*)

LADY ANNE. But, Miss Sands, there's no reason why you should leave. You can talk with Mr Reid here. (*Gathers up the wool-work , and exits.*)

REID. Ellen, we're alone ... You've come to speak to me on an important matter.

ELLEN. Yes; and I'll not linger in the purely personal matter of the transference of your affections to Lady Anne, though that too must be settled. You've ceased to love me?

REID. I'll waste no time in excuses.

ELLEN. That's right – the mere fact.

REID. I have.

ELLEN. Ah, you love her, and will never care for me again. (*She sits down, buries her face in her hands, struggling with her emotion.*) An over-mastering passion, the plea of every libertine. Oh, that you should have lied to me so – the utter vileness of it.

REID. I didn't lie to you. When I told you last week that I loved you, and that you could trust me, I thought I was speaking the truth. I was mistaken.

ELLEN (*getting up*). After all, you're under no obligation to love me; we're free to choose, and I suppose to rectify our mistakes. It must be so, only – only –

REID. I thought it was only for the sake of the cause that you cared for me.

ELLEN. Did she say so? There are as many ways of loving as of living. She loves as she lives. I love as I live. (*Dashes a tear aside.*) And for the sake of this new love you have abandoned not only me, but the cause itself?

REID. No. It was the desperate policy you've pursued in the present strike that destroyed my belief -- a policy that has brought men and women and children to the verge of starvation, that will probably end in riot, violence, murder – a policy that if pursued will reduce

44

the world to a desert, and change civilised man back to a barbarian.

ELLEN. Even that were better than the present system should endure.

REID. It is those very opinions that have produced a change in mine.

ELLEN. Are you sure, John?

REID. We're sure of nothing. It were vain to argue about motives – human motive is inscrutable. You've come on a matter of urgent business?

ELLEN. Yes, on the most urgent business.

REID. Then why have you not spoken before?

ELLEN. I hesitated.

REID. You hesitated. You undecided!

ELLEN. You're gravely concerned in it ... But I must tell you. There's a rumour of a large sum of money having been sent to the strike fund. The letter that contained the cheque was directed to you. It has been suggested that you suppressed the cheque so that you might more easily persuade the miners to return to work.

REID. Who's my accuser? No matter; do you believe him?

ELLEN. I cannot believe such a thing of you.

REID. Then why do you ask?

ELLEN. Because your life will be in danger if the rumour proceeds further.

REID. A word from you'll quench it at once.

ELLEN. Exactly; and it is for the authority to speak that I come here. A word from me is sufficient, and that word shall be spoken if you say that the rumour is false.

REID. I can ask no favour from you. We're fighting on different sides.

ELLEN. Deny it; for if you do not –

REID. You'll have to denounce me –

ELLEN. I shall have to say that you declined to deny it, which amounts to the same thing.

REID. And you'll do this?

ELLEN. I must.

REID. Then – Ellen –

ELLEN. Hush; the time has passed for denial. A moment ago I should have taken your word ... Now I cannot. And so for her vicious sake you detained money that was sent to save men and women and children from famine.

REID. It was for their sake I detained it. Is it worse to suppress a cheque that you know must lead to utter destruction than it is to tell men that books have been kept falsely and urge them to persevere in a mad endeavour which you know must end in their ruin?

ELLEN. Which I know!

45

REID. Which the slightest exercise of common sense must tell you will lead them into irretrievable disaster; and you did this for the sake of theories which, when put to the test, may prove as vain as the wind. You lied to them for the sake of your theories – I held my tongue for their welfare; which of us is the greater culprit?

ELLEN. I do not believe those books; in the way of man's regeneration there are many pitfalls.

REID. There are indeed, and I'm not the only one.

ELLEN. We've not come together to discuss, but to act. Immediately your treachery is known your life will be forfeited – you must fly the town.

REID. They shall listen to me, I will save them. Justice and good sense shall triumph. I'll go to them whom you say are waiting to assassinate me, and in the market-place I'll confute you and your friends, who would lead them on to their ruin.

ELLEN. Do not go to the market-place if you value your life.

REID. If I carry the men with me my life will become of value; if I fail, I may as well perish at their hands as any other way.

ELLEN. I shall not help you – you go at your peril.

REID. I do not ask your help. (*Exit.*)

ELLEN (*speaking like one in a dream*). He's gone to his death. I cannot save him. He detained the money for her sake. (*She turns and goes out slowly. The* FOOTMAN *enters a moment after with a lamp. He places it on the table, looks to the wicks, draws curtains, goes back to lamp. A minute and a half elapses; then a knocking is heard at window opening on to lawn.*)

FOOTMAN. Who is there?

STEINBACH. Baron Steinbach; open at once. (*The* FOOTMAN *opens window. Enter* STEINBACH *dressed in a long travelling overcoat.*) Where's her ladyship?

FOOTMAN. I think her ladyship is in her room.

STEINBACH. Then send to her, and say that I'm waiting to speak to her on a matter that does not admit of delay. (*Enter* LADY ANNE.) Oh, here is Lady Anne. (FOOTMAN *withdraws.*) I was just sending the footman to you with a message that you were to come to me at once.

LADY ANNE. What is it? What has happened?

STEINBACH. The town is mad with famine, the men's leaders are losing all control, wild threats are being uttered, and at this moment a riotous feeling may begin. I've telegraphed for a detachment of soldiers; it is doubtless on its way here. In the meantime, in the meantime – (*Looks at his watch.*) It will not arrive for at least two hours yet.

LADY ANNE. But he? Where is he? Where are they?

STEINBACH. Who?

LADY ANNE. John Reid and Ellen Sands; they were here a short time ago. Have they gone?

STEINBACH. Reid passed me at the bottom of the garden. He was calling to the people. Crowds followed him. I asked a passer-by what was the meaning of it. He said Reid was on his way to the market-place to address a meeting.

LADY ANNE. So she's succeeded in persuading him; she's won him over, and he's gone to betray me.

STEINBACH. Gone to betray you! What do you mean, Anne?

LADY ANNE. I'd better tell you all. When John Reid came here last week to examine the books, he left the library convinced that the men's demands were impracticable, Ellen Sands arrived with a letter; that letter contained a cheque for £2000.

STEINBACH. And for your sake he suppressed the fact of the arrival of the cheque, intending to acknowledge it when he had persuaded the abandonment of the strike and the men were once more safely in the mine.

LADY ANNE. It was not for my sake, but for theirs that he suppressed the cheque.

STEINBACH. A specious sophistry, but one which not even he would have accepted had it not received the endorsement of your love.

LADY ANNE. You wrong us both.

STEINBACH. It may be as you say. Events have, however, proved too strong for him. So that was the way you tried to arrange things? My dear, my dear Anne, you had much better have confided in me. My advice alone will prove valid.

LADY ANNE. So this man has gone.

STEINBACH. To be torn to pieces in the market-place.

LADY ANNE. They may listen to him; he may carry them with him.

STEINBACH. He can only have gone there to explain the excellence of his intentions.

LADY ANNE. You do not believe –

STEINBACH. It matters not what I believe, but if he confesses that he detained that cheque his life isn't worth three minutes' purchase ... To think that a man should be such a fool – vanity – belief in his eloquence ... Ah! what's that? Crowds still going to the market-place. We shall be able to watch the effect of his oratory from this window. (*Draws the curtain.*)

LADY ANNE. Not at this hour.

STEINBACH. The moon is up. (*Throwing open the window.*) The market-place is as bright as the day. All the town seems to be there. I think they have let him get on the platform; but it is difficult to distinguish detail ... Have you a pair of opera-glasses?

LADY ANNE (*snatching a pair from the table*). Yes, there's one. Is he on the platform?

STEINBACH. Yes, I think so.

LADY ANNE. Do they listen?

STEINBACH (*altering the glasses*). The light is deceitful, and these glasses are not very suited to my sight.

LADY ANNE (*snatching the glasses from him*). Then give them to me.

STEINBACH (*coming down stage*). Can you see?

LADY ANNE. Yes, perfectly. (STEINBACH *sits in arm-chair.*)

STEINBACH. Your friend doesn't seem to be wanting in courage. It requires no small pluck to face a mob like that ... and with such a tale. How can he hope? Imagination, courage, but no brains ... Do they listen?

LADY ANNE. I do not know ... tell me, will they kill him? Yes, they are listening to him. (*Turning from the window.*)

STEINBACH. I'm glad of it. I've no reason to wish him well, but such a death!

LADY ANNE (*turning to the window*). But now there is a movement amongst the crowd; it seems to threaten him.

STEINBACH. Then he's doomed. The first blow's struck, and nothing can save him.

LADY ANNE. They crowd round the platform! Can we do nothing to save him?

STEINBACH. I see that you're still in love with him.

LADY ANNE. You needn't be in love with a man because you don't wish to see him torn to pieces under your very eyes. They have not struck him yet. But why does he remain? Ah, he's fighting now. But he overpowers the brute, and has thrown him from his platform.

STEINBACH. There's plenty more behind that ruffian. Once they're blooded they'll have at him and tear him like hounds a hare.

LADY ANNE. He's retreated; they've driven him into a corner. (STEINBACH *gets up and takes* LADY ANNE *from the window.*)

STEINBACH. Anne, this is no sight for you; come away.

LADY ANNE. See if they've killed him. Here, take the glasses.

STEINBACH. You saw them drive him into a corner of the square, whence there is no egress. It is vain to think further about him.

LADY ANNE. I do not speak so cruelly, and he went there to betray me.

STEINBACH. I did not mean to be cruel. What a death, what a reward for his labours! He gave up everything for them.

LADY ANNE. Yes, everything. This is shocking. Oh, that I ever came here!

STEINBACH. You're trembling . . . This has unnerved you. We must go away at once.

LADY ANNE. Take me away.

STEINBACH. We must escape at once.

LADY ANNE. Escape!

STEINBACH. At the railway station we shall be safe. My yacht is at Southampton. My villa on the Italian coast is at your service should you not care to remain in England.

LADY ANNE. To leave here defeated, scouted the reputed mistress of a socialist.

STEINBACH. My dear Anne, we should never show our hearts, nor any volatile fragment of our hearts, outside of our own society.

LADY ANNE. Oh! this is disgraceful. It was cruel of him to betray me.

STEINBACH. He sacrificed you to his honour, and we've seen how the populace appreciated the sacrifice. Come, Anne, come . . . go for a wrap, and let's get away at once.

LADY ANNE. Flight!

STEINBACH. You shall be revenged. Tomorrow the mine will be under military protection. Non-unionist labour shall be imported, cost what it may, and you shall dictate your own terms. Now go for a wrap, and let us go away at once. (*Exit* LADY ANNE, *right.* STEINBACH *looks at his watch. He goes to the window.*) Crowds coming this way . . . If that fellow should have escaped, he'll be sure to come after her...Then we shall have the town down upon us; the house will be pillaged. (*Returning, left.*) Anne, Anne, I beg you to hasten. (*Enter* LADY ANNE, *wrapped in shawl.*)

LADY ANNE. I'm ready. Come, let's lose no time. A multitude seems to fill the street . . . I'm frightened. If you weren't here what should I do?

STEINBACH. You treated me shockingly, but I was determined to win you. (*They go towards the window that leads on to the lawn. Enter* REID, *torn and haggard.*) Have no fear. In a week we shall be in Italy.

REID. So you are going away with him? (LADY ANNE *and* STEINBACH *turn round.*)

LADY ANNE. You escaped the mob, then?

REID. I escaped the mob.

LADY ANNE. Are you hurt?

REID. Mortally, though hardly a blow reached me.

LADY ANNE. We were watching from that window, and we thought that we saw you killed.

REID. I escaped by a miracle. A door was suddenly opened – I fled through it; it was closed behind me – I know not by whom. I fled through the house, climbed some walls, dodged the crowd through some back streets ... I've come back to find you leaving with Baron Steinbach.

LADY ANNE. Why did you betray me?

REID. Did I betray anyone but myself?

LADY ANNE. And after betrayal and broken promises you returned here expecting –

REID. Forgive my poor expectations – they are my last. So you are going away with Baron Steinbach?

LADY ANNE. I am flying for my life ... If Baron Steinbach were not here –

REID. You could not look to me for help? Truly you could not.

LADY ANNE. You cannot remain here. You'll be taken and torn to pieces. You must escape.

STEINBACH (*coming down the stage*) Lady Anne is right, you must escape; it is too horrible.

REID. Spare me your pity, Baron Steinbach. Spare me that. You've won on every side. Be satisfied with your victory.

STEINBACH. You misunderstand me. I intended no insult. Let our former antagonism be forgotten. Let me help you –

REID. I do not need your help or anyone's. I'm no coward, and will meet my fate as it should be met.

STEINBACH. We do not doubt your courage, but it cannot avail you against numbers. If you leave this house you'll be killed. But you're safe here, and at daybreak you can escape. I'll see that help is sent, and afterwards – (REID *looks at* STEINBACH. STEINBACH *turns from* REID *to* LADY ANNE.) Anne, we must go away. (*He looks once more at* REID.)

REID. Think no more of me. That is the greatest kindness.

STEINBACH. But you'll do what I say? You'll remain here till daybreak?

REID. Yes, I'll remain here.

LADY ANNE. And at daybreak you'll escape?

REID. I shall escape.

STEINBACH. Lady Anne, come away. (REID *sinks into a chair.*) Come Lady Anne, come.

LADY ANNE (*from the window that opens on to lawn*). Will he escape?

STEINBACH. He says so. Come, I insist. (*Exeunt* LADY ANNE *and* STEINBACH. REID *watches for a moment.*)

REID. They have gone. They have gone away together. (*Goes to window, left. Listens, and comes down the stage.*) There is no time

50

to lose; they have discovered that I am here. (*Puts bottle on table.*)
(*Enter* ELLEN.)

ELLEN. They've tracked you here. The house will soon be surrounded.
You must escape at once.

REID. And you came here to warn me?

ELLEN. Yes.

REID. Thank you.

ELLEN. Escape, escape while there's yet time.

REID. Escape. Why should I escape? For why?

ELLEN. For her sake.

REID. I escaped the mob only to find her leaving for Italy with Baron
Steinbach.

ELLEN. So she deceived you.

REID. No, I am the deception, the only deception, and that deception is
about to cease.

ELLEN. You mean suicide?

REID. Yes, escapement from self. I put it to you – you're a sensible girl,
Ellen, and you don't lie. You'll not deceive me. Remember that you
once loved me.

ELLEN. Yes, I once loved you.

REID. Thank you for those words. Now listen. I have lost all. I have
betrayed the woman I loved, and I have been betrayed by her. I've
betrayed the woman who loved me. I have lost not only her love but
her respect. Worse than all, I've lost honour; never again can I look
the world in the face. Belief in the cause is gone too – everything
is gone – I stand a moral bankrupt. In such juncture of circumstances
man must escape from self, I ask you is this not so?

ELLEN. I cannot see that you could ever find happiness again in life,
either for yourself or others.

REID. That is how I feel, Ellen. I suppose all suicides feel the same . . . I
would have been better if I'd gone down fighting . . . The brutes, I
still feel their foul breaths on my face, and their foul hands. I
abandoned my own class for their sake, but I never could assimilate
my life with theirs. I'm not of any class or of any convictions. Why
should I remain?

ELLEN. No, no, you must not do this.

REID. What would you have me do?

ELLEN. Escape at once . . . No, at daybreak

REID. Skulk out of the town at daybreak, and live face to face with my
dishonour. Ellen, there is but one thing to be done. (*A pause, during
which* ELLEN *struggles with her emotion.*)

ELLEN. It is very terrible, but I suppose it is as you say. (*Pause.*) Have you the means?

REID. Yes. It appears that about a year ago her old favourite dog had to be poisoned. This remained.

ELLEN. So the poison came from her. She's the world's poison. (*Pause.*) They're all about the house. They'll break in soon ... But they shall not kill you.

REID. I'm safe from them. A moment and it is done. (*Pause.*) You'll forgive me the pain I've caused you. You'll forgive my want of faith. You'll forgive everything? You'll try to remember when my worst faults press hardest on your memory that I honestly desired the light, and that I sought although I did not find.

ELLEN. All is forgiven to the dead.

REID. Goodbye, Ellen. (*Kisses her on her forehead.*) Goodbye. You must not remain here. (*He leads her to the door.*) Goodbye, Ellen. (*Exit*). (*He looks at poison. He goes to the cabinet, gets some water, dissolves the strychnine, and comes down the stage, the glass in his hand, with his back partly turned to the audience; he raises the glass to drink; as he does so, the curtain falls.*)

CURTAIN

THE BENDING OF THE BOUGH

A COMEDY IN FIVE ACTS

BY

GEORGE MOORE

CHARACTERS

JOSEPH TENCH,	*the Mayor.*
JASPER DEAN, DANIEL LAWRENCE, THOMAS FERGUSON, VALENTINE FOLEY, RALF KIRWAN, JAMES POLLOCK, MICHAEL LEECH,	*Aldermen of the Corporation*
JOHN CLORAN,	*the Town Clerk.*
GEORGE HARDMAN,	*Lord Mayor of Southhaven.*
MISS MILLICENT FELL,	*His Niece, engaged to marry* ALDERMAN DEAN.
MISS CAROLINE DEAN, MISS ARABELLA DEAN,	*Maiden Aunts of* ALDERMAN DEAN.
MRS POLLOCK,	*Wife and First Cousin of* ALDERMAN POLLOCK, *Sister of* ALDERMAN LEECH, *and Cousin of the* DEANS.
MRS LEECH,	*Wife and First Cousin of* ALDERMAN LEECH, *Sister of* ALDERMAN POLLOCK, *and also Cousin of the* DEANS.
MACNEE,	*Caretaker of the Town Hall.*
A PARLOURMAID	*at* ALDERMAN DEAN'S *House*
A WAITER	*at the Hotel.*

Several Town Councillors, People, &c.

54

THE BENDING OF THE BOUGH

ACT I

The Meeting Hall of the Corporation. MACNEE *sets down a large bucket in front and then begins leisurely to sweep the floor.* JOHN CLORAN *enters carrying some papers.*

CLORAN (*with importance*). What are you doing here, Macnee? I'm expecting the Corporation every minute.

MACNEE. I'm sweeping the floor for the Corporation.

CLORAN. You should have finished long ago.

MACNEE. Has the Corporation never been behind with its work?

CLORAN. The Corporation has never been more hard-worked; the Corporation will be engaged this morning with most important matters; and the most important resolutions will be passed.

MACNEE. What are the resolutions about?

CLORAN. I'm too busy now to explain.

MACNEE. I think you'd find them hard to explain.

CLORAN. That'll do. It isn't my business to argue with a man like you.

MACNEE. Ah, you're a proud man to be Town Clerk, but I can tell you this Corporation you think so fine isn't respected much in the town.

CLORAN. You are, no doubt, a sound authority as to the feeling of our town.

MACNEE. I'm in the way of hearing the many, and, believe me, if you don't begin to do the people some good, none of you will long remain where you are.

CLORAN. Oh indeed! I suppose your associates, the proletariat, are discontented because there is not more unanimity among the members of our Corporation. Well, what do you expect? You don't suppose that where there are so many men of equal intelligence, ability and push that they will sink their individual opinions to follow the opinions of one of their number who is no better than anybody else.

MACNEE. How long have they been tearing each other in pieces, I should like to know. When will they begin to think of the good of the town?

CLORAN. All their opinions are for the good of our town ... But what

55

we want is somebody who will offer a superior opinion. We want a leader – a man whose superiority will unite us in the best interests of our town. And we shall find him, if we haven't found him already.

MACNEE. You mean young Mr Jasper Dean?

CLORAN. The very man. He has been elected alderman for a ward, and today he is to take his seat here for the first time as a member of our Corporation.

MACNEE. Well, he's a good deal spoken of; they say he is a great scholar.

CLORAN. He carried all before him at Oxford. He has one thing in his favour.

MACNEE. What is that, Mr Cloran?

CLORAN. He is a very fine gentleman and comes of a good old family.

MACNEE. There are too many fine gentlemen already in this country.

CLORAN. Yes, but I hear the members coming in.

MACNEE. I must be going. They don't want to see the people here. (*Exit carrying his bucket*).

CLORAN. He is always trying to push himself forward! I am sure he would like to sit with the Corporation. (*Enter* ALDERMAN JAMES POLLOCK *and* ALDERMAN MICHAEL LEECH.)

POLLOCK. A dangerous man. I tried to get the Corporation to give him the sack.

LEECH. He was in quite a good position once; it was politics that brought him to this menial work. That's so, isn't it, Cloran?

POLLOCK. Isn't the Mayor here yet?

CLORAN. No, Alderman Leech, he is very late today.

POLLOCK. Any news, Cloran?

CLORAN. Not a word, Alderman Pollock.

POLLOCK. Nothing about our claim against Southhaven?

CLORAN. Only a letter received this morning which I shall lay before the Corporation. But it leaves matters pretty nearly where they were, sir.

LEECH (*to* POLLOCK). Ferguson has to some extent succeeded in forcing us to pursue this matter.

POLLOCK. Today he is to bring on a resolution to start our steamers again, regardless of our agreement. If Southhaven takes action against us for breach of contract we are to answer by a counter-action for non-fulfilment of contract.

LEECH. No-one will support such a resolution. It would mean involving the town in two costly lawsuits.

POLLOCK. And lose us our connection with Southhaven. (ALDERMAN

RALF KIRWAN *enters*.) We are talking about Alderman Ferguson's resolution.

LEECH. That, in defiance of our agreement with Southhaven, we shall start our line of steamers again. Do you believe that anyone in his senses will support his resolution?

KIRWAN. I do not think the resolution a wise one at the moment. But what matter? As well as another it will supply fuel for dissension.

LEECH. If you do not believe in municipal life why do you come here?

KIRWAN. I often ask myself that question. I suppose because hope is undying, and every time I come here I come believing that the miracle has happened, that we shall find a leader waiting us.

CLORAN. Gentlemen, gentlemen! Ah, gentlemen, I declare there is not one of you but is entitled to lead.

KIRWAN. No, Cloran, there is not one among us who can lead, and among the failures I include myself.

CLORAN. But you have hopes, Alderman Kirwan. Report says that you speak highly of young Mr Dean, our new alderman.

POLLOCK. It appears that he has taken up all your ideas enthusiastically.

LEECH. It appears that you have found a disciple at last.

POLLOCK. But why should he succeed with your ideas better than you've succeeded with them yourself? No, Kirwan, he won't do, there is not the stuff of a leader in him. You agree with me, Michael?

LEECH. I do indeed, James. He is nothing particular. And we ought to know, aren't we his relations?

POLLOCK. The only thing I ever heard in his favour is that he has become friends with Hardman, and is going to marry his niece – an excellent connection.

KIRWAN. What you put to his good account I put to his bad, so you see we think as differently on this as on other subjects. Yes, he distinguished himself at Oxford, and the great man learns only what he wants to learn, the mediocre man can learn what others think he should learn. Oh, there is a great deal to be said against Dean. (ALDERMAN VALENTINE FOLEY *enters*.)

FOLEY. Good morning, good morning. Now tell me what you think of Ferguson's resolution. I am not sure that I approve of it, but it is full of interest. Quite a sensational resolution, I'd like to see it supported even if it is not carried. Oh, for a little more unanimity, for some kindly feeling, avoidance of personal attack even when we disagree!

KIRWAN. But the last number of your paper, Foley, contained an attack against every one.

FOLEY. You read my articles in the *Denouncer:* they were all mine, the whole of the back page was mine. What did you think of it?

KIRWAN. I thought that you were an advocate of union.

FOLEY. So I am, but not of union with traitors. The sense of our wrongs fills me with indignation, but to right them all I would not hold out my hand to any one with whom I could not entirely agree.

CLORAN. The last number of the Denouncer was a glorious one, full of fury against the enemies of our town. The people say that you have a mission.

FOLEY. Do they? (*Pause.*) I always felt that I had a mission.

POLLOCK. What is your mission?

FOLEY. No man can define his mission, you must feel your mission (*looking round*); it must be a terrible thing not to feel that you have a mission.

KIRWAN. You're a journalist, Foley, to the finger-tips, which are inky. You exist in the day, in the very hour.

FOLEY. And what is life but an accumulation of days and hours?

KIRWAN. In the eyes of most people it is no more. Would that those who believe this would act up to their theory. The mission of this day, if it has a mission, is surely the settlement of our claims against Southhaven.

LEECH. So far I will go with you. That it is impossible not to be indignant at the manner in which our seaport has been ruined at the advantage of Southhaven.

FOLEY. And yet you and Pollock have voted against every measure for re-establishing the line of steamers which Southhaven has filched from us.

KIRWAN. Filched? No; we agreed to sell our steamers. The accounts rendered by Southhaven are not satisfactory – cheated if you will. I like to preserve these nice differences – a cheat is not a thief.

POLLOCK. Even in joke we should not use such words against our neighbour, nor do anything that might injure our neighbour.

LEECH. There are so many interests involved, you know.

KIRWAN. Certain members of our Corporation hold shares in the Southhaven line.

FOLEY. This raises a very interesting question. Don't you think that our duty towards ourselves and our duties towards the State would make an excellent subject for an article?

LEECH. And our duties towards our families.

FOLEY. True, true, I am glad you mentioned it.

KIRWAN. There would be no difficulty in considering the collective interests of the town if one had not one's old particular desires and those of the lady upstairs to consider too.

POLLOCK. You're a bachelor; all reformers are bachelors, all extreme reformers have been bachelors.

FOLEY. The State and the family are for ever at war: the summer of the State is the winter of the family – two forces always at war.

POLLOCK. I only hold a few shares in the Southhaven line. I should not mind running the risk of reducing their value if I could only feel that our dear neighbours were not going to suffer.

LEECH. Quite so. What should we be without our neighbour, our rich neighbour? And is it not nearly sure that if we insist on the fulfilment of the bargain we made with Southhaven we shall lose as much as we gain?

KIRWAN. Here we love our neighbour – well, not more than ourselves, but much better than we love the interests of our town.

LEECH. Kirwan, do you mean to say that the Corporation doesn't consider the best interests of the town? that, having regard for their own private interests, certain aldermen do not press the claims that our town have against Southhaven?

KIRWAN. For many reasons the claim is not pressed – for social reasons, for pecuniary reasons; and the principal reason of all is because we are hopelessly divided, because we have not found a leader.

LEECH. There are plenty of leaders. Our friend here (*pointing to* POLLOCK).

KIRWAN. Plenty who desire to lead, but no leader.

LEECH. The question is whether we should insist in demanding one pound of flesh – the clause is vaguely worded, you admit that, Kirwan.

KIRWAN. I see that you wish to abide in the good wishes of Southhaven; you prefer her good wishes to the pound of flesh. (*Enter the* MAYOR *and* ALDERMAN THOMAS FERGUSON.)

MAYOR. Well, of course, Alderman Ferguson, you may bring forward your motion; but I fancy it will meet with a good deal of opposition.

FERGUSON. I will carry it in spite of opposition.

KIRWAN. That is what every mover of contentious matter thinks.

FERGUSON. Alderman Kirwan again criticises. Why doesn't he come forward with a proposal himself?

KIRWAN. None of us could make a proposal that the others would not tear to pieces; they would gather about it like hounds about a fox.

FERGUSON. And so you spend your time thinking, Alderman Kirwan?

KIRWAN. If I've thought well, I've done everything that is required.

FERGUSON. We want action.

KIRWAN. If I've thought well, some one else will act well. (*Enter* ALDERMAN DANIEL LAWRENCE *and* JASPER DEAN *followed by other aldermen and several town councillors. Then the public crowd into the place allotted to them.*)

LAWRENCE. My dear Jasper Dean, I haven't seen you for a long time – how well you are looking! I never saw you looking so well in my life. I am delighted you have become a member of our Corporation. We want men of your position and education – yes, we want your Southhaven ideas.

DEAN. I never met with any ideas in Southhaven. It was here that I met ideas for the first time. (*He lays his hand on* KIRWAN'S *shoulder.*)

LAWRENCE. I am sorry you don't think better of Southhaven, you know our interests are so inseparably connected. (*The* MAYOR *and the Corporation all now take their places.*)

MAYOR. Mr Cloran, will you read the minutes of the last meeting?

CLORAN. Yes, your Worship. (*Reads from a large book.*) 'At the last regular meeting, present the Worshipful the Mayor Alderman –'

FERGUSON. That'll do. Let us get on to the business of to-day.

LAWRENCE. Really, Alderman Ferguson –

MAYOR. Order, order!

FOLEY. What is the good of taking up our time by reading all those minutes?

KIRWAN. They might have been read in less time than this dispute has taken.

ALL. That'll do. Enough.

CLORAN. Then I am not to read them, your Worship?

FERGUSON. Of course not.

MAYOR (*looking around*). Well, I suppose not.

CLORAN. Names of aldermen present and minutes taken as read. (*Laughter, during which he hands the book to the* MAYOR.)

MAYOR. Is it your wish, gentlemen, that I sign these minutes which Alderman Ferguson won't have read?

LAWRENCE. It is most illegal.

FERGUSON. Oh, illegal be hanged!

KIRWAN. Sign them, sign them, and let us get to work.

MAYOR. Well – I suppose I must. (*Signs the minutes in the book.*) Mr Cloran, have you written, as directed, to the authorities in Southhaven?

CLORAN. Yes, your Worship, in accordance with your resolution at last meeting, I wrote and have received this answer from the Town Clerk.

MAYOR. Well, read it then. Silence, gentlemen.

CLORAN (*reading the letter*). 'SIR, – In reply to your communication, in which you demand on the part of your Corporation a definite answer from our Corporation to your repeated claims, I am directed

60

by our Corporation in the first place to remind you that it is very unusual for us to state definitely beforehand the course of action which we may eventually deem prudent to pursue. Our Corporation wish you to understand that our well-known integrity (*laughter*) and generosity in our dealings with other bodies have hitherto rendered such a demand as yours hurtful and superfluous; and that we might have been led to expect from the unanimity of interests which exists between our two towns a complete disappearance of all doubt as to the possibility of our acting in any other than in a just and generous spirit towards you. Finally, I am expressing the very general feeling of our Corporation when I now demand of you such trust in this matter of dispute as past experience should warrant you in bestowing upon us, and remain, &c., &c'.

FERGUSON. We will certainly give that pack of rogues such trust as experience warrants us – which means just no trust at all.

KIRWAN. Our position is not advanced one jot by that letter.

FOLEY. They will never pay this money unless they are made to.

LAWRENCE. The Southhaven Corporation is at least as honourable as our own, and I am sure that they will pay anything that is really due.

MAYOR. May be so, but that letter is a most evasive letter.

LAWRENCE. Southhaven never disappoints one's just expectations.

FERGUSON. Well, I hope they won't disappoint yours, that's all.

LAWRENCE. What do you mean, sir?

FERGUSON. Don't you expect the appointment of solicitor to the Southhaven Corporation, which is now robbing us? For how long have you not been sniffing after it?

LAWRENCE. How dare you, sir! Mr Mayor, I protest, I protest in the name of my honourable profession – (*Uproar and cries of 'Place-hunter!'*)

MAYOR. Order, order! (*Continued uproar.*) Order, order! At this rate we shall never finish, and there are some of us who want to catch the four o'clock train. Let us now proceed to discuss what action we shall take in reference to the letter you have just heard read. What are your opinions as to the line of action we should adopt?

LAWRENCE. Mr Mayor, I submit that this is an affair in which we ought to proceed with the greatest caution. (*Murmurs and applause.*) We cannot foretell what may be the consequences if we rush into any rash action. Our substance and our safety, I may say, depend upon our neighbour. Are not our savings invested in the very line of steamers with which some mischievous persons among us propose to interfere?

POLLOCK. Very true. No one of any standing would wish to interfere with the line of steamers.

LEECH. Yes, it would be a disreputable thing to do, and at the same time fatal to our interests.

LAWRENCE. Of course it would; but, to put the question of our interests altogether aside, think of the regard and gratefulness we are bound to feel for a great town like Southhaven.

LEECH. To be sure. I forgot that. That is far more important than our mere interests.

FOLEY. I repudiate it altogether! What have we to be grateful for? I should like to know.

LAWRENCE. All fashion, all society, all culture comes from Southhaven. I ask, What would Northhaven be without Southhaven? Our wives and daughters, their season, what would become of it? Have these things not to be considered?

KIRWAN. We have exchanged our arts, our language, and our ancient aristocracy for shoddy imitation.

FOLEY. Mr Mayor, I intended to support Alderman Ferguson's resolution, that we should answer this letter by the purchase of several ocean-going steamers. At the same time I feel it my duty to move that those holding shares in the Southhaven line shall be compensated.

FERGUSON. Compensation! That would be putting a premium on dishonesty.

LEECH. Explain, explain!

FERGUSON. Mr Mayor, one moment –

FOLEY. I am in possession of the meeting.

FERGUSON (*shouting*). Mr Mayor, I have some observations to make. (*There are cries among the Corporation and people for* FERGUSON *and* FOLEY. *Those for* FERGUSON *preponderate; and* FOLEY *sits down.*)

MAYOR (*thumping the table*). Silence! Silence!

FERGUSON. Mr Mayor, this matter before the Corporation would be easily settled if only we could agree to one thing – the restoration of our line of steamers.

LAWRENCE. You want to ruin us by severing our connection with our Southhaven neighbours, who can carry our goods better than we could ourselves.

DEAN. Mr Mayor, may I say a few words?

MAYOR. Certainly, Alderman Dean. Silence, gentlemen, please.

DEAN. Mr Mayor, if one so new at municipal business as I am might presume to advise gentlemen so experienced, I would suggest that each of us should keep more strictly to the question before us.

KIRWAN. Hear, hear.

DEAN. We have really nothing to do with any question except whether we shall decide or not decide to enforce the payment of what is due to us. Each man among us may fight for whatever he wishes when the thief has been run down. (*Cheers.*) The matter is very simple, and I am glad that you all seem to be of my opinion.

LAWRENCE. Not all, by any means, Alderman Dean.

FERGUSON. Yes, all except a few place-hunters.

KIRWAN. Is our town to surrender every advantage for the sake of a few officials? (*Cheers.*)

DEAN. Mr Mayor, we have nothing to do with officials. What interest can it be to us whether this or that official, however excellent, is or is not making money by our connection with Southhaven? Every town, every people, every race that has ever risen to greatness has asked one first question of its public men and of all other men who belong to it, 'Are you for us or against us?' The answer can only be yes or no.

LAWRENCE. Alderman Dean, I'm afraid you are not a sound politician. I thought you were a different man, sir.

DEAN. My thought is for the good of this people as a whole. Has not this people become a proverb, a symbol of poverty as it were, and does it not call us to its help? (*Cheers.*) If you will listen to me with patience I am sure that we shall agree upon a policy. Our ancestors were ready to endure to the utmost for their convictions. Cannot we agree together to do and to endure the little that is required of us?

LAWRENCE. Well, what is this policy? what is this grand discovery?

DEAN. That each man should, for the moment, put aside every question that divides us, and above all that we should pass a general act of oblivion as it were, and forget our private quarrels, however justified (*cheers*), till this great work has been completed. (*Cheers.*)

LAWRENCE. We are far too independent for that.

DEAN. It is because we are becoming so independent that we understand the necessity of being united. (*Cheers.*) We are discovering that we can only escape from dependence on petty interests and petty animosities by sharing in the greater life of our race and of our town. We must cease to think of ourselves as individuals, and think of ourselves as so many members belonging to the body of our town.

FERGUSON. Very true – very true.

DEAN. It is very encouraging to know that you agree with me. Well, then, admitting that I am right, how ought you to meet the present crisis? What is our public capacity? We are the Corporation of a northern town, situated on a western coast on the brink of a natural harbour; and, until a few years ago, we enjoyed the fruits of this good position. Our town was a most important packet station, it had full control of its own dealing with the world at large; it was independent of outside help or hindrance. But we sold our steamers to Southhaven, a large and prosperous town many miles further south, for a certain advantage, including sums of money that have been paid and a much larger sum that has not been paid. In past times, and we are all (no matter what our party) agreed upon this, the mainly Celtic people of this town and countryside were oppressed, killed, and pillaged by the mainly Saxon people of that more wealthy and powerful town, but this is a commercial age, and it has been found sufficient to cheat us. The clause in our agreement referring to the harbour dues is loosely worded, but we have taken counsel's opinion, and it has been held that our case is a good one; but this case has not been pressed because some think that if we did press it Southhaven might say, Take back your line of steamers and return those advantages and those sums of money which we have given you. Others hoped for posts in that wealthy municipality, or had vested money in its line of steamers. It has also been suggested that certain not very clearly defined social advantages which we are supposed to derive from our connection with Southhaven might be taken from us, and I have reason to believe that strong social influence has been exerted to prevent our claim from being pressed. Our women folk are particularly open to such influences, they understand better than we do the value of class prejudice and family interest. I have now sketched in outline the main facts of our case against Southhaven, and I think I have included nothing with which a single member of this Corporation will disagree.

LAWRENCE. Mr Mayor, I do not agree to it. I agree to nothing.

DEAN. I will not question now the wisdom of the sale of our steamers. I will not go into the question whether or not we should, so soon as the money has been paid, close our agreement with Southhaven, and start our steamers again, as we have a right to do. Several of my colleagues and I myself do not agree with my friend Mr Kirwan and with the majority of the members of the Corporation on this point. We have been opposed, for reasons which I need not enter into here, and we are still opposed to, the agitation for re-establishing our line of steamers. But we are all agreed, the most extreme of every section is agreed, that we should be paid our rightful percentages on the harbour dues of Southhaven.

LAWRENCE. Indeed, sir, what is really owing ought to be paid. We are all agreed to that, but what is it that is really owing?

DEAN. To hear Alderman Lawrence admit even so much is satisfactory. For many years Southhaven evaded the issue by furnishing no accounts. When the accounts were at last forced from her, our accountants perceived that she owed us a very large sum of money. It is most important, too, that, although Southhaven contested the results our accountants came to after an exhaustive examination, the accountants that she herself called in, after they had carefully checked every item, corroborated our accountants on almost every detail.

LAWRENCE. But all the Southhaven accountants did not. There was one man who held out, who disputed the admission of certain items.

DEAN. What would the evidence of one man against the evidence of ten amount to in a court of law? (*Hear, hear and a cheer from the crowd at the back.*) Well, Mr Mayor, we have made several appeals to our rich debtors for payment. In what spirit has she received our appeals? We have all heard her Town Clerk's letter to-day. Is it a candid letter? Is it the answer of a town that wishes to act justly? Are we to be thus put off and played with while our town is impoverished by defalcations? (*Tremendous cheers.*) No, sir, we will not consent to such treatment. After all, what have we but our town? Do we not stand or fall together? If she is ruined shall not we – yes, every class among us – be ruined too? (*Hear, hear.*) We must cast to the winds the deference to Southhaven that makes us weak, and, above all, we must sink our personal and our class differences. We have only to agree upon taking legal proceedings, and the law will do the rest.

FERGUSON. I'll unite with any one on that.

SEVERAL VOICES. We are all with you! We are all ready to unite!

DEAN. I am overjoyed to hear it, for I look upon it as so necessary to obtain this subsidy that although, as you know, I am opposed to the restoration of the packet station and have always with my family been a staunch supporter of our connection with Southhaven; still, if the authorities of that port evade the law by any means and deny us justice and cast us back upon civic ruin, I for one do solemnly declare that I am prepared to advocate the buying of new vessels and to run them in defiance of all existing agreements. (*Tremendous and prolonged cheering and enthusiasm.*) Mr Mayor, I beg to move that immediate legal proceedings be taken for the recovery of this debt of so many years' accumulation.

FERGUSON. I second that resolution. (*Cheers.*)

LAWRENCE. Mr Mayor, it is with very considerable pain that I have listened to the able speech of my respected and cultured young friend, Alderman Dean. I feel it is a disadvantage to all respectable people in our town and a disadvantage to his own family that such rare abilities as his should not be used in a cause more fit for the approbation of right-thinking people. Indeed, my ears could hardly make me believe it when I heard him wonder to such an extent from right principles as to advocate action so discourteous towards a Corporation whose friendship is of paramount importance to us. (*Murmurs.*) I sincerely trust that our Corporation will do nothing to alienate the sympathy of our wealthy neighbours. (*Uproar.*)

SEVERAL VOICES. Put the resolution! Put the resolution!

LAWRENCE. Shall I not be listened to?

FERGUSON. We have heard too much from you long ago.

LAWRENCE. Mr Mayor, I protest. (*Uproar, during which he is forced to sit down.*)

POLLOCK. It is very extraordinary how Jasper has brought the Corporation with him.

LEECH. Most extraordinary – because he really hasn't much in him, you know.

POLLOCK. I think his arguments quite wrong. However, I suppose we cannot go against such an unanimous burst of opinion.

LEECH. Oh no – besides he is one of the family, and it wouldn't look well if we took an active part in opposing him.

MAYOR. Let all who are in favour of the resolution say 'Aye'.

SEVERAL VOICES. Aye! Aye!

MAYOR. The contrary say 'No'.

LAWRENCE. No! (*Laughter.*)

MAYOR. The 'ayes' have it (*taking out his watch*). We shall catch the four o'clock train after all. (*Laughter and wild excitement. Several gather with congratulations around* JASPER DEAN, *while all move out of the room.*)

END OF ACT I

ACT II

Drawing-room in JASPER DEAN'S *house.* MISS CAROLINE *and* MISS ARABELLA DEAN *are seated by an afternoon tea-table.*

ARABELLA. So the day has come at last, Caroline, and our task is ended. Jasper is now a man. To-day he enters public life and he is going to be married.

CAROLINE. Quite so, Arabella. But I'm anxious for him to be here to meet Miss Fell. I told him not to be later than three.

ARABELLA. So the little boy who came to us sixteen years ago when our poor brother died is now a man, and passes beyond our keeping?

CAROLINE. Not beyond our influence, I trust, our teaching will survive in him.

ARABELLA. It is strange to look back upon it all – our bickerings about what he should eat and what he should wear, when he should get up and when he should go to sleep. It was a pleasant task, and I'm sorry it is ended. And what he should learn too. That was your department. Now we shall never quarrel any more over him. You will never accuse me again of ruining him with too much indulgence, and I shall never say that you are ruining him with too much severity. (*Enter* MRS BESSIE POLLOCK *and* MRS SARAH LEECH.)

CAROLINE. She has not arrived. But come in. She does not like the sea and is coming round by train; she missed the connection at Rossborough, but she telegraphed that she was coming by a later one. We're expecting her every minute.

ARABELLA. We were talking about dear Jasper. In a moment like the present one looks back; the simplest things seem so wonderful, and we wonder how it all happened.

MRS LEECH. You have every reason to be satisfied with the result.

CAROLINE. He distinguished himself at Oxford, and I began his education. I taught him to read and write, and before he went to school I learnt a little Latin so that I might teach him his declensions and verbs. Did you see his article on conciliation in the *Denouncer?* Alderman Foley thought very highly of it.

MRS LEECH. But is it true? may we venture to ask if there is anything in the rumour that Jasper's marriage will not be the only marriage in the family?

CAROLINE. Since you do not put your question directly, it is clear that you think it an impertinence.

ARABELLA. I am sure that Sarah did not mean to be impertinent.

CAROLINE. I used the word in its strict grammatical sense. If Sarah wants to know what I think of Mr Foley, I will tell her that I think him an estimable man whose literary knowledge should be of great use to Jasper.

MRS POLLOCK. Jasper I think you said went to school at Southhaven. Now what do you think of their schools?

CAROLINE. A Southhaven accent is essential, and if a boy does not quite pick it up he acquires a sort of ante-accent, which is the next best thing.

MRS LEECH. But at school Jasper gave trouble. There was some talk of insubordination.

CAROLINE. We don't pretend that in bringing Jasper up we reached perfection. We sincerely hope that your own boys will turn out as satisfactorily.

ARABELLA. Then he went to Oxford?

CAROLINE. Oxford is most important; Oxford weens a boy from local influences, and teaches him to act with his class and to consider the interests of his class and his family.

MRS POLLOCK. And to-day is the fruition of all your teaching and love.

CAROLINE. I hope I have rendered him fit to take a leading part in public life, Bessie.

MRS LEECH. If he is really all you wanted to make him he will never take the lead anywhere.

CAROLINE. Really, Sarah?

MRS LEECH. I only meant that your teaching will not qualify him to lead the popular party. You know what they say, that he has fallen under the influence of Kirwan, and has adopted all his ideas.

CAROLINE. Jasper is safe against Kirwan's influence, and will not be carried away by the enthusiasms so common in this country.

MRS POLLOCK. You're pleased, of course, at this marriage?

CAROLINE. You know who she is – niece of George Hardman, Mayor of Southhaven, which they say owes us all this money.

ARABELLA. We're most anxious to become acquainted with her; that is why Jasper has asked her to stay with us.

CAROLINE. She is very much admired; quite a notable figure in society, and very rich. (MRS LEECH *and* MRS POLLOCK *get up to leave.*) No, don't go. She cannot be long now, and Jasper will be sure to bring back James and Michael after the meeting, so she will be introduced to quite a number of the family.

MRS LEECH. We're all cousins. I am my husband's first cousin, and sister to Bessie's husband, so what relation is Jasper to me?

CAROLINE. Don't let us go into cousinship and aunts, it will never end. (*A knocking is heard at the street door.*)

MRS POLLOCK. There she is. (*The* MAID *enters.*)

MAID. Miss Fell. (MISS MILLICENT FELL *enters, exit the* MAID.)

CAROLINE (*to* MILLICENT). We are delighted to see you, my dear.

MILLICENT. Thank you, you are very kind. (*To* ARABELLA.) How do you do?

ARABELLA. These are our cousins – Mrs Bessie Pollock and Mrs Sarah Leech.

MILLICENT. How do you do? How do you do?

MRS LEECH. (*aside to* MRS POLLOCK). That cloak is the latest fashion. They're all wearing them at Southhaven. Do you like it?

ARABELLA. Jasper says you have a great interest in this northern town and country, Miss Fell.

MILLICENT. Oh, yes. I was always interested in your northern landscape even before I knew Jasper. Your old castles, your legends, your romance and your wit is a welcome relief after the solid prose of commercial Southhaven.

ARABELLA. We are so sorry that Jasper is not here to meet you. We were only just saying so when you arrived.

MILLICENT. Where is Jasper?

CAROLINE. He is at a meeting of the Corporation. You have no idea of the political success he is having. I wonder if you will approve. It all turns on –

MILLICENT. You must tell me about it. I need hardly say how interested I am in all his work. (*Enter* ALDERMAN JAMES POLLOCK *and* ALDERMAN MICHAEL LEECH.)

CAROLINE. James, this is Miss Millicent Fell.

MILLICENT (*to* POLLOCK *and* LEECH). How do you do? How do you do?

POLLOCK. You must find our town, Miss Fell, rather poor-looking after your handsome, opulent town.

MILLICENT. No, indeed. After the manufactures of Southhaven the picturesque beauty of your landscape comes upon one's eyes very pleasantly.

LEECH. I am glad you think so. But in my eyes prosperity is an essential part of beauty.

MRS POLLOCK. Have you come from the Corporation, James?

POLLOCK. Yes, yes. The proceedings are finished. (*Aside to* MRS POLLOCK.) It is all decided. We're going to begin an action against

Southhaven.

ARABELLA. I wonder Jasper isn't here.

POLLOCK (*laughing*) Oh, Jasper; he has been carrying all before him.

CAROLINE. Why, what has he done?

POLLOCK. He has succeeded in uniting us all for once. He leads the whole Corporation.

LEECH. Yes, it seems a wonderful thing; but he has done it. I am sure no one would ever have thought he could.

MILLICENT. I always knew he only wanted an opportunity to prove himself great.

ARABELLA. He is great.

CAROLINE. Arabella, such undue expressions of admiration only tend to render their object ridiculous.

MILLICENT. Oh, I hate reservations in admiration. Why cannot one say a man is great when we feel that he is?

MRS POLLOCK. I wonder you should say that. In Southhaven I've always found every one so reticent.

POLLOCK. You have, doubtless, had many opportunities, Miss Fell, of judging the abilities of Jasper.

MILLICENT. Yes. We have been acquainted for some time. We met at Oxford. My cousin, George Hardman, junior, was a friend of his there. He brought him during one vacation to stay at his father's the Mayor's house. That is how I first met Jasper.

CAROLINE. You always live at Southhaven with your uncle the Mayor, don't you, my dear?

MILLICENT. Oh, yes – he is like a father to me.

MRS LEECH. Ah! – (*There is a noise of voices outside.*)

ARABELLA. Here is Jasper coming. (*Enter* ALDERMEN JASPER DEAN *and* RALF KIRWAN.)

DEAN (*At the door, to* KIRWAN). That's just it; the man who is at once polite and firm is irresistible in diplomacy. Diplomacy is but a union of the two qualities. (*Perceives* MILLICENT *and advances.*) Oh, Millicent, so you have come at last. I hope you had a pleasant journey.

MILLICENT. You know I hate the sea; the railway was more than usually tedious; we missed the connection at Rossborough. But here I am. Jasper dear, I hear that you have made a most successful first appearance in public life.

DEAN. There is every hope of success. This is my friend Alderman Kirwan.

KIRWAN (*bowing*). He has exceeded our wildest expectations, Miss Fell.

DEAN. I am indeed so fortunate as to have all the people with me.

70

MILLICENT. I hear that you carry every one with you.

DEAN. I am glad that my success coincided with your arrival in Northhaven, that you were here to congratulate me.

MILLICENT. It was fortunate, was it not? But I don't know yet what has happened.

ARABELLA. Yes, we are dying to hear the story of your triumph.

MILLICENT. Do tell us, Jasper, how it all happened. What was it that led to your success?

DEAN. I thought you all knew that to-day the Corporation were to consider our claims against Southhaven.

MILLICENT. Oh, I have heard my uncle often speak about that. But he says there is nothing in your claims.

DEAN. He says that, does he?

MILLICENT. Yes – why, Jasper?

DEAN. Because to-day our Corporation had to deliberate over a letter on this subject from the Town Clerk of your uncle's Corporation.

MILLICENT. I suppose this letter explained all the bearings of the case.

CAROLINE. What did you say, Jasper, to succeed so wonderfully in uniting every one?

DEAN. I explained that we had a legal right to the payment of our claims and urged that the law should be set in motion.

KIRWAN. It seems very simple, doesn't it?

POLLOCK. Yes, indeed; and the wonder is that no one ever before could do what he has done.

DEAN (*turning to* MILLICENT). Until now every one was at variance.

MILLICENT. That has always been so in Northhaven.

KIRWAN. It could not be otherwise; the many various attractions of the larger town distract our interests from our own town.

DEAN. Yes; and, Millicent, the great public enthusiasms which once moved our people have faded in recent years, and when public enthusiasms are faded, men care for nothing but their private hatreds and their miserable private interests.

CAROLINE. But that is a foolish thing to say, Jasper. A man must look after his private interests and the interests of his family. I am sure you are with me on this point, Miss Fell.

KIRWAN. It is all these private interests that have ruined our town, and because of them nobody who did not come from outside all our cliques could unite us.

DEAN. Yes, that is true; but, Millicent, you must not suppose that this town is worse than other towns on account of its squabbles. It is as all other towns are when the fire burns low. It is a little image of the world. (CAROLINE *is about to intervene*.) Very likely I'm wrong,

71

aunt, but that can't be helped.

CAROLINE. Why can't it be helped?

DEAN. Come, Kirwan, to the study, I want to show you a rough draft of a letter for our solicitor to send to Southhaven; but I'm forgetting. (*Looks at* KIRWAN.) Here is the man.

KIRWAN. My dear Jasper, I do not wish it.

DEAN. Here is the man. He preached in the wilderness and what he preached has come to pass, though no one heard him. It is a mistake to think that words are lost if they do not fall into the ears, for even those thoughts survive and have influence that never find their way into words. A thought is a spiritual thing.

CAROLINE. My dear Jasper, what do you mean?

DEAN. Something that he has taught me to understand. Listen to him, and you will all understand. Say something, Kirwan, tell my Aunt Caroline your ideas. She is most anxious to understand.

CAROLINE. I understand very well, sir, you're going to take advantage of some vaguely worded clause in an agreement to bring an action against Southhaven, and alienate every respectable person from our town. To talk about preaching in the wilderness is merely the usual rhetoric of the county. Ideas! what you are after is a sum of money.

KIRWAN. The significance of the fact, the sum of money which is owed to us, should be understood. This sum of money is a symbol, behind it there is something more, far more, precious than the material prosperity that the money will bring; the material prosperity we want and sorely, for we want to liberate the mind and we can only do that through the body. This money will be the liberation of many ideas which poverty holds in slavery, and the ideas thus liberated will urge the race to its appointed destiny.

DEAN. Aunt Caroline, I hope you've understood that the one thing of moment is the cause itself, that the cause is above us all, and behind every action; and that we can only be happy when we are in union with the cause, for the cause is our real selves, that part of us which shall not pass away. (*Turning to* KIRWAN.) And the destiny of the race, tell them what that is.

KIRWAN. My dear Jasper, these are questions that we find interesting to ponder, but we must not intrude them upon the drawing-room. These ladies will excuse us. Come, show me the letter that you speak of! (*Exeunt* DEAN *and* KIRWAN.)

LEECH. Well, Caroline, Jasper seems to be coming out of his shell.

CAROLINE. I should say that he seems to be trying to get into Kirwan's shell.

LEECH. You kept him shut up so long in your own shell, Caroline, that

72

it is not surprising that he has got into the first empty shell he came across.

MILLICENT. But you would not call Kirwan's an empty shell, would you?

MRS LEECH. I should call it a shell that has been long looking out for a boarder.

MILLICENT. A shell, I should say (to somewhat change the metaphor), that has been long loaded but into which Nature omitted to put a fuse. Jasper is the fuse.

MRS LEECH. I'm tired of Kirwan's ideas and hope Jasper will explode them all.

MILLICENT. I was amused at the interpretation he gave to the sum of money; not only the money was nothing, but the benefit that the poor would gather from it was nothing. Beyond the gold there was a light, a supernatural light; I think he suggested the light of Paradise. But it may have been merely Tir-nan-og shining behind a sum of money.

LEECH. Very admirably put. Your quick wits see through the glamour of the Celt.

MILLICENT. I do not want to depreciate what Jasper has done, but if the issue were a noble one I should be better pleased.

POLLOCK (to LEECH). His was certainly a very flagrant bid for leadership.

LEECH. We could all have been leaders if we had not hesitated.

POLLOCK. We did well to hesitate, but I must be going. Goodbye, Michael!

LEECH. So must I. Goodbye, James. (*Exeunt amidst general leave-takings* ALDERMAN JAMES POLLOCK *and* MRS POLLOCK, ALDERMAN MICHAEL LEECH *and* MRS LEECH.)

CAROLINE (to MILLICENT). Now that they've all gone will you tell me what you think of this matter? I will come and sit down by you.

MILLICENT. Well, every one seems agreed that Kirwan has obtained an extraordinary influence over Jasper; and I don't like that.

CAROLINE. Yes, but what interests me more for the moment is the effect that this sudden resolve to carry our claim into the law courts will have upon the people of Southhaven.

MILLICENT. Mr Alderman Kirwan's visions will irritate and no doubt alienate our town if he tries to carry them into effect in a law court.

CAROLINE. But does not this strike you as being very serious?

MILLICENT. I really don't know; I suppose it is since you say so, but I have no knowledge of political matters. Perhaps you'll think it silly, but I'm disappointed that the agitation should be more Kirwan's idea than Jasper's idea.

CAROLINE. Jasper has never been the same since he met that man. If Jasper had not met you before he met Kirwan –

ARABELLA. Really, Caroline, you are going too far. I'm sure that Alderman Kirwan has never sought to influence Jasper except in political matters, and even in that direction you exaggerate his influence.

CAROLINE. Have it so, Arabella, have it so; but I think I ought to warn Miss Fell. Moreover, I think that Mr Hardman ought to be told of the political situation, and I would suggest that Miss Fell should write to him.

MILLICENT. I think that Jasper would resent any interference. Don't you think so?

ARABELLA. I certainly think so.

CAROLINE. If these movements are not checked at once there is no saying how far they will go.

ARABELLA (*to* MILLICENT). Would you not like to come to your room?

CAROLINE. Then I'll take the responsibility on myself. (*Enter* MAID.)

MAID. Alderman Foley, Miss. (*Enter* FOLEY. *Exit* MAID.)

CAROLINE. I hope, Valentine, that you have not lent your aid to this abominable agitation which will unite all parties in Southhaven against us? (*Exeunt* MILLICENT *and* ARABELLA).

FOLEY. Well, you see, Caroline, that popular enthusiasm runs so high; one's emotions overrules one's reasons, and I really do feel that –

CAROLINE. I shall telegraph the facts of the case to Mr Hardman. (*She goes to the table, writes the message.* FOLEY *waits in the middle of the stage.*) Here it is, Valentine. Take it at once to the office. (*As he goes out the Curtain falls.*)

74

ACT III

The same as last act, JASPER DEAN'S *drawing-room. Enter* DEAN *and* KIRWAN. *Voices heard cheering* DEAN *in the street.*

DEAN. My name is upon their lips, but it is you they are cheering.

KIRWAN. Very likely. The man who cheers never knows whom he is cheering. (*Enter* MACNEE.)

MACNEE. I spoke to you at the door, sir, but you did not hear me. I hope you'll excuse me for having followed you upstairs.

KIRWAN (*aside to* DEAN). You know this man, I introduced you to him just now.

DEAN. Well, I hope all is going well for the meeting, Macnee?

MACNEE. It was about that that I wanted to speak. I've sounded them, sir, and you can reckon all the clubs. It will be the biggest and the most determined meeting ever held in the town, sir.

KIRWAN. You've seen about the posters.

MACNEE. Yes, sir; any further orders?

DEAN. No; I feel I can leave everything to you.

KIRWAN. Thank you, my man. (*Exit* MACNEE.)

DEAN (*throwing himself into an armchair*). At last a quiet half-hour in which to live. I got up this morning seeing the day before me as a long battle in which my will went out to conquer numerous enemies, sometimes drawn up in battle array, and sometimes one by one in single combat.

KIRWAN. This is public life. How does it strike you?

DEAN. The first thing that strikes me is a sense of unreality; my real self is not here. Macnee, who has only just gone out, seems to me like something I have dreamed.

KIRWAN. I love their simple minds and their mysterious sub-conscious life – the only real life. To be with them is to be united to the essential again. To hear them is as refreshing as the breathing of the earth on a calm spring morning.

DEAN. But they understand nothing of our ideals – that man, for instance.

KIRWAN. The earth underfoot does not understand our words, but it understands as we may not. So it is with the people.

75

DEAN. I envy you your deep sympathies and their sudden simplifications of the world.

KIRWAN. Unfortunately I have not the magnetism that moves the people.

DEAN. I often wonder why your love and sympathy, which are much deeper than mine, should not reach them, should not appeal to them, as readily as mine.

KIRWAN. It is for that very reason; your appeal is stronger because you are not of the people; you are the romantic element outside them, the delight they follow always.

DEAN. Looking at you I often wonder how it is that the whole world does not know of you. It seems to me to be a pity that you have decided that the world shall not know you. You name is always on my tongue – I talk about you, I tell people how wonderful you are.

KIRWAN. And their answer is, What has he done?

DEAN. Sometimes.

KIRWAN. I could have done many things. I could have written, I dare say, but perhaps after all literature is a temptation. It is a pleasure.

DEAN. And yet it was from your writings I learnt that although our country can do without any one of us, not one of us can do without his country.

KIRWAN. All begins in a sense of the boding sacredness of the land under foot. I think I have made that clear.

DEAN. The sacredness of the hills I understand; but the people are alien still.

KIRWAN. If you understand one you are very near to understanding the other. The landscape is the visible image of the mind of its people, created by the imaginations of the race.

DEAN. For all is thought, all proceeds from thought, and all returns to thought, the world is but our thought.

KIRWAN. And the thought of our ancestors.

DEAN. When I talk with you, Kirwan, life seems to widen, the horizon seems lifted, it is thrown back. I was struck the other day when you told my aunt, who did not understand you in the least, that the question we are now agitating is not merely the payment of a debt of money, but a step on the way, on the long road which leads –

KIRWAN. Whither the race is trending.

DEAN. But the destiny of the race, what does that really mean?

KIRWAN. That which is you, which is me, and which is leading us. It is a quality which never ceases among us; each of us bears his spark of the magical power; now and then a spark blazes up into a flame, and the fire fades down to a spark; but the last spark always remains.

DEAN. It was from you that I heard these things for the first time, and

76

I had only to look within myself to see that they were true. I used to think that material prosperity, that long, settled life, all the things they have at Southhaven, were the only important things. But for a long time back, before I met you, I was conscious of a vague disquietude – that was how the change began in me, in a vague disquietude. I tried to convince myself that it was I who was at fault, and I struggled with my feelings, I battled with my heart, but without avail; I had to give way at last; and once I let myself go, my life, like a tree released from rocks and planted in natural soil, shot up, and as leaves my thoughts lifted themselves and saluted the sun. It is such joy to allow the truth into one's mind, to think for one's self, to be true to one's self. It was like a sudden change of light, and all that had seemed right was suddenly changed to wrong, and what I had thought despicable became right and praiseworthy.

KIRWAN. Over there if one shuts one's eyes all is pitch blackness, but here, if one shuts them, there is still light.

DEAN. And the things which I had thought beautiful grew vile, small, and the whole world trivial and black and barren as a handful of gravel.

KIRWAN. You were dissatisfied even with the earth under your feet; the air was empty of supersensuous life. We are lonely in a foreign land because we are deprived of our past life; but the past is about us here; we see it at evening glimmering among the hollows of the hills.

DEAN. We miss that sense of kinship which the sight of our native land awakens in us; the barren mountains over there, so lonely, draw me by their antique sympathy; and the rush of the river awakens echoes of old tales in my heart; truly our veins are as old as our rivers. But if I had not met you, Kirwan, I should have known nothing of these things. What should I have been if I had not met you? I dare not think. I should have lived without a dream in my heart, like Aunt Caroline. You remember the seemingly accidental way we met, yet when I met you I seemed to have always known you, and what you said seemed to be just what I was waiting to hear.

KIRWAN. Everything comes to him who waits. However narrow the circle of our lives we need not wander beyond it, to meet all we need. I did not seek you in Southhaven, I waited here at the foot of these northern mountains, and you came inevitably.

DEAN. You expected me, then?

KIRWAN. I expected some one.

DEAN. But you are not satisfied, not altogether. You sometimes think I am a wanderer, a will-of-the-wisp whose course is zigzag, and that I will light up the way but for a moment.

KIRWAN. Our lowlands are full of these merry gentlemen, and our skies are full of meteors.

DEAN. Yes indeed, yes, indeed; we all begin by thinking we are fixed stars, and then begin our erratic courses; we know not why or whither we wander, we were born to wander perhaps. Kirwan, I want to tell you about myself, I want to open my heart to you so that you who are wise may tell me what I really am.

KIRWAN. I have received many confidences, many have opened their hearts and with an unreserve that would surprise you.

DEAN. Faith is what I need; outside of faith no life exists, unbelief is an empty gulf. I have discovered that. And it is that I may get faith that I seek you so constantly, it is for this that I watch, and that I listen; and the desire of faith in me is so great that my very pores open like thirsting flowers when you speak. It is faith that ennobles, and those who have not faith are conscious of their baseness and of the baseness of life. When I am with you, Kirwan, all seems true, holy, and worthy, but when you leave me to myself, when I live among worldlings, the beliefs you have inspired within me die like the leaves and flutter away.

KIRWAN. As you become the voice of the people the personal voice which you dread will die out of your heart.

DEAN (*looking up*). Ah ... The instincts of Macnee are surer than reason, and we have to take up the great national chain to free ourselves from the little chains of personal interests. Life is a strange intricacy of chains.

KIRWAN. There are only two chains, the material and the spiritual. I have always told those who come to tell me how interested they are in spiritual things, that there is but one way to attain the spiritual, and that is by sacrifice.

DEAN. I'm thinking that if I am to become a leader of men, and give effect to your teaching, I must believe at once in the self-sufficiency and in the destiny of our race. The immediate influence behind me is you, I am your tool; other influences are behind you, and you are their tool. I am called to perform a task and to perform it I need not believe much in myself; I am nothing, but I must believe in the sacredness of the land underfoot; I must see in it the birthplace of noble thought, heroism and beauty, and divine ecstasies. These are souls, and in a far truer sense than we are souls; this land is the birthplace of our anterior selves; at once ourselves and our gods. Our gods have not perished; they have but retired to the lonely hills; and since I've known you, Kirwan, I've seen them, there, at evening; they sit there brooding over our misfortunes, waiting for us to

78

become united with them and with each other once more. You taught me to understand these things; and I think that I do not misinterpret your teaching.

KIRWAN. If the moment has arrived, you will suffice. Your speech which carried the Corporation with you and your speeches to the people do not convince me so much of your individual capacity as that the moment has come, and that you really are part and parcel of the movement of a nation. Your ideas are merely personal, it is Macnee's ideas that are universal and valid.

DEAN. Some day I shall believe as implicitly as you do in the great unity of things; I wish to feel when I look at the stars shining, or the flowers growing, that all is a great harmonious song, singing through space and through the ages; and that each race has its destiny; and that as no race has looked so long and so steadfastly through the shells of things out into the beyond, as our race, that it will be the first to attain this supreme end; we know the end is union with something beyond, though words may not further define it; we feel it throbbing always like a pulse within us. But, Kirwan, I should have met you earlier. The truths which you have spoken have not fallen on barren soil, but they have not taken root yet, and I fear every moment lest the wind should come and blow them away. (*Enter* MILLICENT.) Oh, Millicent, here you are. I wish you had come a little sooner, the conversation has been so interesting, Kirwan has been saying most interesting things.

KIRWAN. I think that on this occasion you have done most of the talking yourself, Jasper.

DEAN. I was but repeating the ideas I learnt from you. It is a joy to me to hear them spoken. When you do not speak them, I have to speak them myself lest I should forget them.

MILLICENT. Jasper is very modest. Even when he speaks quite original ideas he willingly attributes them to some one else. But on what subject were you saying such interesting things that it was a pity I was not here to hear them?

DEAN. We were talking of the spiritual destiny of the Celtic race, because of its spiritual inheritance it is greater than any other race; and we were talking too of the necessity of faith, if we would see anything but baseness in life. But one cannot enumerate. It was perhaps the emotion in us that made us think what we were saying was interesting. Set down in cold print our conversation would seem ordinary enough.

MILLICENT. I know how interested you are in such subjects, Jasper, and some of the emotions of which you speak still linger in your eyes.

79

Then I heard Mr Kirwan speak of these things the other day.

DEAN. He only said a few words.

MILLICENT. But you had told me about your friend, and in a measure I know his ideas, and I spent this morning reading the Cuchullin epic. The description of Cuchullin at the ford is most moving. Even the horse, the grey of Macha, refuses to be harnessed for the last battle, and when he reproaches it, it comes weeping tears of blood.

KIRWAN. You have read the tale aright. It is an emotion that comes straight out of the heart which is the essential quality of our literature. There are a thousand tales told by greater tellers, but there are no tenderer tales in the world than ours. The Cuchullin epic is full of tenderness so deep that the deadliest conflicts are softened by it. Cuchullin laments over the fallen Fardia with as passionate a grief as Dierdre over Naisi; this tenderness enters into every tale; it is the thread on which all are strung. But I should hardly have thought that Southhaven would appreciate this quality.

MILLICENT. Southhaven is not all of a piece, there is tenderness there as here. Do you not think that with time and with modern means of communication race characteristics must soften down? After all there is but one race – humanity.

KIRWAN. Humanity is over and above, but I believe that each race has its destiny, and that a destiny may be spiritual or material.

MILLICENT. But with inter-marriage these wide differences disappear.

KIRWAN. Only in so far as that the spiritual dissolves the materialistic race. The Franks settled in France in hundreds of thousands, but the stronger genius of the Celt easily melted the inferior, and France is as Celtic to-day as she was before the Saxon invasion, and it is the same here. (*Pause.*)

MILLICENT. I wonder if I shall become absorbed? Jasper, do you think you are equal to the task? (*To* KIRWAN, *who has got up to go.*) Why are you going?

KIRWAN. I feel I'm in a harsh humour, I always go when I feel it coming upon me.

DEAN. But where are you going? When shall I see you again? There are many things I must see you about.

KIRWAN. You'll find me at my lodgings. I must go, I have some pressing work to finish by this evening.

DEAN. Why not write in my study? you will find everything you require and no one will disturb you.

KIRWAN. It will save time, thank you.

MILLICENT. He seems indispensable in your life. I don't think I should like to give my room, where all my papers are, to any one to make himself at home in.

DEAN. I have to talk to him about some business presently. He lives such a long way off and he will be more comfortable there. And then I like to have him in the house; while he is here the atmosphere seems purer, brighter.

MILLICENT. And while you are talking to me, you will be thinking of how soon you will be able to get back to him.

DEAN. Millicent! You are not jealous of Kirwan? You will get to like him as much as I do and his presence you'll find as indispensable as I do. He was a little harsh, I admit that. You see the worst of Kirwan in the first meetings! When I met him the first time he was harsh to me, it was only by degrees that he allowed me to see the beauty of his nature.

MILLICENT. A sort of ugly dog which you end by getting fond of – when he has left off biting you.

DEAN. Yes, there is something of that in Kirwan. But can't you see the sweetness of his nature showing through?

MILLICENT. I think I can see that, given certain conditions, he would attract many. I can see that he was just the man who would attract you at the present moment. You're so different.

DEAN. Really, I've often thought that we're alike. I seemed to discover all that I had been unconsciously seeking in him.

MILLICENT. You're a man of many ideas and you will try them all; he is clearly a man of one idea.

DEAN. You must see him again – you don't wish to?

MILLICENT. Yes, I do. But I don't think he likes me – and I'm sure he's opposed to our marriage.

DEAN. My dear Millicent, Kirwan is a great friend and anxious about my public life; but he would never dream of interfering with my private life.

MILLICENT. Can we separate the two?

DEAN. I don't know. But did you not hear what he said about the inter-marriage of different races, that the weaker race disappears after a few generations?

MILLICENT. My dear Jasper, you're talking ridiculously.

DEAN. It is a fact that those who settle in this country become characteristically Celtic. For it is not a question of race, it is the land itself that makes the Celt; and you will soon begin to feel the fascination of this dim, remote land steal over you. When these tiresome politics are over it will be my delight to teach you our heroic past. We will see together the golden work of the fourth century, and we will stray together round many a ruined porch covered with beautiful scroll-work. And we will sail into the west, and I will show you where Conhullen wooed Schya the queen of warrior women.

MILLICENT. Yes, we'll do all these things, but now you must listen to something more prosaic. I came to tell you that I'm expecting my uncle Hardman this afternoon.

DEAN. Coming to-day?

MILLICENT. You don't seem pleased?

DEAN. You see our business with Southhaven, our claims against Southhaven, make it difficult for me to meet him. Oh, I daresay it will make no difference. What has brought him over?

MILLICENT. Your aunt said –

DEAN. Aunt Caroline still interfering in my life – in my ideas?

MILLICENT. I half agreed, Jasper, that she should send the telegram; in any case I take the entire responsibility. I'm sure it would be well for you to hear what my uncle Hardman has to say before you commit yourself any further in this agitation.

DEAN. When you talk like that, Millicent, you remind me too closely of my aunt Caroline. It makes me think that in marrying you I shall fall into what I am trying to escape from. She never could think of me in any other light than as so much clay which she could gradually mould into her idea of what a man should be; when I came home from Oxford she expected me to be that, nothing more and nothing less.

MILLICENT. And it was this influence so diligently exercised that rendered you susceptible to Kirwan's influence?

DEAN. No doubt it counted largely. It was the inevitable reaction from an education which taught me to consider nothing but class and family interests. At home and at school I was in revolt, and life was so unsympathetic that I thought I was unfitted for life; but since I met Kirwan, since I entered public life –

MILLICENT. You're quite happy. Perhaps, Jasper, you're more fitted for public life than for married life?

DEAN. How so?

MILLICENT. Married life is private life.

DEAN. Yes; but they do not conflict. I should be sorry to think that.

MILLICENT. Tell me, Jasper, what is your idea of life?

DEAN. I see you as the centre of my life, that to which all things lead up and that from which all things shall proceed. I never thought of marrying any particular woman until I met you. But life as I conceived it was always married life, life within the family circle. Why do you ask? Because you thought that I had led a life such as

82

most young men are supposed to lead?

MILLICENT. No, that wasn't the reason. I did not think that.

DEAN. Well, then, why did you ask?

MILLICENT. I don't think that family life is Kirwan's idea of life.

DEAN. You surely don't think that Kirwan — What an idea! A purer man never was born.

MILLICENT. Very likely. But I don't think that life within the family circle is his ideal.

DEAN. True, he never married. I daresay you are right, though I should be puzzled to say why.

MILLICENT. You have spoken on so many subjects, I wonder if you ever spoke on this subject?

DEAN. No, I don't think it ever was mentioned. But I feel you are right all the same.

MILLICENT. Kirwan is no doubt a very clever man, but he is a mono-maniac, he hates women; he has no conception of private life; he has spent his life in hotels and public meetings. But are you prepared to do the same? If you are, you had better not marry.

DEAN. This jealousy of Kirwan is — is unexpected, and quite un-reasonable.

MILLICENT. No, it is not unreasonable; and nothing in this world concerns me more intimately, and I should be a weak fool indeed if I were to let it pass. You are a man of original mind and talent, Jasper, but you let yourself be absorbed by this man; and the strange thing is that it is your pleasure to allow him to absorb you.

DEAN. I should have been nothing without Kirwan.

MILLICENT. Every scholar thinks the same of his schoolmaster.

DEAN. Maybe you're right. I hadn't thought of that. I suppose so. Admiration of the schoolmaster is inherent in us all.

MILLICENT. But in a few years we wear through his ideas, and then he seems paltry enough.

DEAN. And then we get another schoolmaster unless we close our education, and I suppose it is every one's ambition not to do that. But, Millicent, how does my interest in Kirwan's ideas affect you?

MILLICENT. You deliberately put on his soul, and though you will put it off sooner or later, something of it will sink in, will become part of you.

DEAN. And then?

MILLICENT. Then you will see me with Kirwan's eyes, and that I do not wish — I do not intend. I recognise Kirwan as my enemy. His challenge was clear and direct.

DEAN. His challenge!

MILLICENT. Yes; his challenge was very explicit, and he has taught you hatred of my town, of the south, and he has induced you to embark in a lifelong adventure against both.

DEAN. But political questions –

MILLICENT. Do not concern women. That no doubt is Kirwan's theory. There is nothing on God's earth that does not concern women. Our concern may be different from yours, but it is equal. Kirwan is limiting your life to this place. Dear, I want a wider sphere for your talent.

DEAN. But to succeed in Southhaven would mean nothing to me. We are nothing outside of our own race and the traditions and the destiny of the race.

MILLICENT. Those are Kirwan's ideas.

DEAN. It does not matter whose ideas they are. Are they true?

MILLICENT. They are true to him. Are you sure that they are true to you? And if this agitation be pursued we shall have to live here always. I daresay that social life means little to you, or you may have grown tired of it, and when you are tired of public affairs you would like a family circle wherein to renew your energies. But what should I be here? You see, you ask me to give up my pursuits, my friends, everything, my life. And what shall I get in exchange?

DEAN. It is impossible for me to answer that question.

MILLICENT. I did not put the question to embarrass you. The answer is your love. But your love, much as I covet it, is not sufficient. I want your life, Jasper. I want to share it. I cannot consent to be either a sensuality, a housekeeper, or both. Do you understand?

DEAN. Yes, I understand.

MILLICENT. What I say is reasonable, I know I'm right. My heart tells me that I am, and my heart now is the heart of every woman in the world. I will make sacrifice for you, Jasper. 'Thy people shall be my people,' but I will not yield any part of my right to share your life. I will be no fly on the wheel: you must choose between me and Kirwan. I will share you no more with him than with another woman. It would be worse, for he absorbs the best part of you.

DEAN. Do you mean that I'm to give up my friend?

MILLICENT. No, I'm not so unreasonable as that. I only want your friend to take his proper place in your life, that is all.

DEAN. I hardly know you to-day, Millicent.

MILLICENT. How am I different?

DEAN. It is like coming across a hard and unyielding streak in a beautiful piece of satinwood. (*She goes up the stage.*)

DEAN. Are you going? (*She goes to him and puts her hands on his*

84

shoulders.)

MILLICENT. Jasper, we shall always be united.

DEAN. Yes, we shall always be united. I know it. (MISS CAROLINE DEAN *enters.*)

CAROLINE. I'm interrupting an agreeable conversation.

DEAN. Well, perhaps you are, Aunt Caroline.

CAROLINE. Then I'll go away again.

DEAN. No, stay. I've some business with Kirwan. He is writing in my study. I'll go to him. (*Exit* O.P.)

CAROLINE. I came to tell you that your uncle may now arrive at any moment. Did you tell Jasper that I had telegraphed to Mr Hardman?

MILLICENT. Yes.

CAROLINE. Was he very angry?

MILLICENT. No – well, rather, but I told him that I acquiesced.

CAROLINE. Ah, then he forgot. Your hands were on his shoulders, but I could see you were divided. Not about the sending of the telegram, I hope.

MILLICENT. No, not about that. Jasper is greatly changed. I seem divorced from his ideas and his interests, and I had hoped to share them all. Now I cannot enter into his life at all.

CAROLINE. Did you tell him that?

MILLICENT. Yes; I told him that if I was not to share his life that I did not care to marry him.

CAROLINE. And did you tell him he would alienate himself from all respectable people?

MILLICENT. Yes; I said that we should have to live here always.

CAROLINE. Did you say that he would lose all your friends? Did you mention that?

MILLICENT. I mentioned everything, but my first interest in him is himself.

CAROLINE. You don't think that he loves you less?

MILLICENT. I'm sure that he thinks of me differently; now I am merely a joy in his life which he would not willingly be without, but I am no longer his chief interest in life, and I know why.

CAROLINE. You mean Kirwan?

MILLICENT. Yes, and I told him so.

CAROLINE. How did you put it?

MILLICENT. I told him that if he were going to give up his life to Kirwan that he had better not marry. What is so strange is that he delights in allowing Kirwan to absorb him; if he is not speaking Kirwan's ideas he does not care to speak at all. Unless I can win him from Kirwan I shall be no more than a servant in his life, and he, unless

85

he shakes off Kirwan, will be no more than a shadow of Kirwan. I would help Jasper, I would direct his energy.

CAROLINE. You would take Kirwan's place?

MILLICENT. I would prevent Kirwan from taking mine. Jasper is a leader of men and –

CAROLINE. There I think you're mistaken. The natural centre of Jasper's life is marriage, and if Kirwan succeeds in turning him from marriage he is ruined.

MILLICENT. I think he is a leader of men, but I want him to bear forth his own ideas and not Kirwan's.

CAROLINE. You will never induce him to give up Kirwan.

MILLICENT. Then I will give him up.

CAROLINE. Better induce him to give up this agitation.

MILLICENT. I care little about the agitation. I am thinking of my share in his life, that is the problem before me.

CAROLINE. But in winning him away from this agitation you will win him from Kirwan. Kirwan's interest in Jasper is merely a political one, only his country interests him. He has no friend.

MILLICENT. But I have no reason to urge why he should abandon his present politics – no sufficient reason. I am helpless. (*A bell is heard.*)

CAROLINE. Very likely that is Mr Hardman (*runs to window*). Yes, the boat is in; I see them wheeling the mails into the post-office. (*Enter* MAID.)

MAID. Mr George Hardman. (*Enter* HARDMAN. *Exit* MAID.)

MILLICENT. Oh, how do you do, uncle? This is Miss Caroline Dean.

HARDMAN. I received your telegram last night, Miss Dean. Millicent knows all about it, of course.

MILLICENT. Miss Dean consulted me before sending it. I could see that she was very anxious.

HARDMAN. Well, I came at once.

CAROLINE. I hope you don't think that we exaggerated the importance of this agitation?

HARDMAN. It doesn't matter if you did. To-day was comparatively a free day and I was glad of an excuse to get away; the trip will do me good.

CAROLINE. I felt that no one would bring such knowledge of the world to bear on this matter as you.

HARDMAN. It is serious. But there's nothing so difficult in this world that it can't be arranged by practical men, as my worthy friend Alderman Lawrence would say.

CAROLINE. It was a great sorrow to me to find Jasper allying himself to all the needy adventurers of our town.

MILLICENT. They are not all needy adventurers. Several of your own family and Alderman Foley –

CAROLINE. Alderman Foley will regret the support he is giving to this agitation.

HARDMAN. I see that at least on one important particular you are not agreed. I must see Jasper, I must see the others and find out exactly how the matter stands (*Pause*.) (*Enter* MAID.)

MAID. A gentleman who wishes to see Mr Dean, miss. (*Enter* MACNEE.)

CAROLINE. Good Heavens!

MILLICENT. Mr Dean is in the study. (*The maid crosses the stage with* MACNEE, *and opens study door. Exit* MACNEE. MAID *crosses the stage, and exit.*)

CAROLINE. These people are constantly about the house now. (*Pause*). I'm sure you would like lunch, Mr Hardman?

HARDMAN. I started early in the morning, and a sea breeze awakes the appetite.

CAROLINE. Then I'll go and see if I cannot get them to bring up lunch at once. (*Exit.*)

HARDMAN. Now tell me, Millicent, what it is all about, why did Miss Dean telegraph to me? Did she do so at your suggestion?

MILLICENT. Yes, I could see that she was alarmed at the part Jasper is taking in politics. That is one reason.

HARDMAN. And then?

MILLICENT. There is another reason, though I was then only vaguely conscious of it; since I have discovered it.

HARDMAN. Surely not that Jasper is changed towards you?

MILLICENT. Now Jasper looks at life from a different side, so he has changed towards me.

HARDMAN. He has not said that he is.

MILLICENT. No, nor do I suppose that he knows that he is.

HARDMAN. This does not sound very serious.

MILLICENT. But it is; a woman knows everything that concerns her. Jasper is quite different. He seems to have receded from actual life, he seems to live only in abstractions.

HARDMAN. Very solid kind of abstractions – an action at law to extort a large sum of money.

MILLICENT. He has fallen under the influence of Kirwan, and he sees and hears at present with Kirwan's eyes and ears. So I really have ceased to care to marry Jasper. I was telling Miss Dean so when you came in.

HARDMAN. Who is this man Kirwan?

MILLICENT. Jasper is but his mouthpiece, I can tell you no more. I'm very unhappy.

HARDMAN. My dear Millicent...Where is this man!

MILLICENT (*recovering herself quickly*). He is in there, in the study with Jasper. Let us talk of something else. I told Jasper that I had heard you say there is nothing in this claim. Is that so?

HARDMAN. Well, it is just one of those vexations – but, putting aside the public question for a moment, it occurs to me that a large part of your money is invested in house property in Southhaven, and the extra rate that would have to be levied to meet this claim would reduce your income considerably. You have money too invested in our line of steamers.

MILLICENT. I wonder if it ever occurred to Jasper that one of the results of this agitation would be to reduce my income?

HARDMAN (*walking up the stage*). No man in his senses would put himself at the head of an agitation, the first result of which would be to reduce his wife's income. (*Returning to* MILLICENT.) You will speak to him on this subject, you will tell him what I say?

MILLICENT. Of course.

HARDMAN. I knew we should find a way out of the difficulty.

MILLICENT. Now I feel happier; before all was dark and vague. At last I begin to see my way. Thank you, uncle. How clever you are! (*Enter* MAID.)

MAID. Lunch is ready, sir. (*Immediately after enter* MISS CAROLINE DEAN. *Exit* MAID.)

CAROLINE. I hope that you and Millicent together will be able to persuade Jasper.

HARDMAN. Not a doubt of it, not a doubt of it, Miss Dean. The whole thing might be described as a wild-goose chase, and I am hungry enough to eat the wild goose if you have nothing else.

CAROLINE. But what has happened? You looked so serious when you arrived.

HARDMAN. I'll tell you at lunch. Where is Jasper?

MILLICENT. He is in the study and does not wish to be disturbed. (*Exeunt* HARDMAN *and* MILLICENT *and* CAROLINE. *The* MAID *crosses the stage and knocks at the study door.*)

MAID. Lunch is ready, sir. (*The* MAID *returns, exit* P.) (*Enter* DEAN, KIRWAN *and* MACNEE. *Exit* MACNEE C.)

KIRWAN. Whether she be clever or charming is a matter of the hour and the day. What should give us pause is that in accepting her one is accepting life, and life is what we should fly from.

DEAN. Fly from life, how can we?

KIRWAN. Life, always hungry, follows eager to devour us, and only three men, a Hindu, a Greek, and a Jew escaped; the others, the great ones, the greatest ones, lost some part of themselves in the jaws of life. Woman is life in its most typical form, and family life a wolfish pack.

DEAN. How strangely you think, Kirwan! You look to the very end; nothing stays or turns aside your thought.

KIRWAN. We must choose between thought and the conventions. Come, let us go downstairs; they'll be able to tell us if a married man would be justified in setting aside private interests for public duty. (*Exeunt.*)

CURTAIN

ACT IV

A sitting-room in the principal hotel of the town. GEORGE HARDMAN *anxious and restless.* THE WAITER *enters.*

WAITER. Alderman Daniel Lawrence wants to see you, sir.

HARDMAN. He has come at last. (*To the* WAITER.) Show him up. (*Exit the* WAITER. DANIEL LAWRENCE *enters.*)

LAWRENCE. My dear Mayor, I'm so glad to see you. How well you are looking! I never saw you looking better in my life.

HARDMAN. Thank you, Alderman Lawrence, thank you. I am very glad to see you. I hope you are well!

LAWRENCE. As well as can be expected in these anxious times, Mayor.

HARDMAN. Beautiful weather, isn't it? (*Pause.*) You will excuse me sending for you in this hurried way. I wish especially to consult you about the unjustifiable agitation that is going on in this town. You are an able man, Alderman Lawrence – a man of the world and of affairs. You know this town well. Tell me, how do you think this agitation will end?

LAWRENCE. I think it will succeed.

HARDMAN. You do?

LAWRENCE. That is my opinion.

HARDMAN. You are a staunch friend of ours. What is your advice?

LAWRENCE. I advise payment before the law is set in motion; otherwise you will have to pay enormous costs in addition to the original payment.

HARDMAN. Oh, this is impossible!

LAWRENCE. Why?

HARDMAN. No member of our Corporation could propose such a thing without being politically discredited for life.

LAWRENCE. Well, I don't see what else you can do.

HARDMAN. You know this town well, Alderman Lawrence, cannot you think of some device?

LAWRENCE. You set me a most difficult task.

HARDMAN. Just consider. I always maintain that Southhaven has not appreciated your merits as it should have.

LAWRENCE. Now that you have touched upon it, I will say it to you, as

90

a friend, that Southhaven has done nothing to encourage me, considering the extremely unpopular part I play here from time to time in her interest.

HARDMAN. You know the post of solicitor to our Corporation is just vacant. The emoluments are very handsome.

LAWRENCE. I know, my dear Mayor, I know.

HARDMAN. The appointment will surely be given to the lawyer who does the best service to our town.

LAWRENCE. Quite so. I have often thought what a pleasant thing it would be to have that appointment.

HARDMAN. Besides, remember there is a very handsome retiring pension.

LAWRENCE. Yes; I have always considered a pension as the fine flower of an appointment.

HARDMAN. And still with such a prize before you, can you not find a means of winning it?

LAWRENCE. My dear Mayor, how you torture me!

HARDMAN. Come, come, Alderman Lawrence, there must be some way out of this difficulty.

LAWRENCE. Well, really I am put to the pin of my collar. Have you yet seen the Corporation?

HARDMAN. Only a few of them, and then not in a business way.

LAWRENCE. Perhaps it might come to something if you were to meet them in a body?

HARDMAN. Or perhaps one by one – just casually, you know. Who are the most likely to be influenced?

LAWRENCE. You see, popular excitement has risen to such a pitch that not one of them would dare, even if he were inclined, to take your advice. Moreover, the secession of an alderman would make little difference, but if Jasper could be induced to abandon the movement there would be such a scramble among the rest for leadership that everything else would be forgotten.

HARDMAN. Nothing can be done with Jasper. I've never seen any one so determined. Millicent's money is invested in Southhaven house property and in our steamers. I put it to Jasper. I said, 'It is quite impossible for you to continue at the head of an agitation which will reduce the value of her property'.

LAWRENCE. I quite understand; and Jasper, what did he say?

HARDMAN. He spoke of private interests clashing with public interests, and that if each individual case were to be considered the State could not exist, and so on.

LAWRENCE. Ah I think he must be a little mad, I've often thought so.

Such a thing was never heard of before. A crusade to reduce the value of your wife's property! Good Heavens! And then I've always heard that he was deeply attached to Miss Fell.

HARDMAN. I believe he is, but for the moment he is so carried away by popular enthusiasm, he is like a cork on a wave. He was of course very much shocked when I told him, and he said that it made his position very difficult.

LAWRENCE. But he remained firm. Ahem!

HARDMAN. Is there no one who is shaky in his convictions regarding this unfortunate business?

LAWRENCE. There is a certain erratic creature called Foley, who is not of much account, however, except for his newspaper.

HARDMAN. Yes, now I remember, my niece told me that he seems doubtful of the justice of Dean's action, and that she thought she might have influenced him.

LAWRENCE. I have no doubt of it. He is one of those people who have a difficulty in not going over to the side of any sympathetic person they meet. Ferguson says of him that 'everybody he talks to leaves the mark of his five fingers on his face'. If only Miss Fell could see her way – to – well, a little flirtation – ever so little – just a little sympathy in her voice, you know – it might do wonders.

HARDMAN. My dear Alderman, you don't know what you are talking about. My niece flirt with Foley! Quite impossible!

LAWRENCE. Quite so, quite so, I am trying to think of a way out of this difficulty. Perhaps after all it is not necessary. The tender spot in Foley's heart is Miss Caroline Dean's fortune. I think if Dean shows even the least sign of wavering, and above all, if he can suggest some literary or economic idea which will not be injurious to Southhaven, and may help to preserve Foley's good name with the mob, I think he will come over to our side – to Miss Caroline Dean's side. Her politics are fortunately very decided.

HARDMAN. Is he, then, incarnate insincerity?

LAWRENCE. On the contrary, he finds it so easy to be sincere about any idea, that he sees no reason why he should not prefer the ideas which suit his interests best. Why, he is sincerity itself; sincerity is a prevalent vice in this town, and Foley is a striking example. Our public life would be much more continuous if there were more people with sufficient strength of will to say one thing and believe another. (*They walk to and fro.*) Here is an idea! If you were to meet the Corporation in a body you might reason with them, and in the course of the argument the weak spots would begin to appear; you might put your views to them quietly and with tact.

92

HARDMAN. They are as obdurate –

LAWRENCE. I have never seen them so obdurate.

HARDMAN. But this matter, like every other matter, is a question of compromise.

LAWRENCE. If you have anything to propose.

HARDMAN. What would they take?

LAWRENCE. If I could only think of something that you might offer!

HARDMAN. I wish you could. (*They walk up and down thinking.*)_

LAWRENCE. What do you think, my dear Mayor, if you were to – well to buy a house here, and grounds, and to say that you would stay part of the year with them, and spend money in entertaining?

HARDMAN. I'd willingly do that (*looking round*), for I like the place; but I don't think they'd accept my company as an equivalent for the supposed debt.

LAWRENCE. No, perhaps not! (*Sits, and falls into an attitude of thought.*) Anything to be done in the tourist line? Excursion steamers! No, you think not. Very likely not. The opening up of the country! (*Changes his position. Pause.*) Let me see, what are the questions that have been agitated lately? There has been, among other things, a good deal of talk about a tramway line running from the centre of the poorer parts of the town. What do you think of that?

HARDMAN. I should be very glad to supply the capital. Ah! if they would accept a tramway, if that could be arranged! That's a very happy thought of yours, my dear Alderman! And I can send them some cart-loads of seed potatoes – an early kind, you know – for those impoverished nursery gardens to the west of your town.

LAWRENCE. That will do nicely, my dear Mayor. Potatoes do not stir up any dangerous fermentation of ideas. The tramway is very much needed, and you could weigh the certain advantages of the tramway with the risk of long legal proceedings. After all, nothing is certain in law. Now let me see, the Corporation is sitting at present. Supposing I were to go now, and ask all the members to meet you here when their business is finished?

HARDMAN. Or do you think it would be better if I were to go and meet them? What do you think?

LAWRENCE. Oh no, that would be too public and formal. The meeting ought to be friendly, convivial – you understand. You know all our Corporation, don't you, my dear Mayor?

HARDMAN. Yes, I think I have met them all.

LAWRENCE. And have no doubt come to an opinion as to their abilities. There is Ferguson, a lawyer: he considers himself a veritable Blackstone on legal procedure. He and Foley have always been at each other's throats, and the marvel is how Jasper ever induced them to unite in a common policy.

HARDMAN. I quite understand.

LAWRENCE. Kirwan you know about. He is at the bottom of the whole mischief. It was he who set Jasper's imagination aflame. He is a compound of literature, patriotism, and belief in what he calls the spiritual inheritance of the race.

HARDMAN. Nothing to be done with him?

LAWRENCE. Nothing. Pollock and Leech support Jasper because the second cousin of one married the third cousin of Jasper's mother, and they take the opinion of the family, and like to support what they call their class.

HARDMAN. The weakest point is the natural antagonism of Foley and Ferguson. I see, I see. (*The* WAITER *enters.*)

WAITER. The Misses Dean. (*Exit* WAITER.) (*Enter* MISS CAROLINE *and* MISS ARABELLA DEAN.)

CAROLINE. Mr Hardman, how is your dear niece? How do you do, Alderman Lawrence? (HARDMAN *goes to the* WAITER *and speaks to him in dumb show.*)

LAWRENCE. How do you do, Miss Dean? How well you're looking! I never saw you looking better in my life.

CAROLINE. Don't say that, Alderman Lawrence, I feel ten years older. I am sure I'm looking wretched, and not without sufficient reason. This has been a terrible blow to me, as you may easily imagine. After all my teaching – no one ever was brought up more carefully than Jasper – to see Jasper turn against his family and his class. Oh, it is very sad! Within the last few days my whole life seems to have crumbled before my eyes.

LAWRENCE. Kirwan –

CAROLINE. It was all his doing. He is the origin of it all. Don't mention the man's name. I abhor the man himself – his literature, his politics, and his religion, if you can call such beliefs as his a religion.

ARABELLA. Our life since Millicent left us has been most wretched.

CAROLINE. Jasper does not speak to me when we meet; we sit down to meals in silence. I must say, though, that Arabella has supported me; she had the strength to tell Jasper that although she would always love him, she could not entirely approve of an agitation which would reduce the value of Miss Fell's property.

ARABELLA. It is this that Jasper feels most sorely; if it had not been for this he would not have cared –

CAROLINE. If he never spoke to another respectable person. And that odious man coming about the house! Alderman Lawrence, can you not help us?

LAWRENCE. That is exactly what I'm trying to do, Miss Dean. I'm going to bring the Corporation here for a conference with Mr Hardman.

CAROLINE. If they would only listen to reason! But I've lost hope.

LAWRENCE. I've great hopes of success. (*Exit*).

CAROLINE. How is Millicent? Shan't we see her?

HARDMAN. Won't you sit down, Miss Dean?

CAROLINE. I'm so excited and worried that I'm better standing up. But Arabella might like to sit down. Well – I'll sit down. I should like to see Millicent.

HARDMAN. She is in her room. I don't think she is feeling very well. Perhaps you will excuse her.

CAROLINE. She knows it was not our fault.

HARDMAN. She knows that.

CAROLINE. The mistake was her leaving us. If she had only remained I am sure she would have succeeded in winning Jasper over. You see, we know Jasper better than you can know him. You and she take Jasper to be a determined strong-minded man; he is not in the least that.

HARDMAN. I've noticed no signs of weakness in Jasper; there is more grit in him than I thought. He is against me, I do not approve; he is as wrong-headed as you like, but he is not weak.

ARABELLA. He is deeply attached to Millicent; there can be no question about that.

CAROLINE. Yet he is more than ever determined in his politics. For her to leave us was a mistake; I'm convinced of it. She ought not to have broken off her engagement.

HARDMAN. But what else could she do? She was asked not only to give up all her friends, her social position in Southhaven, but also to consent to lose a considerable portion of her property. Really, Miss Dean, I don't think that I need insist further.

CAROLINE. I know all that; but if she had remained with us she might have persuaded him.

HARDMAN. He did not flinch, he told her to her face.

CAROLINE. I know, I know. But if Millicent would consent to marry Jasper she would soon get her way with him. Once he was removed from the influence of this maleficent Kirwan –

HARDMAN. The risk is really too great; I could not advise such a course.

ARABELLA. I've always thought that I understood Jasper, but in the last few days he speaks with a strange voice that I do not recognise at all.

HARDMAN. Quite so; I confess I was taken by surprise.

CAROLINE. Jasper is a rich man. Unless the loss to her property be very considerable he could compensate her.

HARDMAN. Only by diminishing his own income.

ARABELLA. Caroline and I would make sacrifices.

CAROLINE. My dear Arabella, our incomes would not suffice, and Jasper would not allow us. (WAITER *enters*.)

WAITER. Alderman Jasper Dean. (*Enter* DEAN.)

DEAN. Oh, I do not find you alone. You have invited the Corporation to meet you, and I thought that I would come over before our business was finished. I did not expect to meet my aunts here.

CAROLINE. We will go.

ARABELLA. Jasper, have you come to see Millicent?

DEAN. Yes, I hope to see her.

HARDMAN. Millicent is in her room; she is not very well to-day and does not propose to receive visitors.

DEAN. I hoped, Mr Hardman – I came here in hopes –

ARABELLA. We too came here in hopes. How can you expect a girl to marry you when you are doing everything you can to deprive her of her property?

DEAN. That you, Aunt Arabella, who have always been kind, should turn against me at last! (*He repulses her.*) Mr Hardman, you are a stranger, and will understand better than my relations. I feel keenly the difficulty of my position; it is most painful; it is almost unbearable.

HARDMAN. My dear Jasper, I easily guess that you must suffer, for I know that you're fond of Millicent; I may say even that I appreciate the pluck you are showing in very trying circumstances.

DEAN. Thank you for that. That is the first word of sympathy (looking at his aunts) I have had.

HARDMAN. The worst of it is that you are sacrificing your life for no object.

DEAN. No object! Ah, if you knew! But you look at life from a different side.

HARDMAN. You enter your house like a rioter, and having thrown your furniture out of the window you stand there surprised to find that you have not changed the face of the world. We change nothing. The enthusiasms which have lit your imagination will pass away; soon you will be sitting over the embers. I have invited your Corporation to meet me. I intend to try to arrive at some sort of compromise; if you oppose me you will go to the wall; for I'm appealing to the grosser instincts which are always with us, which are the world we live in. (*Enter* WAITER.)

96

WAITER. The members of the Corporation are below, sir.

HARDMAN. Very well; show them up. (*Exit* WAITER.) Well, Jasper? You're undecided.

DEAN. No, I'm not undecided. There's always a right and a wrong way, and the wrong way always seems the more reasonable. (*Enter* ALDERMAN DANIEL LAWRENCE, ALDERMAN JAMES POLLOCK, ALDERMAN MICHAEL LEECH, MAYOR JOSEPH TENCH, ALDERMAN RALF KIRWAN, FERGUSON, VALENTINE FOLEY, *and various Town Councillors, the Town Clerk,* JOHN CLORAN. *The* WAITER *brings in tray with glasses, &c.*)

LAWRENCE. My dear Mr Hardman, I suppose it is superfluous for me to introduce our respected Mayor and Corporation?

HARDMAN. Indeed, we are no strangers, gentlemen, you are welcome. How is Alderman Ferguson, my courteous friend? – ah, a noted authority on municipal procedure too. And here is the new journalism – Alderman Foley, how do you do, sir? Ah, Alderman Kirwan, the beginning of modern Celtic literature. (*He shakes hands with other members.*) How do you do, Alderman Leech? Gentlemen, won't you have some refreshments? (*They help themselves largely to liquor.*) (FOLEY *comes down stage to speak to* MISS CAROLINE DEAN.)

CAROLINE. I am sorry, Mr Foley, that you have taken a pronounced part in this agitation.

FOLEY. My dear Miss Dean, I do not pretend that it is an eternal truth. But there is some truth in everything, though the truth of to-day is not always that of yesterday.

CAROLINE. Truth is not a thing of to-day or to-morrow.

FOLEY. There are the eternal verities, to be sure; but they are not the business of the newspapers. Our ideas are borne in upon us like the leaves on the wind; we express them; we have to think of the need of the moment. Popular feeling is to-day for this movement, to-morrow it may be against it.

ARABELLA. But we should not change our practice of life.

FOLEY. Our practice of life is, alas! often mean enough, but the intolerable is not to have large and noble views of what life should be and to expound those views in language as – as –

ARABELLA. As eloquent as space will allow.

CAROLINE. At all events I hope you will give a fair hearing to the proposals Mr Hardman intends to make, and you will come to see me soon I hope.

FOLEY. I shall have much pleasure. (*They shake hands.*)

CAROLINE (*going up the stage and meeting* MR HARDMAN.) Goodbye,

Mr Hardman; I came here in the hopes of inducing my nephew to abandon an agitation which every one must see is entirely unsafe. I regret, Mr Hardman, that my influence has proved of no avail. Arabella, are you coming? (*Exeunt* MISS CAROLINE *and* MISS ARABELLA DEAN.)

HARDMAN (*coming down the stage*). If you have made up your minds to decline every proposal whatever it may be, I will not weary you with any one. Let us talk of other things. I hear that the year promises to be an excellent one.

KIRWAN. You press alms upon us, whereas we desire only that you should pay your debts.

FOLEY. I am here as a representative of the Press, gentlemen, and it would be impossible for me to decline to hear Mr Hardman's proposal. I hope that Mr Alderman Ferguson will see the unreason of saying he does not agree to proposals which he has not yet heard.

FERGUSON. Alderman Foley is very quick to jump down my throat, I only meant that nothing short of our strict rights would satisfy me.

HARDMAN. I suppose you mean that very little short of your strict rights will satisfy you, for compromise enters into all human affairs.

FERGUSON. Nothing but our strict rights.

HARDMAN. Even the law courts cannot give you what you believe to be your strict rights. The costs will be enormous, even if you win; and the law is proverbially uncertain.

FERGUSON. Upon a point of law, sir, I can assure you that you have no case; and upon a point of law these gentlemen will be guided by me.

HARDMAN. I wished to discuss this matter quietly among ourselves. I assure you that there are arguments.

FERGUSON. Everything that can be said has been said; is not that so, Dean?

DEAN. I think so. But if Mr Hardman has any offer to make, I shall be glad to hear it.

HARDMAN. I should like to hear Alderman Foley's opinion upon a little matter which Alderman Lawrence and myself were discussing this morning. The town is in eminent need of a new tramway leading to the quarter of the poorest people. and it would be a great benefit to them. Now, it seems to me that –

KIRWAN. What you say, Mr Hardman, is quite true; the tramway is wanted, and it would likewise prove an excellent investment for Southhaven capital.

HARDMAN. If it is in that spirit my proposals are met, it would be useless for me to proceed further. (*Looking in the direction of* FOLEY.) Alderman Foley, without desiring you to commit yourself to an opinion, I hope I can rely on you for a fair statement of my proposal. The people should know my offer.

FOLEY. I should be wanting in my duty to the public if I were to allow my private feelings to prevent me from publishing every matter of news.

KIRWAN. But, Alderman Foley, I thought we had all agreed on the one line of action.

FOLEY. I shall place the matter impartially before my readers. The interests of the Press must be safeguarded.

HARDMAN. I am glad to see that Alderman Foley is not of your opinion on the question of compromise, and you may be sure that not a few of your townspeople will blame you for neglecting the solid interests of your town.

KIRWAN. Alderman Foley has shown no sign of wavering that I know of, and it would only matter to him if he did. Our townspeople are solid behind us, as will be seen at the great mass meeting at the Town Hall to-morrow.

HARDMAN. Then what further boon? I offer to supply the capital of the tramway, and Mr Lawrence proposed this morning that I should take a house and grounds and spend part of the year with you. But I should like to hear Mr Jasper Dean's opinion. Does he believe that compromise is impossible?

DEAN. I've really nothing further to add. I think Mr Alderman Ferguson touched the root of the question when he said that he did not believe it would be possible to compromise this matter. Your offer of the tramway convinces me he is right. As Mayor Tench has said, we stand by the finding of the accountants.

LAWRENCE. But the accountants were not all agreed that certain harbour dues should be charged.

DEAN. That is a point of law on which we have had the best advice. (*Turning excitedly to* HARDMAN.) We are resolved to fight this to the end.

LAWRENCE. I am sure, gentlemen, that with patience this discussion will lead to an amicable settlement.

TENCH. Did you ever see the Corporation so united before? As for the tramway, we shall have plenty of money to build that for ourselves, when we have been paid what is owed to us. Won't we, Alderman Dean?

DEAN (*absently*). What? Yes, of course.

LAWRENCE. Take my advice, and come to terms when you can. A change of affairs might happen that would upset all your calculations. Then you might find yourselves in a worse state than ever.

FERGUSON. I must be going too. Goodbye, Mr Hardman. Your cigars are excellent!

HARDMAN. Your demands are outside the pale of practical politics.

KIRWAN. That is your answer to all our demands.

LAWRENCE. Oh, my dear Mr Hardman! Oh, my dear colleagues of the Corporation, where are you going? Where are you going?

TENCH. I am afraid, Mr Hardman, we cannot stay any longer.

HARDMAN (*as the Corporation are bowing and departing*). Well, gentlemen, I hope we part good friends, in spite of all differences in opinion. I will see you downstairs. (*Exeunt all except* DEAN *and* KIRWAN.)

KIRWAN. The choice was difficult, but you proved equal to the task of choosing.

DEAN. Shall I regret?

KIRWAN. No, you will not regret, but while the blood is young it will cry out. Miss Fell is the temptation that Southhaven sent you, and she sends to each some insidious temptation. Southhaven is always beside us to tempt us in our moments of weakness. No sooner do we become united behind any man than she comes to him with her hands full of bribes. (*Enter* MILLICENT.)

MILLICENT. I heard that you were here. But you are engaged – it doesn't matter.

DEAN. But Miss Fell. (*To* KIRWAN.) Miss Fell wishes to speak to me. I'll see you presently. I'll call for you on my home. (*Exit* KIRWAN.)

MILLICENT. I did not like to go away without seeing you. My uncle told you that I could not see you.

DEAN. Yes; I understood that you did not wish to see me.

MILLICENT. But I changed my mind. I felt that I must see you.

DEAN. And, Millicent, I felt that I must see you.

MILLICENT. Tell me about the meeting. I can see there was no compromise. You would yield nothing. (*They sit on two chairs half way up the stage facing the audience.*)

DEAN. As Kirwan says, there are but two ways, the right and the wrong, and no compromise is possible.

MILLICENT. So we are parted.

DEAN. There is no reason why we should be if –

MILLICENT. Let us not go over it all again; all that can be said has been said.

DEAN. Alas. And our happiness is a mere matter of money – money which neither of us cares much about; and yet this money puts me in a wretched plight.

100

MILLICENT. That I may lose a few hundred pounds or all I have got matters nothing compared to –

DEAN. To what?

MILLICENT. To the fact that you do not love me enough. This money we could do without, but I cannot marry a man who has resolved that his life shall be Kirwan's apparitor and satellite. My friends, my pursuits, my family, I can give up, but I cannot give up myself; and am I not an inheritance of ideas which you hate, which you used not to hate, but which you have learnt to hate? Everything divides us, and yet we're very dear to each other.

DEAN. That is the misery of it.

MILLICENT. Ah, if you had never met Kirwan!

DEAN. I should be quite different, no doubt, and many things which lie heavy on my heart would pass by lightly enough.

MILLICENT. My uncle, who is a clever man, compared you to a rioter who breaks into his own house and, having wrecked it, looks out of the window surprised to find the world exactly the same as before.

DEAN. He said the same to me, and from his point of view the image is a striking one.

MILLICENT. He said you were following a chimera.

DEAN. Do we not all follow chimeras, he as much as I? Is it so sure that the material world which he follows is less chimerical than the spiritual truths which I strive to follow?

MILLICENT. I do not trouble about such things, I only know that –

DEAN. At all events we have no proof that spiritual truths are illusory, whereas we know that the world is.

MILLICENT. Yes, it slides like sand under our feet, even I have perceived that.

DEAN. The difficulty in life is the choice, and all the wonder of life is in the choice.

MILLICENT. Between what?

DEAN. The world within us and the world without us. You are the world that is outside of me, I am the world that is outside of you. (*Pause.*) Do you understand?

MILLICENT. Yes; I think I do. (*Pause.*)

DEAN. Now tell me of what you're thinking, Millicent.

MILLICENT. I was thinking how we think of all these things, and how we act just as if we hadn't thought of them at all. So this is the end. It was to part like this that I met you at Oxford.

DEAN. Ah, the day I met you as you sauntered across the sunny old quadrangle, that Sunday morning!

MILLICENT. And the day we went on the river! We rowed by the ruins

101

of Godstone nunnery where fair Rosamund ended her days. We talked of her strange beauty and looked across the yellow meadows.

DEAN. That happy day! My soul was in all the air. I felt that something had befallen me – something momentous, something that would never happen again. Millicent, we cannot part. You said the other day that we were united. I feel that we are.

MILLICENT. You say so now (*they get up*), but to-morrow you would regret it –not to-morrow, perhaps, but sooner or later. Kirwan has shown you the way, and your feet have begun to travel the way which it would be a lifelong regret to turn back from. You would feel at the end of the journey that you had not walked in life, but alongside of life.

DEAN. I shall be unhappy whichever is my choice.

MILLICENT. I don't wish to ruin any one's life, nor do I wish any one to ruin mine.

DEAN. To ruin your life!

MILLICENT. Yes; I too have a life to ruin, though I am only a woman. Can I not see you five years hence looking across the table at me, even at your children, and regretting that you had sacrificed your country for them? Go to your country, it shall not be said that I have robbed it.

DEAN. I am not equal to the sacrifice. I cannot forego the joy of you, Millicent.

MILLICENT. You think so now. To-morrow your heart will rejoice secretly in your escape. (*She is about to go.*) Here is my uncle. (*She goes out by one door as* HARDMAN *and* LAWRENCE *enter by another.*)

HARDMAN. Well, Jasper, I hope that Millicent has convinced you that as you have only one life to live you had better live it.

DEAN. That we should live our lives there can be no question, but in which direction we may live them the most fully is a question which neither she nor I have been able to settle. (*Exit.*) (*They sit down on the same two chairs.*)

LAWRENCE. What has happened? (HARDMAN *shrugs his shoulders.*) One has given way, but which? We're in their hands; they hold us in the hollow of their hands.

HARDMAN. Perhaps neither has given way.

LAWRENCE. One must have given way. The yielding one is the hinge on which the world swings. My idea that you should meet the Corporation wasn't a bad one, was it? (HARDMAN *doesn't answer.*) Do you think that Jasper will give way? It is generally the woman that yields. And if she yields my appointment is lost. (*They get up.*)

102

HARDMAN. The appointment may yet be yours. Goodbye for the present, my dear Alderman. (LAWRENCE *goes out and* HARDMAN *stands looking after him.*)

CURTAIN

ACT V

The same as in the Second and Third Acts. MISS CAROLINE DEAN *and* MISS ARABELLA DEAN *discovered talking,* KIRWAN *standing at the back of the stage.*

ARABELLA. From the beginning I thought that you were inclined to overdo it; not only were the hours of study, but the very hours of recreation were arranged by you.

CAROLINE. Wild nature is abominable; beauty and morals are cultivation. You train a tree, you train a horse, why should you not train a child?

ARABELLA. He was bound to break through your severity. I don't think he was right, Caroline, but a man of genius gets loose somehow –

CAROLINE. Jasper is not a man of genius.

ARABELLA. Jasper is very young. We do not know what he will become –

CAROLINE. There will be no becoming; he will remain what he is for a while, and then deteriorate.

ARABELLA. I daresay you think, Caroline, if it had not been for me you would have succeeded.

CAROLINE. You never helped me, you always gave way to him; I have myself heard you urge him to follow his own inclination.

ARABELLA. We are divided on the question whether we can mould a soul, or if, without our aid and despite our hindrance, a soul takes the shortest cut to its own destiny.

CAROLINE. It must be right to teach what we believe to be right; and the proof of this is that we all teach. Our teaching may be a benevolent neutrality like yours, a general go-as-you-please, or a disciplined teaching like mine; but in either case we teach.

ARABELLA. Yes, teaching seems as essential to teacher as to pupil. I daresay you are right, Caroline.

CAROLINE. I at least think that I am right, and you have no clear convictions –

ARABELLA. I have no clear convictions on this point, perhaps; on no point are my convictions as clear as yours. (KIRWAN *comes down on the stage.*)

KIRWAN. I beg your pardon for interrupting you, but time is flying. I'm

104

afraid he'll be late.

CAROLINE. You are very forgetful, Alderman Kirwan; can you not remember that my desire is that he shall not go to this meeting?

ARABELLA. Do wait a little. Do wait, he will be disappointed if he misses you.

KIRWAN. The meeting has begun, and it is a matter of vital importance that he should be there.

ARABELLA (*rising*). Where can he be? His study door is locked, he must have gone to the meeting, for he is nowhere about the house.

KIRWAN. It is very strange.

ARABELLA. Wait a little longer, unless you think you know where you can find him.

KIRWAN (*to* CAROLINE). Let us differ amicably, Miss Dean, since we must differ. I believe all your fears to be groundless, and that the result will prove them to be so even to you. But the man who loses his opportunity, loses himself. (*He goes up the stage.*)

CAROLINE. Arabella, why did you ask him to stay? You have no consideration for my feelings. (*She gets up,* ARABELLA *detains her.*)

ARABELLA. He's Jasper's greatest friend.

CAROLINE. Jasper looks to him as a god, and drinks down every word he utters as eagerly as if he were listening to a divine utterance.

ARABELLA. Kirwan is the first man of ideas that Jasper met.

CAROLINE. Really, Arabella, I understand you no longer. At the University –

ARABELLA. I don't think that Jasper was ever interested in learning, it was something else that interested him in Kirwan.

CAROLINE. Something else! What else? hatred of respectable people and a preference for abominable folklore to Greek culture. All our labours in vain, my early teaching and the teaching of the most learned professors in Southhaven wasted!

ARABELLA. But, Caroline, you have never read our Gaelic literature. I have been with him on his quests.

CAROLINE. Yes, taking down ridiculous stories from the lips of old croning women sitting by peat fires.

ARABELLA. You have not heard his explanation of the value of these old wives' tales as you call them. All literature begins, he says, in such tales. For no man originates - a nation does that just as the earth produces the marble the sculptor carves.

KIRWAN (*comes down the stage*). I cannot wait any longer; the meeting has begun.

ARABELLA. What shall we tell Jasper?

KIRWAN. I don't think there is anything to tell him. It is clear that he does not intend to go to the meeting. He has put his faith in the joys of the flesh and the world.

ARABELLA. Will he be the unhappier for that?

CAROLINE. He thinks too much of happiness; he should rather try to consider what is right for him to do.

KIRWAN. For once we find ourselves in agreement, Miss Dean (*turning to* ARABELLA). Tell him nothing. Yes, tell him that I will not reproach him.

ARABELLA. Thank you, Alderman Kirwan, thank you.

CAROLINE. And what are you going to do, Alderman Kirwan – nothing?

KIRWAN. I am going to the meeting to see the disaster. I am a collector of broken causes.

CAROLINE. You are going there to lead, this is your opportunity.

ARABELLA. No one can take Jasper's place. You will be beaten, Alderman Kirwan.

CAROLINE. Really, Arabella, you begin to strain my patience.

KIRWAN. She understands better than you do, Miss Dean. I cannot lead. My opinions are too well known, and when I write them or speak them people merely say 'There is Alderman Kirwan again, how many years has he been saying that now?' and they yawn and talk about something else.

CAROLINE. But Jasper merely expressed your ideas.

KIRWAN. I know that, but that was just what was wanted, a new man to speak old thoughts, that is what the world always wants.

CAROLINE. I don't understand.

KIRWAN. I daresay you don't; but I say that in losing Jasper we have lost everything. The very strength of personality that makes union so hard among us might have made us a great people if he but dared to lead us. He preferred – well, goodbye, Miss Dean, goodbye. (*Aside as he goes out.*) He might have been remembered in times to come, we should have told our children about him. (*Exit.*)

CAROLINE. We're saved, we're saved.

ARABELLA. But if he succeeds in leading after all and Hardman is defeated?

CAROLINE. Oh! what do I care as long as it is not Jasper who defeats him, and we are safe with our Southhaven friends and with respectable people here. Jasper will now be able to take the lead in respectable causes.

ARABELLA. Respectable causes! is a cause ever respectable?

CAROLINE. What do you mean, Arabella? You are as enigmatical as our unfortunate nephew.

ARABELLA. It would seem to me that a cause is lost when it becomes

106

respectable.

CAROLINE. Did you hear Kirwan say that, Arabella? It sounds like one of his acute observations.

ARABELLA. No, I did not hear Kirwan say that, but I daresay it is one of the things he would say.

CAROLINE. You never hear me expressing any one else's views.

ARABELLA. No, I will say that for you. You bring people round to your views. It seems that you completed Alderman Foley's conversion yesterday.

CAROLINE. He saw, of course, that I could not consent unless he joined the respectable party.

ARABELLA. Yes, Caroline; but I wonder if Jasper will look favourably on the alliance.

CAROLINE. Alderman Foley's grandfather, I have reason for knowing, was in a much better position than Valentine's father, and as for Jasper, it would ill – become him to criticise me after having done all he could do disgrace his family. Had it not been for my influence Alderman Foley might have remained on the popular side.

ARABELLA. It would not matter, everything depends on Jasper. Do you intend to tell him?

CAROLINE. Of course he'll know some day. (*Enter Jasper.*)

ARABELLA. Oh, Jasper, Alderman Kirwan has been here looking for you.

DEAN. That was he whom I heard talking.

ARABELLA. I tried your door; it was locked.

DEAN. Yes, I locked the door; where is he?

ARABELLA. He is gone to the meeting.

CAROLINE. I persuaded him to go there and lead in your absence.

ARABELLA. Aren't you going, Jasper? (*He walks to the window and looks out, and returns like a man uncertain of his next action, worried and nervous.*)

DEAN. What did Kirwan say?

ARABELLA. He seemed distressed that he did not find you; he believed so entirely in you, Jasper. I asked him if there was any message he could give you, and he said there was none.

DEAN. Did he say anything else?

ARABELLA. I don't remember anything else. Ah! he said that you were not to be afraid, that he would not reproach you. He was very kind

DEAN. He's always that. He knows that I shall reproach myself. Did he say anything else!

CAROLINE. I cannot understand the attention that is paid to his slightest word; every word is treasured up like a pearl examined, looked at from this side and that, and then put away to be quoted on some future occasion.

DEAN. Kirwan is the noblest of men, and every word that falls from his lips should be treasured up. His words are pearls indeed, but unhappily they sometimes fall where pearls proverbially fall.

CAROLINE. Jasper!

DEAN. I'm not thinking of you, Aunt Caroline, I'm thinking of us all. (*Sitting down.*) Oh! Kirwan, that you should have begotten so unworthy a disciple. (*Getting up.*) That I should be able to see so clear, and should be so unable to act. I'm like a hound in a leash. I strain at the thong, but it does not break, and I am choking.

ARABELLA. You will make yourself ill, dear; shall I fetch you a glass of water?

DEAN. No, no. I was speaking in metaphors. It's ridiculous to give way like this, but when one speaks of Kirwan I'm overcome, that is all.

ARABELLA. Let us not speak of him, then.

DEAN. On the contrary, let us speak of him! If we cannot act like him, we can at least admire. All his life he has sacrificed the world to his ideas, and to do that is holiness. To see the right way and to follow it always without wavering is the sublime life.

CAROLINE. I know that in your opinion, Jasper, I am a very inferior person, but you cannot accuse me of wavering in my ideas.

DEAN. Alas! Aunt Caroline, you never had an idea in your life. You mistook worldly advantage for ideas.

CAROLINE. Then if you're so sure of what is right, why don't you go to the meeting? However wrong my ideas may be, I have not abandoned them; in that at least I have the inestimable advantage of resembling Alderman Kirwan.

DEAN. Yes, you are steadfast, whereas I am a weak creature that errs. But I do not blaspheme, I do not deny the truth as you do. But, Aunt Caroline, let us not reproach each other; let us rather pity each other. You see a little clearer on one side than I do; perhaps I see clearer on another side when I look towards Kirwan, my master, whom I am too weak to follow.

ARABELLA. But, Jasper, you seem terribly distressed. Do you think it would make you happy to go to this meeting?

DEAN. Yes, in the long run, years hence, but the entanglements of the moment hold me.

ARABELLA. Dear Jasper, tell me about it; it has to do with Millicent has it not?

DEAN. Yes, it has to do with her. I promised her not to go to this meeting, that is all! It doesn't sound sufficient for this fuss, but life is, as you know, a trivial affair, and we are trivial beings … I'm going with her and Hardman to Southhaven. We shall be married and –

ARABELLA. You will be happy.

DEAN. Happy! Ah! I have chosen the delight of the passing hour; I've not known how to do the one needful thing.

ARABELLA. What is that?

DEAN. To sacrifice the passing hour to the idea. I wonder how all this will seem to me ten years hence?

CAROLINE. It's at all events satisfactory that you are not going to disgrace your family for the sake of feelings which you may never live to experience.

DEAN. I know well which is the honourable course; but this obsession, this intolerable obsession! Oh, if I could throw it off! (*A sound of tumult is heard outside in the streets, and he goes to the window.*) The streets are moving. Numbers must have failed to get into the hall. Kirwan told me there would not be room for every one. (*Coming down the stage.*) Kirwan has the will and not the power, I have the power and not the will. The shallow and the light-souled are always the chosen of the people, and the shallow and the light-souled betray the people, because they are as God made them. (*Turning away from the window.*) It is now too late.

ARABELLA. Then let us try to forget. Let us have done with thinking. Let us be happy. You're going away to-night; we shall not see you again for a long while.

DEAN. If it had to happen again I should act as I have acted. We do not make ourselves, and however weak we are we have to put up with ourselves; the burden is not of our choosing. Not only have we to bear the burden of our real selves, we have to bear that of our acquired selves, and that is the heaviest burden of all. That is the burden that I now bear, the burden of early contradictions of my inclinations, and the imposition of ideas which were not mine by nature, or sufficiently akin to me to become mine.

ARABELLA. But, Jasper dear, you have no cause of complaint against me. I always wished you to develop yourself according to your inclinations, which were always good and pure.

DEAN. Yes, dear aunt, you were always sympathetic, and had it not been for you I should have left home long ago. Perhaps it would have been better if I had.

CAROLINE. Then neither was right. But since you have discarded my advice and repudiated my teaching I do not see how I can be held accountable for your failure.

DEAN. I would not shift the blame upon any one. I'm thinking it out, that is all. Kirwan was the first noble mind I ever met, the first brain and

109

energy, and my hope in myself is based on the fact that I was attracted to him at once. So much good there is in me. Yes, I recognised and acclaimed the true, the noble, the steadfast, the holy. So I cannot be entirely bad. But the influence of years is not shaken off at once, and I fell back into materialism; I am powerless to rise out of it for the moment; it will take years for me to free myself, but later on, years hence, I will come back and prove myself a worthy disciple. Tell Kirwan that Aunt Arabella.

ARABELLA. I will tell him; but, Jasper dear, you make us feel very sad. Years hence is a long while. May we not smile now? You're going to marry the girl you love. Come here and sit by us, and let us talk about her.

DEAN. Yes, I love Millicent, and I would do well to love her, for I have nothing but Millicent now.

CAROLINE. I'm sorry, Jasper, that my influence has forced you into marrying the girl you love, for that is the charge against me.

DEAN. My business now is to make Millicent happy, and I'll think no more lest I should fail in that as in other things, so let us sit together as you say, and talk of happiness and wedding bells. (*He sits beside them.*)

CAROLINE. I have to tell you, Jasper, that I have promised to marry Alderman Foley.

DEAN. Alderman Foley!

CAROLINE. Do you not approve?

DEAN. I'm in no mood for questioning any one's desires. I am outside of my real self, and you may tell a fellow-sufferer why you were tempted into this marriage.

CAROLINE. Alderman Foley has been devoted for years, and this is the recompense of his devotion.

DEAN. A very splendid way of putting it. I wonder you do not add that this is how you propose to redeem the family from the disgrace I have brought upon it.

ARABELLA. Enough of recriminations. It is well known that everybody objects to everybody else's marriage.

CAROLINE. I do not object to Jasper's. It is Jasper who objects to mine.

DEAN. Well, aunt, I hope you'll be happy. You ought to be, for I'm sure there is no shadow of doubt on your mind that you have done the right thing. (*Sounds of tumult in the street, the women run to the window.*)

ARABELLA. The meeting must have broken up, there is a great crowd. The crowd with the band is going towards the other crowd, and there is Alderman Kirwan running.

CAROLINE. Do you know, Arabella, I think he is running away from the crowd. I believe he is coming in here.

DEAN. I cannot bring myself to meet him, I could not look him in the face. I will go. Do not say I'm here. And you, Aunt Caroline, try to be as little triumphant as possible. The victorious should pity the vanquished, to do so adds lustre to victory. (*Exit.*) (*Enter* KIRWAN *with coat torn and hat broken in. He sits down in deep depression.*)

KIRWAN. Miss Dean, excuse this hasty entrance. The maid had the door open watching the crowd and I came straight up. I had to escape them – they would have killed me.

CAROLINE. Oh, Mr Kirwan, I hope you're not hurt! (*He shakes his head.*) –

ARABELLA. But won't you tell us about the meeting?

KIRWAN. Oh, like many another meeting, tumult among the many, a few in despair.

CAROLINE. But was not a leader chosen when Jasper's absence was discovered?

KIRWAN. In spite of my own better judgment I tried to unite them for a common end, and Ferguson accused me of keeping Jasper away to make myself the leader, and then they all wanted to be leaders and so the row began. (*Furious tumult outside and sounds of glass broken, stones are thrown through the window.*) The mob is chasing the Corporation up the street.

CAROLINE. Mercy! We shall be murdered. Where are the police? (*The bell rings.*)

ARABELLA. Who are these coming in? (*Enter* ALDERMAN FERGUSON *torn and bloody,* ALDERMAN POLLOCK *rather drunk and excited, and* MICHAEL LEECH *and* MAYOR TENCH, *their coats soiled and torn. The stage begins to darken slowly.*)

FERGUSON. It is some consolation that though I have not become leader myself, I have kept every one else from leading.

POLLOCK. The day will come when the people will require common sense, then they will think of the old stock, they will come to Alderman Pollock. Hurrah for Alderman Pollock!

TENCH. Come over here, James, and sit down, I'm afraid you're not very well.

FERGUSON. Where is Jasper? Why was he not at the meeting?

CAROLINE. I hope you're not hurt, Alderman Ferguson!

FERGUSON. If only Jasper had a thimbleful of courage I should not be in this plight. But I knew he was no good after yesterday. To think of these fools wanting to be leaders! That such mice should be ambitious!

ARABELLA. Who was it that hurt you? May I get you something?

FERGUSON. Thank you, I feel rather faint. (ARABELLA *rings; the* MAID *enters.* ARABELLA *gives her order; the* MAID *enters immediately after with tray and glasses.*)

ARABELLA. And you, Alderman Pollock, you will have something too?

POLLOCK. Yes, thank you, I think I will. It happened as we were trying to get outside. That ruffian Macnee was cheering for Kirwan and I ventured to ask him a question.

FERGUSON. And his arguments were decisive.

POLLOCK. He pushed me, I fell, and the others walked on top of me. I always said he was a dangerous man, and warned the Corporation against employing him. I fancy I'm bleeding somewhere. (*He pulls up his sleeve and examines his arm.*)

ARABELLA. And you, my dear Mayor, how did it happen? You have lost your hat?

TENCH. Yes, I lost it at the top of the stairs; it fell off and rolled down the steps.

POLLOCK. I had no chance whatever.

TENCH. Would you mind telling me if there's a cut here at the back of my neck, it feels a bit sore?

CAROLINE. I will get some sticking-plaster in a moment if you require it. But Alderman Ferguson is going to tell us how it all happened.

ARABELLA. Tell us how it all happened.

FERGUSON. I had no sooner got possession of the platform than I was attacked by an organised body of the greatest blackguards in the town. I believe they were sent there by Lawrence, though he did not dare to show his face. I had to oppose you at the meeting, Kirwan, but if you will advocate a restoration of our line of steamers we can work together.

KIRWAN. We can do nothing without a leader.

FERGUSON. That is indeed true. When will Providence send us a leader? (*Cheers for* LAWRENCE *outside.*)

KIRWAN. The people are cheering Lawrence – listen! (*They all listen.*)

POLLOCK. Lawrence is the leader of the people. It is his voice they like, and I like to hear it myself when I am drunk.

KIRWAN. I believe that is he walking at the head of the mob. How has this popularity come about?

FERGUSON. When Jasper Dean deserted us the mob turned like a greedy pike and swallowed the first bait.

KIRWAN. Then the tramway has been accepted as an equivalent.

FERGUSON. That or the residence. Oh, that residence! I can see all the plush footmen and the matrons and their charges making obeisance

112

to the largest export trade in the world. (*A ring. Enter* ALDERMAN FOLEY.)

CAROLINE. I hope you're not hurt, my dear Valentine?

FOLEY. My dear Caroline, thanks to you, I found myself once more with the majority. Alderman Lawrence has carried all but the most extreme of the people with him. You've no idea of the ovation he's receiving; the town will be lighted up, and a banquet is preparing. He told me to tell you and your sister that he expected to have the pleasure of your company.

FERGUSON. We would like to hear how you were persuaded to the other side.

FOLEY. That is a matter for the next number of the *Denouncer.* I've no fear whatever but that my readers will approve of my conduct. At all events as much as your supporters seem to have approved of yours. (*Turning towards the others.*) After some friends had gone among the people and explained matters a little Alderman Lawrence addressed them from the pediment of the statue of Patriotism in front of the Town Hall, and told them how he had arranged to lay down the tramway from the centre of the city to the poorer quarters which has given us all so much trouble. Mayor Hardman has promised to find the money.

FERGUSON. Tell us about the residence. What office are you going to take in that establishment?

FOLEY (*answers* FERGUSON *with a glance, then turning to the others*). I then addressed the people. I told them that the Aldermen of Southhaven would bring their wives here during the summer and spend a little money among them, and that Mr Hardman might be induced to live amongst us occasionally.

CAROLINE. You've given an excellent account of these proceedings, Valentine. Now, will you tell us where are Mr Hardman and Millicent?

FOLEY. They are at the Railway Hotel waiting for Jasper. After the banquet Jasper is going with them to Southhaven. I do not expect my friends here to agree with me, but I hope that in time they too will learn what I have learnt, that the State is founded on such happy lives as Jasper's and Miss Fell's will be, that our private interests are the foundation of the State, and that he who does the best for himself does the best for the State in the long run.

KIRWAN. You've quite caught the master's accent. With one's eyes shut one would swear it was he who is speaking.

FOLEY. And you? You will go on repeating the same ideas for another ten years and then the end. Since I have known you, you have not

113

acquired a single new idea. (*Turning to the others*.) I have the pleasure to announce to you all that I'm going to be married. Miss Dean and I have decided to make our engagement public.

KIRWAN. Let nothing disturb the happiness of this evening. (*The stage continues to darken*.) Let all the bitterness, the dregs of our late folly, be forgotten among us; we are all at peace now.

FOLEY (*to* CAROLINE). But where is Jasper? His presence is essential. I hope he will not disappoint this meeting of friends. Is he at home, Miss Dean?

ARABELLA. I'm afraid to venture out in the present condition of the street. You said that Alderman Lawrence had invited us to supper. You will use your influence, Alderman Foley, to protect us.

FOLEY. I'm afraid that that would strain my influence, great as it is, and for an insufficient end. Those who want to restore our line of steamers are always dangerous; we can go out through the back door. Come, Miss Dean, and come Miss Arabella Dean, let us delay no longer. The supper will be getting cold.

CAROLINE. Valentine, give me your arm!

FERGUSON (*to* KIRWAN). This marriage at all events cannot lessen Alderman Foley's reputation for austerity. Come, Pollock. (*He rouses him*.) Don't you want any supper?

POLLOCK. Yes, indeed I do! Alderman Pollock will always drink the health of the happy bride and bridegroom. (*He goes out clinging to* FERGUSON, TENCH *follows limping*. KIRWAN *remains alone on the stage*. JASPER DEAN *enters from the other side. The stage is in twilight*.)

DEAN. Kirwan ...I hoped to get away without meeting you; but we cannot escape our punishment. But, Kirwan, you who see deep into the heart, can you find nowhere an excuse for me? Kirwan, have you never been in love?

KIRWAN. Yes, and I have been faithful to my love.

DEAN. I understand. All men are not as high and as steadfast as you, Kirwan. You must judge others by a different standard. I have failed, I know, but is my failure irreparable? Is there nothing for me to do now except to be happy?

KIRWAN. There is an antiquarian society, you might join it, and advocate the preservation of our antiquities. But if I were you, I would not vex my mood with anything except the matter in hand. You've chosen to be happy, be a success in what the world calls success.

DEAN. But the cause I have abandoned, is it lost for ever? Can I not return?

KIRWAN. The cause is not lost, but the next opportunity will come to a

114

new man.

DEAN. Goodbye, Kirwan! (*He turns to go. Turning back.*) And you, what are you going to do?

KIRWAN. For the moment our hopes are ended, our ideas gone by. What remains now? I will go home and write a violent attack on some personal friend; if I do not I shall not be in the fashion.

DEAN. On me?

KIRWAN. Oh no, not on you; nor does it matter on whom, so long as the attack be bitter.

FINAL CURTAIN

THE COMING OF GABRIELLE

A COMEDY

BY

GEORGE MOORE

PEOPLE in the PLAY

MEN
LEWIS DAVENANT, a man of letters living in a provincial town.
SEBASTIAN DAYNE, his cousin and secretary.
JIM GODBY, a sailor, second mate of the Hannah Maria
MR MEYER, a translator of Mr Davenant's works.
LORD CARRA, a sportsman.

WOMEN
LADY LETHAM, an admirer of Mr Davenant's works.
MARTIN, a parlour-maid.
GABRIELLE, the Countess von Hoenstadt

ACT I. takes place in Mr Davenant's Drawing-Room in Rockminster, ACT II. in the Library at Claremont Villa, and ACT III. in the same place as ACT I.

AUTHOR'S NOTE
This comedy does not seem to me suited exactly to the present time; it would be better to throw it back a few years into the sixties or eighties – in other words, into the crinoline or bustle period.

THE COMING OF GABRIELLE

ACT I

LEWIS DAVENANT'S *drawing-room.* SEBASTIAN *is discovered when the curtain rises bidding good-bye to a visitor. He rings. Enter* MARTIN.

SEBASTIAN. Are there many people in the parlour?

MARTIN. I think there are still five, sir.

SEBASTIAN. And the sailor, is he still there?

MARTIN. Yes, sir; he refuses to leave.

SEBASTIAN. I suppose there's nothing for it but to see him. (*A moment after* MARTIN *announces* MR GODBY.)

GODBY. One has to wait for the tide, but one gets into port at last. (*On catching sight of* SEBASTIAN.) Ah! I suppose you've been waiting for the tide, too?

SEBASTIAN. I am always in port, and often wishing the tide would take me out of port. You see, Mr Godby, I'm Mr Davenant's secretary.

GODBY. I'm glad to hear it, for you'll be able to tell me if Mr Davenant is coming down.

SEBASTIAN. He may come down.

GODBY. What do you mean by "he may come down"? To-day is 'is at 'ome day, ain't it?

SEBASTIAN. I didn't say that Mr Davenant wouldn't come down.

GODBY. But he must come down to receive 'is visitors.

SEBASTIAN. He begged of me, in his unavoidable absence –

GODBY. Unavoidable?

SEBASTIAN. You know, Mr Godby – or perhaps you do not know – that Mr Davenant is exceedingly busy just now. He feels that he must make some alterations in the play that is going to be performed at Vienna, and as soon as you have left, and all the other gentlemen and ladies in the parlour, he will ask me to copy the new text; and whilst his valet is packing up his trunks he will be walking up and down the room, back and forth, meditating further changes ... I beg you to believe, Mr Godby, that we have not a moment to lose.

GODBY. I don't understand much of all you're saying. I only know I've been told that he's always at 'ome Tuesdays.

SEBASTIAN. Martin was wrong to say as much. Mr Davenant does receive visitors on Tuesdays sometimes – I may go so far as to say generally, but to-day he is very busy. I've spoken to you of the alterations he is making in his play, and, of course, there is his luggage, which, although in the hands of a capable valet, requires Mr Davenant's personal supervision. But as I am his secretary, I may ask if you have come on literary business, to speak to him about one of his books, or about *Elizabeth Cooper*, the play. You've heard about it, no doubt.

GODBY. Heard about it! My wife never talks of nothing else but Elizabeth Cooper.

SEBASTIAN. Ah! then it is about *Elizabeth Cooper* that you wish to see Mr Davenant?

GODBY. I must see him. I have come up from Southampton.

SEBASTIAN. I'm really very sorry, Mr Godby. Your wife is only one among thousands who would like to speak to Mr Davenant about his famous novel, and in the unavoidable absence of Mr Davenant I beg that you will tell me –

GODBY. Tell you my business, young man! Now, is it likely? – or didn't you 'ear me say that I'd come up from Southampton?

SEBASTIAN. That's nothing of a journey, Mr Godby – a mere matter of a couple of hundred miles. People come much farther than that to see Mr Davenant.

GODBY. Do they, now? and go away without seeing him, maybe? But I'm not one of them crew, and when I tell you that I was spliced three weeks come Tuesday, and 'ave come up here on the wife's business, you may bet the last shot in your locker that I am pretty keen to see Mr Davenant, and mean to speak to him as man to man.

SEBASTIAN. To speak to Mr Davenant as man to man!

GODBY. Them's my sailing orders, and it needs no spy-glass to see that you ain't got a wife, Mr Secretary, else you'd know without my telling that none but a fool would go out on his wife's very particular business and return home with nothing more interestin' to tell her than that he had seen Secretary.

SEBASTIAN. Mr Davenant is engaged in making certain alterations in his play –

GODBY. I've heard enough of those alterations.

SEBASTIAN. His valet is packing his luggage –

GODBY. I've heard about the luggage –

SEBASTIAN. Our time will be completely occupied till the carriage comes to take him to the station. I do hope you will understand how impossible it is for Mr Davenant to see you; and as there are three other people waiting to see me in the parlour, you will excuse me, Mr Godby.

GODBY. I shall wait. (*He goes out.* SEBASTIAN *rings. Enter* MARTIN.)

SEBASTIAN. How many, Martin, did you say were in the waiting-room?

MARTIN. Two gentlemen and a lady, sir, are all that are left.

SEBASTIAN. Show the lady up. (*A few moments after* MARTIN *announces* LADY LETHAM, *a young and pretty woman about thirty, of almost ecstatic gaze and gait.*)

LADY LETHAM. So this is his room – the room in which he writes! Letters, books – his books, and the books he reads! Pictures, manuscripts in the cupboards, no doubt. Oh! I beg your pardon, sir; I did not know anybody was here. You're waiting for Mr Davenant?

SEBASTIAN. I am his secretary. Won't you sit down? I am at your service.

LADY LETHAM. Mr Davenant will come down presently?

SEBASTIAN. Mr Davenant leaves for Vienna this evening to attend the rehearsals of his play *Elizabeth Cooper*, which is to be produced, as I daresay you have heard, at Vienna.

LADY LETHAM. So *Elizabeth Cooper* is going to be played at last.

SEBASTIAN. Yes; and the performance will be a great literary event. Mr Davenant's Continental reputation is growing day by day. You've read the novel?

LADY LETHAM. The book is always by my bedside. But I have not heard of the play. You see, I've just come up from my country home far away in Westmorland, where we live, my husband and I, in a peaceful, almost pastoral retreat within view of beautiful mountain ranges. I should like Mr Davenant to see our landscape, for I'm sure it would inspire him. I have described it in my letters, and as you are his secretary you have perhaps heard my name – Lady Letham.

SEBASTIAN. Mr Davenant will be so sorry to miss seeing·you.

LADY LETHAM. Could he not spare a few minutes?

SEBASTIAN. He would like to, but if he did he'd certainly miss his train.

LADY LETHAM. He must not do that. I am staying, not many miles from here, with my sister, Lady Ewhurst, at Charming Dean, and shall hope to see Mr Davenant when he returns.

SEBASTIAN. You spoke of some letters that you wrote to Mr Davenant. If you'll allow me, I will look out your name. (*He goes to the writing-table and turns over the papers.*) You wrote to him on the 22nd of last month, and again on the 25th. The third letter – I am sure there was a third, but I cannot lay hand upon it.

LADY LETHAM. I thought I put 'Personal' on the envelopes.

SEBASTIAN. That is just why I read your letters. I read all Mr Davenant's personal correspondence.

LADY LETHAM. Oh! How is one, then, to correspond directly with Mr Davenant?

SEBASTIAN. You must write to him on post cards.

LADY LETHAM. But on a post card it is impossible to explain –

SEBASTIAN. But on several –

LADY LETHAM. It seems to me, sir, that you're laughing at me.

SEBASTIAN. I hope, Lady Letham, that you do not think me guilty of such impoliteness?

LADY LETHAM. No, not exactly laughing at me; I exaggerated. Quizzing, perhaps?

SEBASTIAN. I beg of you, Lady Letham, to believe that no such thought entered my mind. It is about *Elizabeth Cooper* that you wish to speak to Mr Davenant?

LADY LETHAM. Yes; but since you assure me he is busy –

SEBASTIAN. Lady Letham, I assure you.

LADY LETHAM. I will promise not to detain him for more than a few minutes. Say that I will not detain him for more than five.

SEBASTIAN. I should be delighted to oblige you, Lady Letham, but I beg you to believe that I dare not approach him just now. He is in the room above us, walking to and forth, chewing his words. Believe me, it will be very much better –

LADY LETHAM. For me to write another letter? But will you promise me to see that he receives it and that he reads it?

SEBASTIAN. On the word of honour of his cousin, Sebastian Dayne.

LADY LETHAM. Thank you, Mr Dayne. On thinking it over, it seems to me that I might do worse than to confide to you my little project. Mr Davenant has not written a long work for some years. He publishes a volume of delightful stories now and then, and some critical articles from a new and original point of view, altogether delightful –

SEBASTIAN. Profound.

LADY LETHAM. True. But are you not of my opinion that it is regrettable that he does not apply himself to a long work? Perhaps he is doing so; you are his secretary, and can tell me. We, his admirers, are waiting for a long, long work from Mr Davenant.

SEBASTIAN. May I ask, if you have a suggestion to make, if you have in mind a theme that you would like Mr Davenant to treat.

LADY LETHAM. I am afraid, Mr Dayne, that you still continue in your quizzical humour, and that you are under the impression that you are talking with some innocent little blue-stocking come up from her country residence in Westmorland. If that be so, I assure you you are mistaken. I am no blue-stocking; I do not care for the colour. My stockings are rose. (*She lifts her skirts and exhibits some pretty ankles and legs.*) Blue stockings and floss silk will never collaborate with Mr Davenant. No, I'm not a blue-stocking. I think I've already told you that I live amid woods within view of a range of mountains, and my idea is this: that these natural landscapes of mine and my husband's might inspire a great work. You understand what I mean, Mr Dayne?

SEBASTIAN. Yes, I think I understand. But, you see, Mr Davenant never writes; he dictates.

LADY LETHAM. Then he must bring you with him. (*Turning from* SEBASTIAN *and looking round the room.*) But what a delightful life you live with him in this room, and in the intimate recesses of his soul, following every turn of his thought!

SEBASTIAN. Mr Davenant's thoughts are very dear to me: but in this world nobody, it would seem, is ever satisfied with his lot. I should like to have some time for my own thoughts – a wish so ridiculous for a secretary to entertain, I admit, that I regret sometimes I did not follow my father's advice and study for a fellowship. My father is a professor of the University; he wished me to study for a fellow-ship, but I had seen so many men wear their brains away in pursuit of a fellowship – running second for it, later turning up third, fourth, fifth and then giving up the hopeless struggle – that I said to my father: 'Fellowships are much more difficult to get to-day than they were in your time; I must think of something else'. He was angry – fathers always are angry with their sons –and my mother asked Lewis Davenant, who is my cousin, if he would give me this job.

LADY LETHAM. If you wish for time for your thoughts to mature in, you must have thoughts worth writing down. Are you a poet or a novelist?

SEBASTIAN. A poet – a volume of verses –

LADY LETHAM. I'm sure they're charming: they couldn't be else. You'll come with your cousin and spend a few weeks or a few months in my Westmorland castle! – the longer the better. Literature will occupy him in the mornings, and in the afternoons we shall go for drives; and the evenings will be passed in conversation. You will read me your verses, Mr Dayne?

SEBASTIAN. Is you husband, Lord Letham, also devoted to literature?

LADY LETHAM. To some extent. Till I married him he had hardly read a book.

SEBASTIAN. But you have been married some time?

LADY LETHAM. For so long that it seems that I never was anything else but married. My husband and I are excellent friends. Now, Mr Dayne, that I have confided to you my secret, you will pass it on to Mr Davenant, and will use all your persuasions to get him to accept my invitation? It will give me much pleasure to have you both with me in Westmorland. Good-bye. (SEBASTIAN *rings. Enter* MARTIN.)

SEBASTIAN (*to* MARTIN). There are still two gentlemen in the waiting-room. Will you show one of them up? (*Exeunt* MARTIN *and* LADY LETHAM. *A moment after she announces* MR MEYER.)

SEBASTIAN. I may as well tell you at once, Mr Meyer, that Mr Davenant is very busy making some alterations in his play. His luggage is being packed, and he starts for Vienna this evening. Be seated, I beg of you; I am his secretary, and if you have come to speak to him on any matter concerning literature I shall be glad to hear you.

MEYER. You have no doubt seen, and perhaps examined with some care Mr Krämer's translations?

SEBASTIAN. I have heard Mr Krämer's translations criticised adversely.

MEYER. I do not believe that any writer has suffered more from mistranslations than Mr Davenant. (*Taking some papers from his pocket.*) I will ask you to find a copy of *Elizabeth Cooper* and to follow me whilst I read. You know German?

SEBASTIAN. Not a word, unfortunately.

MEYER. I'm sorry, for without some knowledge of German it will be difficult for me to make plain the faults that my friend, Mr Krämer, has committed. All the same, if you follow me carefully I hope to be able to make you understand that my friend's text is a mess, and nothing else. No other words can express it – a mess, Mr Sebastian Dayne.

SEBASTIAN. But Mr Davenant starts to-night for Vienna.

MEYER. That is why I have come here so that he may know how he has been defamed, and the German language, too, has been defamed, by my friend Mr Krämer. I cannot find words to express the mess that he has made of Mr Davenant's books. It is sad to speak like this of a friend; and if it were not that my admiration is without limit for Mr Davenant, I should not speak. But after much consideration I decided that it would not be honourable for me to conceal the truth from Mr Davenant any longer.

SEBASTIAN. As Mr Davenant does not read translations, he does not suffer much.

MEYER. But Mr Davenant is going to Vienna, and will hear Mr Krämer's mistakes on the stage.

SEBASTIAN. Quite true; I hadn't thought of that. But he leaves to-night, and that is why he is so very busy, and why I am obliged to tell you,

Mr Meyer, that it would be impossible for me to examine the analysis you have made of your friend's translations. If you will leave your manuscript, I will submit it to our German professor at the University, and Mr Davenant will go into the matter when he returns from Vienna. (*He rings.*) Mr Meyer, I shall be so much obliged if you will excuse me. (*Enter* MARTIN.)

MARTIN. There is still one gentleman.

SEBASTIAN. Show him up. (MR MEYER *goes out with* MARTIN.) I see he hasn't left his manuscript. So much the better! The house overflows. (*A moment after* MARTIN *announces* LORD CARRA, *a young man elegantly dressed – a sportsman, one would judge by his appearance.*)

LORD CARRA. How do you do, Mr Davenant?

SEBASTIAN. I am not Mr Davenant, unfortunately. I do not know why I say unfortunately, for very likely it would be stupid to exchange youthful years for literary glory.

LORD CARRA. It would, indeed, Who would do it?

SEBASTIAN. Who indeed? Yet the object of your visit to Mr Davenant is literature?

LORD CARRA. Not to talk to him about his literature. I shouldn't know how to begin, for I haven't read one of his books.

SEBASTIAN. Not one?

LORD CARRA. It is my mother, Lady Carra, who reads his books.

SEBASTIAN. Then you have come, Lord Carra, to express to Mr Davenant the admiration that Mr Davenant's works have inspired in your mother?

LORD CARRA. Not exactly. I have come to ask him to do me a favour, and as you seem to know Mr Davenant very well –

SEBASTIAN. I am his secretary.

LORD CARRA. Then I can explain my errand to you. In one of Mr Davenant's books there is a man called Rudolph, and my mother never ceases to remind me that Rudolph and I are like each other, and that many things that have happened to Rudolph in the story have happened to me.

SEBASTIAN. Rudolph appears in several volumes. Can you tell me in which these unfortunate coincidences occur?

LORD CARRA. I'm afraid I can't. You see, I didn't ask my mother, who would have thought she was frightening me. But it isn't pleasant all the same, to be told that one is following in the footsteps of Rudolph, who, mother says, is making for an untimely end. Now what is going to be the end of Rudolph?

SEBASTIAN. It appears that Rudolph's suicide depends on his meeting with a certain woman with pale eyes and red hair.

LORD CARRA. Couldn't something be done to prevent his meeting her?

SEBASTIAN. Perhaps. I cannot promise, but will use my influence with Mr Davenant. He may be able to devise a different end. He once spoke of bankruptcy. But you wouldn't like that? Could you suggest an end for Rudolph?

LORD CARRA. I should like him to win the Derby.

SEBASTIAN. So should I. We all like a man who wins the Derby.

LORD CARRA. Thank you. You understand my position? It appears that anything Rudolph does influences me to do likewise.

SEBASTIAN. So you have come to the reasonable conclusion that it would be well for you to influence Rudolph?

LORD CARRA. I am much obliged to you for your kindly offer of help. (SEBASTIAN *rings. Enter* MARTIN.) Good-bye, Mr Dayne. (*Exeunt* LORD CARRA *and* MARTIN.)

SEBASTIAN. The 'at home' day is ended, and my cousin can come downstairs. (*He rings a different bell.* DAVENANT *enters, a man of about fifty-two, of good figure, well dressed and well preserved.*)

DAVENANT. It's all settled, my dear Sebastian. I'm not going to Vienna.

SEBASTIAN. Not going to Vienna! – and everything is ready; all the alterations made in the text and the trunks packed! Not going to Vienna! The Austrian capital turned inside out; all the literary aristocracy invited; the chickens killed! I shall have to write twenty letters, and the first night will be a fizzle without you.

DAVENANT. But people do not go to the theatre to see the author.

SEBASTIAN. My dear Lewis, you should not let your humours get the better of you.

DAVENANT. I know, I know; and have been struggling with myself since early morning. At ten o'clock I decided to go, but at half-past ten my resolution began to wane.

SEBASTIAN. But why won't you go? Tell me. Your trunk is packed; I'll take you to the station; a short sea passage, a few hours in the Orient express, and the train will draw up alongside of the platform and you will be met by a crowd of poets, painters and politicians.

DAVENANT. My dear Sebastian, though the crowd were all lawny bishops, it would still be a crowd, crowd or mob. I couldn't face it. And the subsequent proceedings! You spoke of chickens. Chickens mean a banquet, a banquet means speeches, speeches of how art reconciles nations, and how the fact of having German taught in the schools will make England love Germany better, and that the Germans by learning English in their schools will be able to arrive at a better understanding of a nation which, after all, is the same nation, for there is a great deal of Anglo-Saxon blood still in England. After half-an-hour of this nonsense I shall have to rise and talk about Shakespeare, saying that I have not come hither to speak in my own name, but in the name of English literature, of which I am an unworthy representative. Then I or another will have to explain the relations of Art to Nature, that Nature is something more and something less than Art; that Art is not Nature, because it is Art; and that Nature is not Art, because it is Nature; and that the stupendous creations of the artist are no less mysterious than those of God himself.

SEBASTIAN. Charming, delightful; very like yourself, in your best vein; but what about the disappointment on the platform? – for I shall not be able to write to them all. Can't I persuade you that you want a change from this provincial town in which you have chosen to bury yourself? The poets and literati who rise up in your imagination to frighten you will amuse you when you meet them in a café at midnight, and the fuss won't be as disagreeable as you think for. The Viennese ladies will remind you of the old days in Paris, and if I know you at all, Lewis, you will come back to us talking endlessly of this journey to Vienna; it will become one of your most precious memories. You always say nobody has cultivated memory as you have. Go to Vienna.

DAVENANT. But you see, Sebastian, our ages are different. (*Enter* MARTIN.)

MARTIN. Will you see Mr Godby now, sir?

DAVENANT. Mr Godby!

MARTIN. The gentleman that has been waiting to see you for the last two hours.

SEBASTIAN. A sailor.

DAVENANT. The first admirer that the sea has brought me, so far as I know; so whilst you're copying in the corrections, Sebastian –

SEBASTIAN. Then you are going to Vienna?

DAVENANT. (*testily*). I didn't say I was going to Vienna. You always want to bring things to a head. (*To* MARTIN.) Mr Godby wishes to see me, and as I've nothing to do I think I'll interview this ancient mariner.

MARTIN. He isn't an old man, sir.

DAVENANT. Old or young, show him up. He is a mariner, if nothing else.
(*Exit and re-enter* MARTIN *and* MR GODBY.)

MARTIN. Mr Godby, sir.

DAVENANT. I'm sorry you've been kept waiting.

GODBY It doesn't matter, since I haven't had to go without seeing you.

127

DAVENANT. But I'm told you've been kept waiting all the afternoon.

GODBY (*handing* DAVENANT *a book*). Secretary sent me this 'ere book to read.

DAVENANT. (*taking the book*). The Koran! (*To* SEBASTIAN.) I think you might have found a more interesting book for Mr Godby.

SEBASTIAN. Shall I go and copy the alterations?

DAVENANT. If you like. (*Exit* SEBASTIAN.)

GODBY. I asked Secretary for the paper, but he said that you didn't receive newspapers, and that your visitors were always given this 'ere book. (*Handing* DAVENANT *a box of Turkish Delight.*) A little present from Priscilla. She wouldn't leave go of me till I promised to give it to you.

DAVENANT. A box of Turkish Delight?

GODBY. From Priscilla, my wife three weeks come Tuesday. So no more letters and poems, that is what I have come to tell you. If Priscilla had known what you be like, you would have had them all back.

DAVENANT. What I am like?

GODBY. Her notion of the author of – of *Elizabeth Cooper* was a young fellow all scarves and riding breeches. Bless your 'eart! I saw through you when she read out the number of books you had written. I says to 'er, 'Priscilla, it ain't possible; he be a man of past fifty' – that's ten years older than myself; and when I tell you that she thinks me an old 'un, you can judge for yourself what she'd think of you. Now let's get a good look at ye. The very spit of what I told Priscilla you were! A man about fifty or fifty-two; the hair grown very thin on the top; grey about the ears and in the whiskers; getting a bit bluff in the bows and broad in the beam.

DAVENANT. My secretary mentioned that you're a sailor, Mr Godby.

GODBY. Second mate aboard the brigantine the Hannah Maria, at your service. Now come, Mr Davenant, don't you think a man like yourself might employ his time better than by sending letters and poems to a girl like Priscilla?

DAVENANT. I know nothing of what you're talking – absolutely nothing!

GODBY. Well, if you don't know 'er as Priscilla Godby, maybe you know her as Priscilla Jones?

DAVENANT. I don't remember ever having heard either of those names before.

GODBY. You won't deny your own handwriting and your signature at the end of the letters? (*He fumbles in his pocket and hands some letters to* MR DAVENANT.)

DAVENANT. (*after looking at letters*). This is not my signature, as I shall be able to prove to you in a moment. (*He goes to writing-table, takes*

128

up a pen, and writes on a piece of paper.) Will you compare my signature, which you have seen me write, with the signature at the end of those letters? Are they the same?

GODBY. A man doesn't always sign the same.

DAVENANT. Is there any resemblance whatsoever?

GODBY. I can't say there is.

DAVENANT. You mentioned that Mrs Godby had read some of my books?

GODBY. Yes, she has read all your books, and written you many letters. They cannot all have gone astray.

DAVENANT. Mr Dayne answers my letters to correspondents who are not known to me personally.

GODBY. Well, this is a pretty how-de-do! So all them letters aren'*t* yours, but Secretary's?

DAVENANT. That is the only explanation I can think of. But allow me. (*He rings.*) (*Enter* MARTIN.)

DAVENANT. Martin, will you tell Mr Dayne I should like to speak to him? (*Exit* MARTIN.)

DAVENANT. Priscilla Godby; no, I don't remember anyone of that name. Mr Dayne often mentions the names of my correspondents, and I am sure I never heard him speak of that name. But what is the matter, Mr Godby?

GODBY. I'm thinking how Priscilla is going to take this 'ere news. What a squall! She will be took aback, and all standing. It was all right to do a bit of teasing about yer age, telling her you was an old 'un, hair thin on the top and grey about the whiskers, but I can't bring myself to tell her that all them letters which she has been a-treasuring up was not written by you, but by Secretary.

DAVENANT. But why tell her?

GODBY. Supposin' one of these days you was to run across each other?

DAVENANT. In a world composed mainly of unreasonable accidents such a thing might happen.

GODBY. It might indeed.

DAVENANT. But, Mr Godby, I must plead his youth, and that the correspondence was harmless and gave her a great deal of pleasure.

GODBY. It did that.

DAVENANT. So perhaps it would be better for you to tell her that I am not only the ugly old fellow whom you so admirably summarised in three or four telling touches, but an old curmudgeon who received you very uncivilly and told you that his house was overflowing with letters from all sorts and kinds of women, and that to get rid of a packet now and then was – How would you word it, Mr Godby?

GODBY. Like getting the pumps to work. (*Enter* SEBASTIAN.)

DAVENANT. Mr Godby has come for his wife's letters.

SEBASTIAN. Mrs Godby!

GODBY. Priscilla Jones that was.

SEBASTIAN. Priscilla Jones! Priscilla Jones!

DAVENANT. It would be just as well to avoid prevarication, Sebastian, and to come to the point; for it appears of a certainty that you have been carrying on a correspondence with Miss Priscilla Jones, sending her poems – which you had, of course, a perfect right to do in your own name, but not in mine. Really, Sebastian, this last pleasantry of yours surprises me, and in the presence of Mr Godby I beg to protest.

SEBASTIAN. But I told you, Lewis, that Priscilla Jones had written about *Elizabeth Cooper.*

DAVENANT. Very likely, and it may be that I authorised you to write and thank her for her letter. But I did not tell you to continue the correspondence.

GODBY. He sent her poems, Mr Davenant.

SEBASTIAN. She was not your wife when I sent her poems; and if she had been, it seems to me that a poem may be sent to the married and to the single, to the young and to the old – to everybody, except, of course, to people on their honeymoon. Now how long have you been married?

GODBY. Three weeks come Tuesday.

SEBASTIAN. Your wife hasn't received a poem from me within the last three weeks. So I really fail to see the cause of your complaint.

DAVENANT. I too fail to see it, Mr Godby, and I think you will too if you will consider it. Mr Dayne did not know that Priscilla Jones was about to become Priscilla Godby, nor did he send her poems in his own name, but in mine. I am the aggrieved person if the poems were bad ones.

GODBY. I wouldn't say they were bad, though they were only Secretary's.

DAVENANT. Well, then, Mr Godby, may we agree to let bygones be bygones?

GODBY. We may Mr Davenant, and with all my 'eart. All the same Priscilla would like to have her letters back; naught but reasonable in that, now she's married.

DAVENANT. Nothing more reasonable in this world. Sebastian, we call upon you to produce Mrs Godby's letters.

SEBASTIAN. I wish Mr Godby had written to me about this matter before, for it will be difficult for me to produce these letters at once.

You see, Mr Godby, I have been collecting for some time past the letters that Mr Davenant receives from the admirers of his books. We have several letters from the lady you had the pleasure of meeting in the parlour to-day, Lady Letham. She is one of our latest correspondents, but there have been many before her. We have received five-and-twenty letters from Lady Dartry; several from Lady Onger; Lady Cong is represented by five letters. We have letters from many ladies of high position among the French aristocracy. Madame de Belboeuf writes to us frequently, Madame de Coetlogon occasionally. If I remember right, La Marquise d'Osmond is represented by at least fifty-one letters. (*Going over to a casket.*) In this casket, Mr Godby, are letters that would paint my cousin's name for ever memorable even if he had not written any books. (*Opening the casket and taking out three or four letters.*) And these forty-three letters were written by the delicious Gabrielle von Hoenstadt.

GODBY. You pay out your jaw-tackle all right, young fellow, and them fine names come mighty easy off your tongue, but I do not happen to hear the name of Priscilla Jones amongst them. Now if you would be just good enough to see if you could find Mrs Godby's letters at the bottom of this 'ere casket –

SEBASTIAN. Priscilla's letters in this casket, Mr Godby! This casket is reserved exclusively for ladies of title. Even baronets' wives do not enter here.

DAVENANT. My dear Sebastian, I protest, and warmly, against this fooling! Mr Godby has come here on a serious errand. I beg you to put that casket away and attend to his request, which is a reasonable one, that you return his wife's letters.

SEBASTIAN. I mentioned a few names, my dear Lewis, for I wished to bring home to Mr Godby the great volume of correspondence I have to attend to. My time –

DAVENANT. Put down that casket. Your wife's letters, Mr Godby, shall be returned to her. It is quite undecided whether I go to Vienna or not; and as there are many matters about which I have to speak to my cousin –

GODBY. The alterations you're to make in the play?

DAVENANT. Yes, yes; and in my luggage. Your letters shall be returned to your wife as soon as I return from Vienna; and if I do not go to Vienna, they shall be returned at once, within the next few days. And please to understand, Mr Godby, that I'm grateful to you for your visit; it has made known to me certain things of which I was without any knowledge. I shall have to put my house in order, Mr

Godby. (*He rings bell.*)

GODBY. Thank'ee, thank'ee, sir. (*Enter* MARTIN.) I have the honour to bid ye good-afternoon, Mr Davenant, and thank'ee. If you ever wants anything in the farin' line, such as a parrot or what not – at your service! (DAVENANT *accompanies* GODBY *to the door.* SEBASTIAN *crosses the stage in meditation.*)

DAVENANT. Once more, Sebastian, put those letters back into the casket, and try to remember for the future that you're no longer a baby boy. Thirty is a man's age, and men do not indulge in practical joking. (*The men stand and gaze, and then begin to laugh.*) I was obliged to speak a little severely when Mr Godby was here, but I'm not such an old fogey, Sebastian, as not to understand the humour of this correspondence. You didn't say, by the way, that they were my poems, did you?

SEBASTIAN. No, Lewis. The letters were, I assure you, more circumspect than Godby would have led you to think. The poems were sent out of curiosity, for I wished to know how they would strike the ordinary reader.

DAVENANT. Your poems?

SEBASTIAN. Yes, my poems, but –

DAVENANT. But the letters were signed Lewis Davenant. I suppose time must hang a little heavy on your hands in this provincial town, and I'll overlook the escapade, but don't begin another one. I trusted you with my correspondence, and – I'll say no more.

SEBASTIAN. I am truly repentant, sir. It shall not occur again.

DAVENANT. Among the many names you mentioned just now when you were making fun of that poor simple man Godby was a name that caught my ear – Gabrielle von Hoenstadt. You've spoken to me of her before. She has written, it appears, some very pleasant and witty letters, and it is to her influence that I owe the production of *Elizabeth Cooper* at Vienna!

SEBASTIAN. It is indeed to her that you owe it, for ever since she has read the novel she seems to have thought of little else. It is a pity you didn't read her letters. I pressed you to glance through them – a mere glance would have been enough. Listen to this. (*Reading.*) 'I am tired of the rain, and of myself, and of everything except you. I have never heard your voice. I won't see or hear you, for it would be a catastrophe to fall in love with the man in you. I will only be in love with the author'. I cannot understand, Lewis, that you do not recognise her in these few words as one of your own women.

DAVENANT. Speaking to me across the seas. Repeat the lines, Sebastian. (SEBASTIAN *repeats them.*) A perfervid imagination, no doubt – a

132

whimsy, but whether one of the blood or brain, or both, I cannot say.

SEBASTIAN. May I read a little more?

DAVENANT. I'll look into *her* letters myself later. So you recognise her as of the Davenant kin?

SEBASTIAN. As one who might easily fall in love with you.

DAVENANT. She might have in the years gone by.

SEBASTIAN (*turning over the letters*). She writes forty-three, asking you to come to Vienna. Yet you won't go.

DAVENANT. I'm afraid, Sebastian, that your correspondence with Priscilla Jones has turned your head a little, and that your idea for the moment is that the business of every man is to rush across Europe in pursuit of a woman.

SEBASTIAN. Do you never wish, Lewis, to risk everything – to take a header over the cliff's edge?

DAVENANT. A header after a Naiad whom I have never seen, and of whom I only know through a few extracts from letters? (SEBASTIAN *presses the letters on* DAVENANT.) Later I'll look into them.

SEBASTIAN (*returning to the correspondence*). She sends you the name of the hotel where you are to meet her. You are not to go to the Grand Hotel, Hotel Bristol, Krantz, Imperial, or Sacher, for she 'would not caramboler with her brothers and friends *en sortant de chez vous*'. How amusing she is! (*Reading.*) 'You will stay in the Meissal and Schadn to please me'. A mere detail this, but characteristic. You are to send her a note by the hotel messenger, and he will bring back an answer saying she will be with you at a certain hour. And the next day she's going to introduce you to her cousin, with whom you are going to lunch. Could anything be more charming? – and yet you hesitate.

DAVENANT. It is true that I might like her as a friend; but is it worth my while to go to Vienna for a friendship?

SEBASTIAN. But there is an alternative: you might both love each other.

DAVENANT. In that case the disaster would be greater; for what should I do with her at the end of a week? Ask her to come to Paris?

SEBASTIAN. That is exactly how I imagine the adventure.

DAVENANT. Ah! or bring her hither to settle down.

SEBASTIAN. She wouldn't like Rockminster.

DAVENANT. I should have to bid her good-bye at the end of a week, saying: 'Dear Gabrielle, we have passed a charming week together; but as Rockminster is not to your taste, I'll leave you where I found you, looking forward, of course, to seeing you when I return to Vienna'.

SEBASTIAN. If these women knew what a man of letters really is, they would seek their lovers among soldiers, sailors, diplomats, merchants, even doctors –anywhere rather than among men of letters.

DAVENANT. It may be that I might still find some favour in her eyes, but –

SEBASTIAN. In your striped trousers and morning coat I assure you –

DAVENANT. The wise man knows that it would be stupid to attempt to continue his youth; for even if he could do so by the aid of striped trousers and morning coats, he would be robbing life of its variety, whereas by a little act of renunciation he creates a new life quite different from the old.

SEBASTIAN. I have often heard you say a man's love is attracted in the beginning by the eye, and that his pride in her poetry, her music, and her pictures comes afterwards; that these are condiments which he sucks at his leisure; but that a woman's love – I am still quoting you – arises out of her imagination, enabling her to perform miracles, to straighten the hunchback and to raise the dwarf from 4 ft. 6 in. to 6 ft. 2 in., and to answer an impertinent friend who reminds her that her lover has to stand up at table that she did not notice his height before, but now that her attention has been called to it she can see that he is somewhat short.

DAVENANT. And in pursuance of your theories –

SEBASTIAN. Your theory –

DAVENANT. You think that Gabrielle will re-create me out of her imagination, and that I shall appear to her as a dancing faun?

SEBASTIAN. I don't know about the faun, but as a soul of fire certainly; and that you have come to Vienna to speak in the name of England will be a great help.

DAVENANT. I suppose it will, and the laurel crown too will be a help. Germany's idea of art is somebody crowning somebody, and generally a fat woman does the crowning. But, Sebastian, why all this anxiety to pack me up and send me to Vienna? Is it that you want a holiday, and would like to bestow your holiday upon some other correspondent? Is there another? My good wishes in that event; only I beg of you to do your literary courting in your own name, that is all.

SEBASTIAN. No, you're wrong; there is nobody, unfortunately ... By the way, Lewis, Lady Letham called here this morning and asked me to remind you that she hopes you will accept her invitation to spend some time with her in Westmorland. She owns certain ranges of mountains, and these are at your disposal.

DAVENANT. For my inspiration, no doubt. Now what is this new admirer like – her age?

SEBASTIAN. I should say from thirty to thirty-five; very refined, dainty, beautifully dressed, with exquisite hands and feet. She is staying with her sister, Lady Ewhurst.

DAVENANT. At Charming Dean! (*Aside*.) It seems a pity not to try one's luck, just once, she being in the neighbourhood and Sebastian away. (*Aloud*.) So while you are away, Sebastian, I think I shall write to her and ask her to come and see me.

SEBASTIAN. While I am away?

DAVENANT. Well, you see, somebody will have to go to Vienna to look after my play.

SEBASTIAN. Will you send me?

DAVENANT. Why not? Somebody must see that the play is properly rehearsed; you don't know German, but Gabrielle does. Now, let me see, this is the third – no, the fourth of April. I will give you a month's holiday – five weeks, if you like. For you, Sebastian, Gabrielle and her pleasure; for me, long country walks and long evenings with my old friend Ruskin. You will return within a month, and we will begin work again.

SEBASTIAN. What a delicious adventure! What a delicious adventure!

DAVENANT. Mine or yours?

SEBASTIAN. Mine, of course,

DAVENANT. It wouldn't be like you to refuse an adventure, so I'll give you some money. (*He sits at his desk*.) Here is a note of credit on my bank. The journey is an expensive one but it is really necessary that somebody should be by to look after my play. One moment, Sebastian; you will have to travel in my name.

SEBASTIAN. Why?

DAVENANT. Did you not say just now that Gabrielle had created me out of my books with the aid of her imagination? Would you disappoint her? Go in my name, and unite the two temptations – youth and fame – and you'll be irresistible.

SEBASTIAN. Introduce myself to Gabrielle as the author of *Elizabeth Cooper*?

DAVENANT. Why not, since I give you leave? She might love you if you went to her as my secretary, but not – well, not so ecstatically as she will if you go to her as the author of *Elizabeth Cooper*.

SEBASTIAN. But I'm a poet.

DAVENANT. And a very charming poet.

SEBASTIAN. She might like my verses and think me very clever, but she wouldn't believe that I had written all those books and plays.

DAVENANT. A woman in love believes easily. An imagination that is

135

strong enough to straighten a dwarf's back will find no difficulty in adding a few years to your age. She will see crow's-feet around the eyes, and grey hair about the ears. After all, there are only twenty years between us, and my appearance isn't known except to my personal friends; it hasn't travelled in photographs all over the world like those of most authors. By the way, you always write to the photographers who ask if they may add my portrait to their gallery of literary celebrities that I dislike modern photography, and will never sit until the daguerreotype is re-established.

SEBASTIAN. Yes, I write all that – but the question now is, whether I am to go to Vienna.

DAVENANT. Well, then?

SEBASTIAN. I'm afraid I couldn't, Lewis. One day she would find out that I had lied to her, and would hate me and herself for ever afterwards.

DAVENANT. But you don't intend to pass your life in Vienna. A little while ago you called on me to remember that I was sacrificing a memory. Now, in my turn, I will remind you that you said: Nobody in love should be disappointed. The maker of such aphorisms is usually the first culprit. (*Enter* MARTIN *with a packet in her hand.*)

MARTIN. This packet has just come, sir. (*She hands him the packet and goes out.*)

DAVENANT (*on opening the packet*). You cannot guess what is in this box.

SEBASTIAN. Of course I can; something from Gabrielle. I know it's from Gabrielle.

DAVENANT. Gabrielle has sent her portrait and a letter.

SEBASTIAN. Let me see it. Let me see it.

DAVENANT (*hands him the miniature – reading letter*). Only a short letter, in which she tells me what train I am to travel by. Listen, Sebastian. 'I won't wait much longer. I am not ashamed to rush after you, but I very soon will be ashamed of thinking so much of a man without even knowing if he deserves it. It makes me feel what I do not want to be – a little fool'. You see, Sebastian, there is no time to be lost. (*He takes up the box.*) What! another miniature! (*The two men stand looking at* GABRIELLE'S *pictures in the middle of the stage.*)

SEBASTIAN. She is delightful, delicious, divine! (*Looking round at* DAVENANT.) What is yours like, Lewis?

DAVENANT. This one is a full length.

SEBASTIAN. Let me see it.

DAVENANT. I don't think I shall show it to you. No, I don't think that

I ought to show it to you.

SEBASTIAN. But if I am going to Vienna?

DAVENANT. So you're going to Vienna?

SEBASTIAN. Of course I'm going to Vienna. You've given me the money and the holiday. Let me see the portrait.

DAVENANT. You're going to Vienna, and will get the lady.

SEBASTIAN. Let me see it.

DAVENANT. Sebastian, you want everything, but you're not going to get everything.

SEBASTIAN. Now, Lewis, don't spit gall into my cup of bliss.

DAVENANT. Both were addressed to me. By the way, Sebastian, there's no time to be lost; you have only just time to pack to catch the train at Southampton. I see you've already quite lost your head. But I hope you'll not forget my play. You'll write to me at once, and attend all the rehearsals.

SEBASTIAN. Yes, yes! Good-bye, Lewis! (*He goes out.* DAVENANT *looks at one of his pictures; then he opens the window and rings the bell. Enter* MARTIN.)

DAVENANT. If you look through the telescope in the library you will see Jupiter; then you can bring in the lamp.

MARTIN. Yes, sir. (*Exit* MARTIN. DAVENANT *remains at the window, smoking, as the curtain falls.*)

ACT II

SCENE: DAVENANT'S *country house. A room opening out on a large garden. Light summer furniture. A river is seen in the distance. The sun is shining.*

A month later; about two in the afternoon.

When the curtain rises, DAVENANT *and* LADY LETHAM *are walking to and fro –in the garden.* DAVENANT *carries a pruning shears in his hand and is busy cutting roses.*

LADY LETHAM. My hands are full, you really must not cut any more.

DAVENANT. Just *one* more. (*He cuts another.*)

LADY LETHAM. What a beautiful rose, purple, almost black. (*Coming down stage.*) As I was saying, my sister and I were looked upon by mother in the light of lets and hindrances, and were kept in the schoolroom as long as possible, and when she had to bring us downstairs we were given to understand that we must suit ourselves with husbands without delay; two years was the time allotted, convents were spoken of in case of failure, so we just had to take the men that proposed first, and Henrietta and I married tiresome men twenty years older than ourselves. (DAVENANT *points to the sofa and they sit down.*)

DAVENANT. With the usual pleasant results, I suppose.

LADY LETHAM. Pleasant results! I don't understand.

DAVENANT. Don't you?

LADY LETHAM. Oh, I see. You're quite right, for within a year Henrietta and myself were engaged in arranging our own lives, my sister conducting hers discreetly with due regard to appearances, whereas I took every risk, seeming to court disaster, and would certainly have ended in getting myself talked about if –

DAVENANT. If the wise ant had not begged the foolish fly to bethink herself.

LADY LETHAM (*laughing*). Yes, just so. Henrietta sent for me, I've forgotten for what reason, something she had heard. A certain journey to Ireland; it may have been that; and seeing that I was in for a lecture and in hopes of cutting it short, I said: "As we have to go to hell one day, the sooner we get there the better."

DAVENANT. To hell!

LADY LETHAM. I don't mean a theological hell. Henrietta's intention in sending for me was to make plain a truth often overlooked: that it was not absolutely necessary to forget to order one's husband's dinner if one intended to misbehave oneself in the afternoon.

DAVENANT. But your sister's counsel did not influence the foolish fly.

LADY LETHAM. Yes, it did. I think I was more careful; at least, for a time I was.

DAVENANT. And during that time, long or short, your husband had no cause to complain of the housekeeping, and you ceased to leave your letters lying about.

LADY LETHAM. I never left my letters lying about.

DAVENANT. I was speaking metaphorically. You introduced some circumspection into your love affairs.

LADY LETHAM. But I soon broke out again, and the long and the short of it is that, finding myself unable to play what Henrietta would call the game, I sent my lovers away. Henrietta was surprised, but I couldn't do else, being by nature intemperate.

DAVENANT. Intemperate!

LADY LETHAM. I do not mean that I was addicted to drink; if I had been I should have had to choose between total abstinence and continual intoxication. (*Pause.*) You've often asked me to tell you about myself; I have told you, and I think it is time for me to go. (*She rises, and they go up the stage together. In the middle of the stage* LADY LETHAM *stops suddenly.*) You're expecting Mr Dayne back from Vienna?

DAVENANT. Yes, he is on his way back and will arrive to-morrow, perhaps this evening. He may come by the next train from Rockminster.

LADY LETHAM. So our long mornings together have come to an end. You will never dictate to me again.

DAVENANT. Am I not going to Westmorland in the autumn?

LADY LETHAM. I hope so, indeed, but I shall not be able to act as your secretary, not in the mornings certainly; I never appear till luncheon; all the business of the house is transacted in my bedroom.

DAVENANT. Lord Letham's dinner is ordered there.

LADY LETHAM. Yes, and everybody else's dinner. I am afraid you cannot count upon my help. I should only disappoint you, and a man with ideas in his head waiting to have them taken down is apt to lose his temper.

DAVENANT. But after luncheon?

LADY LETHAM. After luncheon we shall go out driving, for you must see the mountain ranges that I told Mr Dayne might inspire you, a suggestion that seemed to amuse him. Is it true that time and place count for little or nothing in the artist's life?

DAVENANT. You must not pay too much attention to what Mr Dayne says.

LADY LETHAM. He told me that all your writing was done by dictation, so I said that I hoped he would come too. And now good-bye. (*She turns up stage.*)

DAVENANT. You will not forget that you're dining with me at Rockminster to-night?

LADY LETHAM. I shall not forget. (*Exit by garden.* DAVENANT *goes out with her and comes back a moment later. He crosses the stage in silence.*)

DAVENANT. Has she her eye on Sebastian, I wonder - on that irresponsible youth who looks forward to telling me his adventures, which means that he is in love with Gabrielle? (*Enter* MARTIN *with a letter,* L.)

MARTIN. Fletcher has just brought this letter, sir. It came yesterday to Rockminster, and, knowing that you weren't returning till this evening, he thought it better to bring it here.

DAVENANT. He did quite right. (*Takes the letter.*) Wait a moment. Sebastian's handwriting. (*He reads.*) This is too much! Really, this is too much. (*After a pause he bursts out laughing.*) What a splendid impertinence. He even wants to turn me out of my own house. (*Reading by fragments.*) 'My dear cousin, my dear Lewis, you are so good, so kind. Lend me Claremont Villa for two days only, and as I am still Lewis Davenant will you oblige me by becoming Sebastian Dayne? We shall arrive –' WE!! 'We shall arrive tomorrow'. To-morrow. When did you say, Martin, this letter came?

MARTIN. (*comes down a little*). Last night, sir.

DAVENANT. Then it's to-day. He may be here ... they may be here at any moment. (*To Martin.*) Now, Martin, listen to me attentively. I can count upon you, I think.

MARTIN. It wasn't yesterday I entered your service, sir, and you know –

DAVENANT. Yes, I know. But to-day, Martin, it isn't on my account, alas! We must make way for the young folk. Now this is what you are to do. Mr Dayne may arrive at any moment, and with a lady. You know that he went to Vienna to look after my play, but I don't think I told you that he is travelling in my name. I can't go into the matter more explicitly, but when he comes you are to call him Mr Davenant. (MARTIN *begins to laugh.*) It would take too long to explain. You are to stay here to look after them. And while they are here you are to speak to Mr Dayne as Mr Davenant. I think I can rely on you. Mr Dayne will not stay more than two days.

MARTIN. And you, sir?

DAVENANT. I must get back to Rockminster. What time is the next train?

MARTIN. The train from Rockminster has just come in.

DAVENANT. And the train back will be going out in a few minutes; I shall just catch it.

MARTIN. But if you miss it, sir, and Mr Davenant should arrive with the lady?

DAVENANT. Then, Martin, I am Mr Sebastian Dayne. I have some books and papers to collect.

MARTIN. I will send them after you.

DAVENANT. You ought to know by this time that I never allow myself to be separated from my manuscripts. (*Exit.*)

MARTIN. (*with a gesture*). So he is to be Mr Dayne for the next day or two. (*The bell rings.*) Well, I never. Here comes the new Mr Davenant, I suppose. (*Exit hurriedly. A moment after enter* SEBASTIAN *and the* COUNTESS VON HOENSTADT.)

MARTIN. Mr Dayne will be down presently, sir. (SEBASTIAN *and* GABRIELLE *come down the stage.* MARTIN *goes out.*)

GABRIELLE. Didst thou not hear her say, 'Mr Dayne'?

SEBASTIAN. Yes, she said Dayne. Lewis must have instructed her in accordance with my letter, saying that as I was still Mr Davenant, I'd be obliged if he would become Mr Dayne for a short while. As the joke began with him he thinks he had better see it through. How good he is, you see how good he is, and before it is too late –

GABRIELLE. I want to see this vieux farceur (how do you say *vieux farceur* in English – old joker?)

SEBASTIAN. You really must not speak of Mr Davenant –

GABRIELLE. Who should be very proud to receive letters from a Vienna lady , and ought to have come himself, and not sent his secretary to make a little fool of me.

SEBASTIAN. I hope you're not sorry, Gabrielle. I'm certain that you wouldn't have cared for Lewis if he had gone to Vienna, would you? Do you think you would?

GABRIELLE. Do I think I would fall in love with a man who would not read my letters? No, never! Come hither and do not frown, but listen to me. Mr Davenant must be punished.

SEBASTIAN. For what?

GABRIELLE. How many times have you asked me that question? And I have answered it always: for having dared to play a paltry prank on me, treating me as if I were a little servant-girl!

141

SEBASTIAN. My dear Gabrielle, Lewis Davenant never saw your letters. If he had, he would have gone to Germany, and – (*He moves forward with the intention of taking her in his arms. She evades him.*)

GABRIELLE. You read him some pages from my letters. You told me so; and still he thought I was a little fool, and perhaps a cocotte. But no. If he had thought that he would have gone to Vienna, for men like Mr Davenant like cocottes much better than Viennese ladies; so it was quite well that he sent you instead of coming himself. Ach! my pictures should have told him I was neither one nor the other.

SEBASTIAN. All the arrangements were made before your pictures arrived.

GABRIELLE. *Mein lieber Gott!* that the man who wrote *Elizabeth Cooper* should have thought that I could mistake his secretary for the author of seventeen volumes! *Mein lieber Gott* sounds better than your God *tout court.*

SEBASTIAN. I don't know whether it does or not. But that door may open any minute and Lewis Davenant walk in; so once more I beg of you to remember that he did not foresee what has happened; he couldn't have.

GABRIELLE. You remind me of a child who would play a prank upon his parents, but gets frightened at the last moment. But I'm not a child; and if you do not want me to go straight back to Vienna, you will tell him the story exactly as we prepared it on the battlements of the castle at Heidelberg, exactly word for word. (*Enter* DAVENANT.)

DAVENANT. So you've come! Your note arrived only a few minutes ago, and after reading it I ran upstairs to get some books and papers, and now I shall only just have time to catch the train; so if you'll excuse me –

SEBASTIAN. My dear Sebastian, you needn't hurry away, for, run as fast as ever you can, you'll not succeed in catching a train that left the station as we came up the road. Gabrielle, allow me to introduce you to my cousin, Sebastian Dayne, also my secretary.

DAVENANT (*bowing*). Have you had a pleasant journey?

SEBASTIAN. Very. We left our luggage at Rockminster, and came on here with just enough for two days. (*To* GABRIELLE.) Dearest, I am sure you would like to go to your room. (*To* MARTIN.) What room have you ready for – for – madam?

MARTIN (*hesitatingly*). The room –

DAVENANT. The room overlooking the river.

SEBASTIAN. That will do splendidly, quite right.

MARTIN. If madam will come with me –

GABRIELLE. I will leave you with your secretary for a little while. (*In a low tone.*) Dearest, I love you! (*Exeunt* MARTIN *and* GABRIELLE.)

SEBASTIAN (*after following* GABRIELLE *a few steps, returns rapidly to* DAVENANT). Thank you, Lewis. (*He takes both his hands.*) I don't know how to thank you. I hope we are not putting you to too much trouble.

DAVENANT (*in very good humour*). Not at all; stay as long as you please, Sebastian. I am delighted to see you. Your letter didn't reach me until ten minutes ago, and after giving Martin some necessary instructions I was just about to run away. But we have no time to lose. Tell me, and tell me quickly, is that Gabrielle?

SEBASTIAN. Didn't you know her? She is very like her miniature. (*Takes the miniature from his pocket.*)

DAVENANT. I hardly saw her – and in a hat! My dear Sebastian, you have managed this affair splendidly. Now, admit! – wasn't it a good idea of mine to send you to Vienna? You appear very much in love with each other. One could see that from the way she turned to look at you as she went out. It is all delightful, delightful! I congratulate you, Sebastian. Show me the miniature. Yes, it's very like her. And now tell me everything in a few words.

SEBASTIAN. It would take too long.

DAVENANT. But I must hear all about it.

SEBASTIAN. You want to know how we met?

DAVENANT. Of course I do.

SEBASTIAN. In the most original way . . . in the train.

DAVENANT (*more and more amused*). No!

SEBASTIAN. I got into the train at Ostend, and within an hour's journey of Vienna, at a station called - I can't remember the name – three ladies and a gentleman climbed into my carriage.

DAVENANT. One was –

SEBASTIAN. Gabrielle returning to Vienna to meet me.

DAVENANT. To meet Lewis Davenant, since it was me she expected – but to meet you, since it is you she loves. But I beg your pardon. Go on.

SEBASTIAN. Well, I was about to say that the gentleman who accompanied the ladies was very distinguished-looking, an old friend of the family, Baron von Allmen is his name. The two ladies, the Countess Bertha von Maurog and the Baronne von Studenberg.

DAVENANT. I see you already possess some knowledge of Viennese society. I suppose you met these people afterwards?

SEBASTIAN. Oh yes, heaps of times.

DAVENANT. Well, go on with your story.

SEBASTIAN. I helped them to arrange their luggage in the racks, and, seeing that I was English, Gabrielle – for it was she – spoke to me in English, and we hadn't been talking together for long before I began to ask myself where I had seen her face – for I had seen it before, of that I was sure: but for a long time I couldn't think where. All of a sudden I remembered the miniature. But it seemed too improbable. The Baron was explaining something to the Countess von Maurog and the Baronne von Studenberg; Gabrielle did not take part in this conversation, nor show the slightest interest in it, and I began to wonder how this was; and whilst I was wondering I caught her stealing glances in my direction, when she thought I wasn't looking.

DAVENANT. Magnetic influence!

SEBASTIAN. You can imagine my feelings. Then I had another inspiration. I took the miniature out of the pocket of my coat and sat openly comparing it with her - rather rude, but in the circumstance it was the only thing to do.

DAVENANT. Delightful!

SEBASTIAN. I saw her blushing, and all of a sudden, with that exquisite spontaneity and charming accent which you will appreciate when she returns, she said: 'You're Lewis Davenant'.

DAVENANT. You were fairly caught.

SEBASTIAN. I assure you, Lewis, that during the journey I thought it all out, and decided to present myself to her in my own name.

DAVENANT. But there was no time? You were taken by surprise, and in a moment it was too late.

SEBASTIAN. Too late, yes; for a moment after she was talking to me of half-a-dozen things at the same time, and introducing me to her friends as Mr Lewis Davenant who was on his way to Vienna for the performance of *Elizabeth Cooper*.

DAVENANT. Tell me something about my play.

SEBASTIAN. I wrote you a long letter about it, and on the evening of the performance, when I was called before the curtain -

DAVENANT. You weren't called before the curtain! I cannot believe it!

SEBASTIAN. Yes; and I made a speech.

DAVENANT. And told them that you had come to speak to them in the name of England?

SEBASTIAN. I said nothing about England on that occasion, but the next day at the banquet.

DAVENANT. Ho, ho! There was a banquet, then?

SEBASTIAN. A magnificent one!

DAVENANT. Your health was drunk in champagne?

SEBASTIAN. Of course.

DAVENANT. You were crowned with laurels?

SEBASTIAN. A crown of gilt laurels, which I hope to show you when -

DAVENANT. Come, come, Sebastian, you don't expect me to believe this nonsense, this grotesque, impossible tale?

SEBASTIAN (*assuming an injured air*). I don't know why you should doubt my word, Lewis. You sent me to Vienna as Lewis Davenant so that your fame might hide my defects from Gabrielle von Hoenstadt. I went, I saw, I conquered. I have brought her back to you so that you may see for yourself; you have seen her. But you don't believe your own eyes; why, then, should you believe my story?

DAVENANT (*taken aback*). Go on with your story, Sebastian.

SEBASTIAN. I'll say no more. A team of dray-horses will not drag another word out of me.

DAVENANT. Come now, Sebastian, I didn't mean –

SEBASTIAN. An incredulous audience damps the story-teller. Moreover, why should I tell it? The lady is upstairs; she will come down presently; you can hear it from her. She may be able to convince you, but, if she can't, I hope you'll not be so impolite as to tell her that she is telling lies.

DAVENANT. When I said I didn't believe, I meant that you had succeeded beyond my expectations. I begin to perceive in you the true, ever-resurgent type – Don Juan in person.

SEBASTIAN. Again you offend me, Lewis! I am no Don Juan, but a devout lover, who will be faithful unto death, whatever happens.

DAVENANT (*looking at* SEBASTIAN *askance*). But the day will come when you will have to tell her.

SEBASTIAN. Lewis, you are very cruel. You sent me to Vienna.

DAVENANT. But you will have to tell her.

SEBASTIAN. Lewis, I can see you are gloating over your joke. (*He turns to go.* DAVENANT *brings him back, and they come down the stage together.*)

DAVENANT. You did not dare to tell her in the carriage on the way to the Museum, as I can well understand, so charming did she seem under her long-fringed parasol. In the Gallery you were surrounded by tourists, and she chattered so pleasantly of the masterpieces that you had no heart to trouble her with a disagreeable piece of news. On another occasion when you were sitting together in a restaurant at dinner the moment seemed most propitious, the confession was on the tip of your tongue; but resolutions vanished at the sight of a mauve scarf wound about Gabrielle's arms and shoulders.

SEBASTIAN. But you have not seen her arms; as white as an angel's, arms and bosom, and as slight.

DAVENANT. Arms that I shall be glad to hear you have grown weary of, for they have been about you for the last time certainly. What! Not yet? So serious as all that, Sebastian?

SEBASTIAN. Every day I am more and more in love with her, and, alas! every hour brings the moment nearer when I must tell her.

DAVENANT. But she loves you for yourself.

SEBASTIAN. I hope so. I believe so, that is.

DAVENANT. You believe; but you have misgivings.

SEBASTIAN. I dread the unpleasant quarter of an hour, Lewis.

DAVENANT. If you get off with a quarter of an hour you'll be lucky. And now I must ask you what excuse you are going to give her for not telling her sooner.

SEBASTIAN. There is no use thinking out what one is going to say, the spell of the moment will put the right words into my mouth.

DAVENANT. But you do not intend waiting till she is seated in the train to bob your head into the carriage window and cry: I am not Lewis Davenant, but Sebastian Dayne, his cousin. That is not the way to treat a lady, surely!

SEBASTIAN. Lewis, you are more than unkind, you are cruel. I know that I must tell her sooner or later. But we're not going to part because I did not write *Elizabeth Cooper*. I cannot believe it; it would be out of all reason for her to send me away for so trivial a reason. Forgive me, Lewis. I intend no disparagement of your book. Come, Lewis, come, you have had many affairs with women, tell me what to do. Pull me out of the scrape you pushed me into.

DAVENANT. Women build a man up out of their imaginations, as you have heard me say on more than one occasion, and the shock when she hears the news will be great, no doubt, but even if she survives it, what then? You will have to part, unless, indeed ... You don't intend to marry her?

SEBASTIAN. We are married.

DAVENANT. (*who up to this point has been amused, immediately becomes serious*). You've married her, and in the name of Lewis Davenant? My dear Sebastian, this is a piece of folly.

SEBASTIAN. We won't discuss that point; our follies are so essentially ourselves that nobody dares to speak of his follies, and as for parting from them –

DAVENANT. You mean that you went through some ceremony of marriage?

SEBASTIAN. No, the marriage was all right. There was a church, a priest, and a book where we signed our names, so I suppose it was all right, but I'm not very well up in the marriage laws.

DAVENANT. Well, my good friend, you will soon have an excellent opportunity of learning them.

SEBASTIAN. You will be able to advise me? Lewis, Lewis, I beg of you.

DAVENANT. I cannot advise you; the situation is really more than I can grasp.

SEBASTIAN. You'll be able to grasp it better if you will –

DAVENANT. The one thing that concerns me now is that you have married her in my name, and I am not a marrying man.

SEBASTIAN. Try for a moment to imagine what my situation was.

DAVENANT. I am trying to think what could have made you do such a ridiculous thing.

SEBASTIAN. You didn't reproach me for allowing Gabrielle to introduce me to her friends as the author of *Elizabeth Cooper*, did you?

DAVENANT. In the train you were taken by surprise, but you weren't taken by surprise the morning you were married. You knew you were going to be married.

SEBASTIAN. I had not the faintest idea I was going to be married.

DAVENANT. Were you married under the influence of a drug or in your sleep?

SEBASTIAN. No, but it was quite unexpected.

DAVENANT. You speak as if you had been caught in a shower of rain.

SEBASTIAN. That is exactly what happened. We went for an excursion to an island in the Danube, a long narrow island with a village running down the middle. We were passing a church and were admiring it. Suddenly Gabrielle said: "How would you like to come into that church and be married to me?"

DAVENANT. Wait a moment. What had you said to lead up to that suggestion?

SEBASTIAN. Vague things; but as she made the suggestion you would not have had me hang back, would you?

DAVENANT. And then?

SEBASTIAN. Then she went into the church.

DAVENANT. With you?

SEBASTIAN. With me, of course, and we found an old priest asleep in the chair. I cried: "Heirat, Heirat," and he took us into the sacristy, where he asked us if we could show him our papers. Gabrielle showed him a visiting-card; he seemed loath to marry us on such slight testimony of our identity, but Gabrielle talked him over.

DAVENANT. You never said a word?

SEBASTIAN. I do not know much German.

147

DAVENANT (*throws up his arms*). Is that how people usually marry in Vienna?

SEBASTIAN. Sometimes.

DAVENANT. However they manage these things in Austria, these marriages in England often end in the law courts.

SEBASTIAN. A man should always be willing to suffer for the woman he loves. I'm ready.

DAVENANT. To go to prison, to cut your throat. If I had gone to Vienna this wouldn't have happened.

SEBASTIAN. Because she wouldn't have loved you.

DAVENANT. I'm not so sure of that. But you must tell her who you are, and the sooner the better.

SEBASTIAN. You think, then, that the moment she comes downstairs I should introduce her to the real Davenant?

DAVENANT. No; not just now.

SEBASTIAN. Perhaps you would like me to leave you to explain to her.

DAVENANT. This is no occasion for levity. It may be that I did wrong to advise you to go to Vienna and to introduce yourself in my name, but I did not tell you to marry her in my name; and now I am leaving.

SEBASTIAN. Don't go, Lewis; stay. She may forgive me if you will undertake to explain to her my youth, my inexperience. No one can explain a situation as well as you can. You have had so much knowledge of life. In your books –

DAVENANT. Once more I must insist on some seriousness. You will have to explain this matter yourself; nobody can do it but you. S-sh! Here she is. (*Enter* GABRIELLE. *Her hair is pinned up in front, but falls over her shoulders.*)

GABRIELLE. You will excuse me, Mr Dayne, for I did not know you were here, and came to ask my husband to make my hair. I am *si maladroite*. I am not able to make my hair alone, and, darling, your parlour-maid is not used to attending on ladies.

SEBASTIAN. She has broken the comb I gave you.

GABRIELLE. The comb that you bought for me at Strasbourg; I am sorry. (SEBASTIAN *arranges her hair.*) Is it unlucky in England to break a comb when you enter a strange house? I hope not. (*Gets up and goes to mirror and then comes back to* SEBASTIAN.) Make it a little higher, dear.

SEBASTIAN. Sebastian, have you ever seen more beautiful hair? Scented, soft as silk; such thick, brown glossy hair, curling like the tendrils of the anise.

GABRIELLE. What is that plant, dear? (*He hesitates.*) You've forgotten;

148

it makes no difference. (*Goes to the mirror again.*) If Martin had been able to make my hair as well as you I should have begun to suspect that mine were not the first little she-feet (*looking at the carpet*) to tread these roses underfoot. Do you say she-feet in English?

DAVENANT. We do not specify the sex, we merely say feet. (*He moves towards the door.*)

GABRIELLE. No, you must not go, Mr Dayne. There are a great many things I should like to ask you about. Are you not my cousin now?

DAVENANT. So I am, and your secretary should you ever require one.

GABRIELLE. I will dictate to you in German. I am sure you know German, Mr Dayne, and it will improve your German to gossip with me. Is gossip right? Do you say gossip in English?

DAVENANT. We say gossip.

GABRIELLE. Just as I have said. I should like to gossip with you. Will you take a chair, Mr Dayne, and gossip in English with me? Now do stay and tell me –

DAVENANT. What would you have me tell you?

GABRIELLE. Of the advice that I am sure you gave to Lewis when my miniature came, for you have had many affairs – I can read it in your eyes, Mr Dayne – many affairs with ladies, real ladies, ladies in society, not cocottes. Now what did you tell him that I was, a little fool or a cocotte, which? Be truthful, Mr Dayne, for I can read your face, for it's an open one.

DAVENANT. When your miniature arrived I said that he was very fortunate indeed to have written books that could bring him presents from such a beautiful woman.

GABRIELLE. Did you say that truly, Mr Dayne? I'm not at all sure, but no matter. What I would like to know is if you think the miniature does me justice. Lewis says that it does not, and I believe he is right. I always look dreadful and *affectée*, or swollen and greedy, on photographs. I do not look so toothachish in reality, do I, Mr Dayne? But I am not going to ask you for compliments; I know you could not do else than tell me that I am very pretty, but that is not what I want to hear. I should like you to tell me if the lady in the ivory is a woman who would deceive her lover, and what terrible revenge she would wreak on him if he were to deceive her. You don't know – how could you be expected to know? You see, Mr Dayne, I am a little stupid sometimes, but I like to be like that. Pay no attention to me, but just go on thinking of what is in your head. Your head is full of Lewis's books, is it not? It must be, since you are his secretary. We were talking about my miniature, and I was about to tell you that it was painted when I was living with my husband. He carried me off from the convent to a castle in a forest, where I never saw anyone but an old nurse and *les chasseurs*, men that came to hunt the wild boar and the deer. It was very tedious, but very romantic, like your Shakespeare. I used to sit at my casement thinking that it was a play of his and myself Desdemona; but she loved her black man, and I did not love my hunter, who never knew a day's illness until he died. That was what his great friend that shot him used to say: Kuno never knew a day's illness till he died. It was an accident, and I will tell you how it happened one of these days, when I am rested, for it is a very long story.

SEBASTIAN. Darling, let me persuade you to go to your room and lie down for a little while.

GABRIELLE. I am not tired. But I cannot tell the accident that my husband met with while hunting in the forest. It sounds too much like William Rufus, and I want to talk about *Elizabeth Cooper*. After my husband's death in the forest I went to live in Vienna, and seeing the same people day after day began to tire me almost as much as the deer and the boars in the forest. It was impossible for me to see them any more, and so I said to myself: 'I will make some new acquaintances,' and went to the library and began to pick out English heroes from Tauchnitz edition. I found *Douglas, Richard Feverel,* later on *Chandos,* and a thousand more, and one day the librarian handed me *Elizabeth Cooper*. The name struck my imagination; it is such a wonderful name, so romantic, so – I can't say all I want to say in English. Ach! it is so tiresome. *Elizabeth Cooper* is so –

DAVENANT. Evocative.

GABRIELLE. So evocative, of course. (*To* SEBASTIAN.) Why did you not give me the word, Lewis? You should always give me the words I want in English. Thank you, Mr Dayne. If Lewis had written a book for Austrian countesses especially he could not have succeeded better. For weeks I wanted to write to him, but somehow I didn't dare, and when his first letter arrived my hands turned as cold as ice and my cheeks burning hot. Is it not a funny thing to have cold hands and a hot face at the same time? A moment after I made gambols and pinched my dog because I was so happy. Tell me, Mr Dayne, was Lewis really a little pleased when I first wrote to him? Did he tell you his first idea about me? I shall never forget what a great impression his first letter made on me. I got it the 7th of November, on a Saturday. Nearly every year something happens to me on the 7th of November. It is a dangerous day for me.

DAVENANT. The Countess speaks exactly as she writes.

GABRIELLE. So Lewis has shown you my letters.

DAVENANT. He read me a few sentences, only a few. But you see my secretarial work enables me to catch the character of a writer in the first words, almost.

SEBASTIAN. My dear Gabrielle, I insisted that Sebastian should hear a few sentences, so overjoyed was I.

GABRIELLE. Don't trouble to excuse yourself, Lewis; I do not mind in the least your having shown my letters to Mr Dayne. In fact, I knew you had done so.

SEBASTIAN. How did you know that?

GABRIELLE. Well, my darling, didn't you tell me one day?

DAVENANT. If I may dare to put a question?

GABRIELLE. Do put questions to me, and I will answer them truthfully.

DAVENANT. Were your imaginations fulfilled?

GABRIELLE. I did not imagine so young a man.

DAVENANT. And if he had been an older man?

GABRIELLE. I think I should have forgiven him for the sake of *Elizabeth Cooper*. I do not like very young men, so you need not be afraid to tell me you are fifty; for I once had an admirer who was sixty-nine. Young men are all *poseurs* or hypocrites. Oh! I have no patience with them! I wish I could throw something to their heads!

DAVENANT. Have you not read any other books by Mr Davenant? Only *Elizabeth Cooper*?

GABRIELLE. I did not buy any more of Lewis's books. I was afraid that they might disappoint me, and I do not like to be disappointed, Mr Dayne; it gives me nerves. When you know me better you will understand how bitterly I resent any disappointment. But I know *Elizabeth Cooper* so well, every scene in it, and I should have visited all the places he has described, only there were reasons that kept me in Vienna. The man who shot my husband was said to be in love with me – which was not true; and my family – But there is no necessity for going into that story now; another time, Mr Dayne. I want now to talk to you about Elizabeth Cooper. It was she who gave me my liberty from Vienna, and so I said to Lewis: 'We must visit all the towns where she and her lover stayed on our wedding journey'. Elizabeth travelled a good deal in Germany, but while I was upstairs changing my frock, making myself look a little tidy, Lewis was telling you of our wedding journey, I suppose. I hope he didn't forget the old priest and the island on the Danube? For a moment I was afraid he would not unite us, but I managed very well, and persuaded him - didn't I, darling? And then the Danube! Lewis had never seen the Danube before. It seems to me so strange, for to go to Germany and not to see the Danube is hardly like going to Germany. He had not seen the Rhine; so I asked him, 'How is it you never make mistakes in German in your books?' and he said that you put his German right always; and that is how I learnt, dear Mr Dayne, that you know German. I took him to the old town that Elizabeth liked so much, and where everything is the same as in the Middle Ages. And thou wilt always remember, Lewis, the terrace on which we sat overlooking the Rhine? Only one thing was wanted for perfection – Lewis does not know German. It was very sad, for I wanted to read poems to him – Goethe's poems and Heine's, and some poems of Schiller's too; but if you had been there you would have helped me to translate them. You speak German, I know you do, and write it well, for there are no mistakes in Lewis's books. So why was it you did not come with him to Vienna? We could have travelled together, us three, so agreeably; for when I was tired of talking to one, I could have talked to the other, making all the people jealous and angry, as they would be at the sight of three happy people living in the world together. It is a pity, Lewis, you did not bring your cousin secretary, for with him to help us we might have come back with a book full of travel. But tell me, Mr Dayne, am I to believe all Lewis tells me that he can only write when you are with him? Is that true?

DAVENANT. Lewis writes his own poetry, but when I am with him he can only write prose.

GABRIELLE. How extraordinary! But if you were to die, Mr Dayne, what would happen to Lewis?

DAVENANT. As well ask me what would happen to me if Lewis were to die.

GABRIELLE. It is truly very strange, and just like life; so I will not ask any more questions, for it is useless to ask questions about life. Don't you think so, Mr Dayne? But you would like me to tell you where we went after seeing the Rhine; we went on to Heidelberg, and from Heidelberg we journeyed to Strasbourg; we travelled all night. But you who have travelled so much, Mr Dayne, do not need that I should tell you the names of all these places we have been to. I would sooner you should tell me what you were doing in this pretty cottage by a river all the time we were away. For one cannot look at a river all day. Have any ladies been to see you?

DAVENANT. Ladies come to see the author, not the secretary. And my time was passed, not in looking on the river, but in hard work, copying out a new book by Lewis Davenant, which I am prone to believe will exceed in interest everything that he has written before, even *Elizabeth Cooper.*

GABRIELLE. You must tell me about this book at once; I am impatient, and I think I said I bitterly resent being disappointed. How, Lewis darling, was it that you never spoke to me of this new book?

SEBASTIAN. We were seeing places and things, and talking about each other; there was no time for literature. A written story is so faint compared with the real story.

GABRIELLE. How modest he is, Mr Dayne, and shy of talking about his work; but he has to talk to you about his work, since you are his secretary. Tell me, was it here in this room that he wrote *Elizabeth Cooper?* Darling, how was it that thou didst not tell me it was here – that I was in the very room in which you wrote your book? You should have stopped me on the threshold, saying, 'There is the table at which I wrote, the chair on which I sat, the inkstand into which I dipped my pen'. All these things are related about Goethe. But the manuscript, where is it? - in these drawers? I want to see it. (*She goes to the table and pulls out drawers and takes out a heap of papers.*)

SEBASTIAN (*crossing a little hurriedly*). My dear, you must not upset those papers.

GABRIELLE. But I am looking for the manuscript of your new book. What is the title of it, Mr Dayne? You must tell me the title of it, Mr Dayne – only the title.

DAVENANT. *Van Birds.*

GABRIELLE. But what does that mean? Birds kept in a van?

DAVENANT. No, the first of the flock, from Vanguard. But you'll not find the manuscript there; it's in Rockminster.

GABRIELLE. Well, let me see the manuscript of *Elizabeth Cooper.*

SEBASTIAN. Why should you want to see the manuscript? You have read the book.

GABRIELLE. But I do want to see the manuscript. And is it not natural that I should like to see the manuscript of the book that made me love you? Mr Dayne, will you try to find the manuscript of *Elizabeth Cooper?*

SEBASTIAN. We have no manuscripts here, I assure you, Gabrielle.

GABRIELLE. Then I will look at your books. (*She gets up on a ladder.*) Here is the three-volume edition, and the six-shilling edition, and the two-shilling picture-board edition. Why there is an *édition de luxe.* I had no idea you had written so many books, darling! How old were you when you began to write?

153

SEBASTIAN. I think I was about sixteen.

GABRIELLE. And now you are twenty-seven.

SEBASTIAN. I shall soon be eight and twenty.

GABRIELLE. And in ten years you have written seventeen books. How very extraordinary! Now which of these is your first book?

SEBASTIAN. My first book was a volume of poems.

GABRIELLE. I am disappointed! I cannot tell you, Lewis, how disappointed I am! Mr Dayne, you will understand.

DAVENANT. Truly, life is full of disappointments. If you will tell me, Countess, in what particular way you are disappointed, I may be able to help you.

GABRIELLE. You are not as clever a man as I thought you were, Mr Dayne, else you would have understood at once that I came to England to inspire a great literature.

DAVENANT. But you found the literature you hoped to inspire already written?

GABRIELLE. Alas!

DAVENANT. He is seven and twenty, and will not stop at seventeen volumes.

GABRIELLE (*still sitting on the top step of the ladder*). Do you think I shall be able to inspire him, Mr Dayne? If you do, perhaps I had better tell you, who are his secretary, the kind of book I should like him to write. Something that no author has yet quite done to my satisfaction. The story about a married couple, but a long, beautiful, might-be-true story. Is might-be-true a real word, Mr Dayne? Well, you and Lewis must try not to be envious when I invent a new word. You see, I don't want the wife to be a saint, nor the husband an angel. I just want them to be man and wife, to quarrel as well as to kiss, to have temptations both. But the end must be a happy one, Lewis. I don't want the *Kreutzer Sonata* over again. And on some children I must insist.

DAVENANT. How many?

GABRIELLE. I don't know how many, perhaps none at all when the story comes to be written. You see, I am always changing my moods and opinions, Mr Dayne. It is amusing, and fatiguing too; it is like changing one's dress a dozen times a day. (DAVENANT *moves up the stage.*) But must you really leave us? Lewis, shall we go to the station with Mr Dayne?

SEBASTIAN. If you want to, dear.

GABRIELLE (*coming down the steps*). Well, let us get our hats. You men keep your hats in the hall. Lewis, will you go upstairs and fetch my hat? (*Exit* SEBASTIAN.)

154

GABRIELLE (*to* DAVENANT). When you asked me if I was surprised at Lewis's youth, I answered – I've forgotten what I answered; it doesn't matter in the least, for I only speak what I mean at the moment, which in most cases turns out to be the opposite of what I really mean. I had expected to see a man of fifty-five at least.

DAVENANT. And you never doubted that you were speaking to the author of those seventeen volumes?

GABRIELLE. I may have doubted at first sight, but not after the first five minutes of conversation, for Lewis talks just as he writes. Don't you think so, Mr Dayne.

DAVENANT. Very like his books – the living counterpart.

GABRIELLE. If you speak like that, Mr Dayne, I shall think you're jealous of your cousin.

DAVENANT. I am jealous of my cousin, but not of his writings.

GABRIELLE. Of what, then, are you jealous – that I didn't invite you to Vienna? Now tell me your age; I had forgotten to ask it before, Mr Dayne. I was born the 6th of September, 18—, so, you see, my age is quite respectable. I'll tell you a secret, Mr Dayne, one that I have told to no one before. When I was born they saw at once I wasn't a boy, and they were disappointed, as a son was wanted; and I was called Gabrielle, for they think in Austria that when a girl is called Gabrielle the next child will be a boy.

DAVENANT. May I call you Gabrielle?

GABRIELLE. If you really like it so much, I shall not be offended. But I am not like any of his heroines, *quelle mauvaise chance.* My eyes are too small and *myope* , and my hair is brown. Do you like brown hair or fair? And does fair mean beautiful or blond? I should have asked these questions before, and also why you kept the miniature in which at full length I am. Tell me, my good Mr Dayne, why?

SEBASTIAN (*entering*). Here is your hat and cloak, Gabrielle, and if you start at once you will catch the train to Rockminster, and Mr Dayne will show you the manuscripts and some pictures well worth seeing, too.

GABRIELLE. But why should I wish to go to Rockminster, leaving you here. I don't want to leave you, Lewis. (*Coming down the stage.*) Now at once I must hear what the meaning of all this may be? You're not jealous because I like speaking to your secretary? (*Exit* DAVENANT.)

SEBASTIAN. Not jealous, but wearied of this mystification which takes in nobody. You do not think that Davenant does not guess that you know he is Davenant?

GABRIELLE. My dear Sebastian, he does not suspect it - no, never.

SEBASTIAN. You said nothing that would lead him to suppose you knew, did you? I wish you had, for the longer the joke is kept up the more angry he will be.

GABRIELLE. I think Mr Davenant already sees that I am not the little fool he took me for. But he must be punished, for everybody should be punished for being stupid.

SEBASTIAN. Ever since we set foot in England you have been talking of punishing Mr Davenant. But how is he to be punished?

GABRIELLE. By being made to feel in love with me.

SEBASTIAN. And if, in making him fall in love with you, you were to fall in love with him?

GABRIELLE. I could never love anybody but you, Sebastian. But where is that dear Mr Davenant? Something must have frightened him away, for he has gone without daring to bid me good-bye. Yet I didn't say anything dreadful to him. Is he easily shocked? One of my friends tells me that he never knew a lady who talked such dreadful things as I do with my eyes, looking so innocently all the while. You must run after Mr Davenant and bring him back, for my walk with him must not be spoilt.

SEBASTIAN. I do not know where to run.

GABRIELLE. Martin will tell us. (*Rings.*) (*Enter* MARTIN.) Can you tell me quickly if Mr Dayne has gone to the station to get the train? Or has he gone to the garden to gather me some flowers? (*To* SEBASTIAN.) How nice of him, for men so seldom like flowers!

MARTIN. Lady Letham called, your ladyship, and Mr Dayne has gone back to Rockminster with her in her carriage.

GABRIELLE. We must pursue them in another carriage.

SEBASTIAN. My dear Gabrielle! Thank you, Martin, that will do. (*Exit* MARTIN.)

GABRIELLE. Is Lady Letham Mr Davenant's mistress? But that cannot be, for you told me, darling, that Mr Davenant was no longer as fond as he used to be of *la femme de trente ans*. Such a *mal chance*! Just as I was beginning to be one in the full sense of the word! Or did Mr Davenant take Lady Letham away because she loves you? And Mr Davenant was afraid I should make a scene. I don't make scenes, not as you do in England; I merely cry, and then my nose gets swollen and I have hardly any eyes. You will not make me cry, darling, by being unfaithful to me? But of what are you thinking? Of some women that you've loved a little? Tell me the truth, dear, and I will forgive you if it was long ago, and if she was not very pretty, nor very young; middle-aged I should prefer it, but not dead, for the dead have a power that the living ones have not. You didn't desire her, and leave her with a baby which you will ask me to adopt? That I shouldn't like doing - no, never; so please don't ask it. But why, darling, are you making such naughty nostrils? You remind me of my husband that was, and, though we are married, you said you would always be my lover.

SEBASTIAN. I am thinking, Gabrielle, that, despite the nonsense you talk – perhaps on account of it – there is nobody in the world for me but you, and I am asking myself if you will follow me back to happiness. We have been happy – say that we've been happy, Gabrielle, for a little while!

GABRIELLE. Yes, Sebastian; but what do you want me to do?

SEBASTIAN. Let us go back to Austria, and to the time when I used to sit at your feet telling you the story of my life.

GABRIELLE. But you have told me the story of your life.

SEBASTIAN. No, no, not all of it.

GABRIELLE. What secret hast thou kept from me, villain? (*Looking round.*) Ach! why did Mr Davenant go away like this?

SEBASTIAN. You were interested in him the moment you came into the room. The most capricious woman in the world. Men are your amusement, your pleasure; the old succeed the young, and the ugly the beautiful. You said you had cold finger-tips and hot cheeks the moment you met me in the railway train, and when you came into the room and saw Mr Davenant –

GABRIELLE. I like Mr Davenant because his eyes are kind and his teeth are so nice, but I had not cold finger-tips and hot cheeks.

SEBASTIAN. Go to Rockminster and be amused for the afternoon. (*Enter* MARTIN.)

MARTIN. Mr Godby, sir. (*Enter* GODBY.)

SEBASTIAN. Godby!

GODBY. Excuse me, ma'am, but, you see, I've been up after these letters afore now.

GABRIELLE. I'm afraid I don't understand.

GODBY. No more did Mr Davenant. You see, it ain't possible for me to go back to Priscilla a second time without them letters, and they promised to let me 'ave them the last time I came up from Southampton.

GABRIELLE. What letters?

GODBY. Why, Priscilla's letters before she and I was spliced. You see, ma'am, it wasn't the fault of the young gentleman; it was Priscilla what commenced the correspondence over having read Mr D'.s books. I 'ave forgotten the name. Give me a moment.

GABRIELLE. *Elizabeth Cooper.*

GODBY. That was the book that fair turned 'er 'ead, and 'e sent 'er heaps of letters and pomes. And now that she 'as become Mrs G., she has been worrying of me to get them letters back. She's afeard he might publish them; she says you never know what these literary gents will do with letters, and this is the second time I 'ave come up from Southampton after them.

GABRIELLE. Was there a poem beginning 'After many days, and after many tears'?

GODBY. Well, ma'am, I can't say there was, though she 'as read them to me often enough. You see, I 'ave no head for poetry. 'After many days, and after many tears,' yer say? There were plenty of tears in the pomes, and sighs and 'earts and kisses.

GABRIELLE. Thank you, Mr Godby, that's all I want to know. Now I'll leave you to settle your business with this gentleman. (*She goes towards the door.*)

SEBASTIAN. Gabrielle, I can explain.

GABRIELLE. I prefer to listen to Mr Davenant's explanation. (*Exit L.*)

SEBASTIAN. (*looking at his watch*). There is a train in a few minutes. She'll just catch it. I must run!

GODBY. Oh no you don't, not till I gets Priscilla's letters.

SEBASTIAN. But they are in Rockminster, my man! Let me go.

GODBY. Not if I knows it. We'll go back to Rockminster together.

SEBASTIAN. If you run we can catch the train.

GODBY. Run! I likes to hear you talk about running, and to a man that has walked all the way from Rockminster. This be the 'ottest day we've 'ad this summer. Run, indeed!

SEBASTIAN. Let me go! Let me go!

GODBY. Pull that bell and ask your parlour-maid to bring me up a glass of ale.

SEBASTIAN. There isn't time for drinking ale.

GODBY. Out of this I don't stir till I gets it! (*The train whistle is heard.*)

SEBASTIAN. There! we've missed the train! (*He rings the bell.*) (*Enter* MARTIN.) Martin, will you bring a tankard of ale and two glasses? (MARTIN *goes out, looking very astonished.*)

END OF THE SECOND ACT

ACT III

SCENE: Same as in Act I.
When the curtain rises DAVENANT *is on the stage in evening dress.*
Enter SEBASTIAN *and* GODBY.

GODBY. 'Ere we are – the very room – 'member it jush as if it was
yesseday. Beg pardon, sir – Godby, second mate on the *Hannah
Maria.* Don't you remember Godby, sir? Came for Priscilla's letters
'bout month ago.

DAVENANT. Yes, Mr Godby, I remember.

GODBY. Well, to make a long story short, shecktery breaks his word –
no letters – Priscilla getting more and more peevish every day. No
letters – 'ave to come up again from Southampton. Shecktery
'broad, self at Claremont Villa; way I go, all sails set, and over'aul
shecktery with his young lady; bit of a squall; shecktery would 'ave
weighed anchor and gone away after her, but I says: 'No, shecktery;
no, shecktery; not this time'. We go back together after a bit of a rest
and a tankard of ale, at your expense, Mr Davennan. Terrible 'ot
day.

DAVENANT. I can see, Mr Godby, that you are suffering from the heat.
Won't you sit down?

GODBY. I'd like to drop my anchor somewhere. (*He sits down on a light
chair.* DAVENANT *rushes forward.*)

DAVENANT. You'll be more comfortable there, Mr Godby. (*Puts* GODBY
into settee.)

GODBY. Thank'ee. Very comfortable chair. But the letters. (*Rises.*) In
that 'ere casket.

SEBASTIAN. No, Mr Godby, there are no letters in that casket. Priscilla's
letters are downstairs.

GODBY. Downstairs. I'll wait here. Shecktery ... letters ... Shecktery
good sort. D'ye 'ear, Mr Davennan? Shecktery good sort. (*He closes
his eyes.* DAVENANT *and* SEBASTIAN *walk aside.*)

DAVENANT. Now, Sebastian, what is all this about?

SEBASTIAN. Martin let this man into the house, and we've been coming
back ever since, from ale-house to ale-house.

DAVENANT. A drunken man in this house, and an Austrian Countess in

159

Claremont Villa. These eccentricities are no doubt very amusing, Sebastian, but I shall have to explain to your father –

SEBASTIAN. Explain what you like. I don't care; I'm done for.

DAVENANT. Is it so bad as that? You have told her and –

SEBASTIAN. Just as I was trying to summon up courage to tell her, this fellow came rolling into the house asking for the letters that I had promised to send him. At the word 'letters' Gabrielle began to grow suspicious, and the garrulous fool that he is, thinking to make matters right, said I hadn't written to Priscilla since they were spliced. What did Gabrielle care whether it was before or after marriage? All that concerned her was the fact that I had sent the poems that I had written to her to this fellow's wife. As soon as she knew that she just gave me a look. You wouldn't believe that so much hatred could come into that face. She picked up her parasol and ran away.

DAVENANT. And you let her go without any explanation?

SEBASTIAN. As I was about to follow her – Is that fellow asleep! (*Snore from* GODBY.)

DAVENANT. He seems as if he were.

SEBASTIAN. He gripped me by the arm and hung on to me, and a few minutes after I heard the train whistle.

DAVENANT. And she went away still thinking she is married to me? You really must go and tell her.

SEBASTIAN. I don't know where she is. (*Enter* MARTIN *with a letter, which she hands to* DAVENANT.)

MARTIN (*to* SEBASTIAN). Shall I awake him sir?

SEBASTIAN. No, no, no-o. (*Exit* MARTIN.)

DAVENANT (*reading the letter*). She is at the 'Three Kings,' and is leaving Rockminster to-morrow. You must go and tell her.

SEBASTIAN. Now? At once?

DAVENANT. Why not?

SEBASTIAN. I do not think I can, Lewis. My last chance of getting her forgiveness would be lost if I did.

DAVENANT. Why should it be lost?

SEBASTIAN. Because I must begin at the beginning, by getting her to forgive me for sending my poems to Mrs Godby.

DAVENANT. You think she looks upon the correspondence with Mrs Godby as the greater offence?

SEBASTIAN. I don't know whether she does or doesn't, but am certain that when we have persuaded her to forgive one offence, the next will come easy. I can't give reasons, but that's how I feel. Neither of us know what she'll think.

160

DAVENANT. That's very likely; but why did you say when *we* have persuaded her?

SEBASTIAN. I should have said when you have persuaded her.

DAVENANT. But I'm only the secretary.

SEBASTIAN. Don't, Lewis, don't. You will help me, I know you will, and you can do so by sending a note round to the 'Three Kings' asking her to come to see you.

DAVENANT. And then?

SEBASTIAN. You will be able to talk her over. The right words will come to you; they always do.

DAVENANT. Would you like me to say that you sent the poems to Priscilla to find out if the British public would like them, Priscilla being the British public in essence?

SEBASTIAN. The very thing, Lewis. I can see you'll be able to manage it all right.

DAVENANT. Would you like me to tell her that I am Lewis Davenant, taking on myself the entire responsibility of sending you to Vienna?

SEBASTIAN. No, I think not. Let us begin at the beginning, and when she has forgiven me the offence (in her eyes the greater offence), put it to her that she should go away with me, it doesn't matter where so long as I get her and myself out of Rockminster, for here –

DAVENANT. Here you are surrounded by relations.

SEBASTIAN. Just so. Will you do this, Lewis? I shall be for ever grateful to you, and the job will not be as hard as it seems. Gabrielle is more sensible than she appears to be at first sight, for all her eccentricity is on the surface, as one soon begins to find out.

DAVENANT. I hadn't thought of it, but I dare say you're right, and that good sense often comes to us in strange clothes, whilst folly, under the dull robes of dignity, finds excellent cover.

SEBASTIAN. I am sure you are right, Lewis, for what you say sounds right. Send a note. She'll come. She won't leave Rockminster without seeing you; and as soon as we are ten miles out of Rockminster I'll tell her everything from end to end without evasion or omission.

DAVENANT. If she stops the carriage and bids you alight?

SEBASTIAN. I don't think she will.

DAVENANT. You speak with assurance. But however fantastic she may be on the surface, or under it, she won't take it lying down when you tell her that she has married the wrong man.

SEBASTIAN. If you will do as I ask you –

DAVENANT. I will; for I must. It was I that pushed you into the snare.

SEBASTIAN. I feel like a fly on a sticky paper, but shall extricate myself if you will help me. I have your promise, you will not tell her anything?

DAVENANT. You have my hand on it. Ring the bell, please. (SEBASTIAN *rings the bell.* DAVENANT *sits down and scribbles a note.*) But she knows your handwriting, Sebastian. You must write the note. (SEBASTIAN *sits at table and writes. Enter* MARTIN.)

DAVENANT. Mr Dayne is writing a note, and you'll have it sent round to the 'Three Kings' at once, Martin . . . The messenger is to wait for an answer.

MARTIN. Yes, sir. (*Exit.*)

SEBASTIAN. I think it will work out all right. You are still Sebastian Dayne, and I am Davenant.

DAVENANT. May I ask how long this masquerade is to continue?

SEBASTIAN. Not for long. It can't. Things have come to a crisis. (*Looking towards* GODBY.) We'd better wake him.

DAVENANT. I'm afraid we shall have some difficulty in getting rid of him. He won't go without his letters.

SEBASTIAN. I'll get him his letters. (*He goes over to* GODBY.) Now, Mr Godby, shake your leg; lift your leg.

GODBY. (*waking up*). Aye, aye, Captain; aye, aye. Blesh my soul . . . blesh my soul, where am I? (*Getting to his feet.*) Misher Davennan. Shecktery. Long walk. 'Eat of the sun. Arlright. Come back for Priscilla's letters. Shecktery, Priscilla's letters.

SEBASTIAN. Priscilla's letters are downstairs, Mr Godby.

GODBY. Very well. Get away close hauled, cargo on board, Priscilla's letters, a glass of ale, Mr Davennan, before starting. Glass of ale does no man any harm.

DAVENANT. You'll give Mr Godby a glass of ale in the parlour, Sebastian.

GODBY. Thank'ee, Captain, drink yer 'ealth. Fine ale in this country; besh ever drunk. One glass at 'Three Fiddlers' – should 'ave been two – two glasses at 'Pig and Whistle' – should 'ave been three – four glasses at the 'Rose and Crown' – should 'ave been five. England's bulwarks is 'er ale. As long as England brews the ale that I 'ave drunk to-day, England will never be anythin' else but merrie England. (Begins to sing.) 'Oh! for merrie England and the merrie days of yore'.

SEBASTIAN. Come away, and we'll drink Mr Davenant's health.

GODBY. Yesh. Misher Davennan's 'ealth, Priscilla's 'ealth, shecktery's 'ealth, everybody's 'ealth. (SEBASTIAN *helps him out. Coming back.*) Won't you join us, Misher Davennan?

DAVENANT. Presently, Mr Godby, presently. (SEBASTIAN *pushes*

GODBY *off.*) (*To* SEBASTIAN). What are you going to do in the meantime?

SEBASTIAN. I'll wait upstairs.

DAVENANT. Lady Letham is dining here to-night.

SEBASTIAN. Lady Letham! Ah! she called the day I left, and hopes you will stay with her in Westmorland. She wishes to show you a fine range of mountains.

DAVENANT. I wrote to her.

SEBASTIAN. But, Lewis, she would prefer to have you to herself, and until I know my fate I shall eat no dinner, and not even then, should it prove adverse. (*Exit.*)

DAVENANT. (*going to the door and speaking to* SEBASTIAN, *who is still on the staircase*). Will you tell Martin that I'd like to speak to her! (*He walks back and forth.*) (*Enter* MARTIN.)

DAVENANT. You did well, Martin, to come up from Claremont Villa.

MARTIN. There was no use my staying on. The Countess caught the train, and Mr Godby said he wouldn't leave till he had some ale. He made Mr Dayne drink with him, and they went away together.

DAVENANT. I know, Martin, I know. But we must think now of what we can give Lady Letham for dinner. I dare say Mrs Coleman will be able to manage a dinner of some sort.

MARTIN. I dare say she will, sir. I know pretty well what is in the house. You can have *soup printanière*, fillets of sole, *vin blanc*, and a spring chicken *en casserole* –

DAVENANT. And a sweet. That will do famously. As Lady Letham does not drink champagne, you had better have a bottle of the best claret warmed for her. The gardener has sent the flowers all right?

MARTIN. Yes, sir. (*She turns to go out, but stops.*)

DAVENANT. Well, what is it?

MARTIN. Only this, sir – are you still Mr Dayne?

DAVENANT. (*pause*). Well, Martin –

MARTIN. You sent round a note to the 'Three Kings,' sir, asking Mr Sebastian's friend to come round here – the Countess von – I never caught the name properly, sir, but who will she ask for?

DAVENANT. She will ask for Mr Dayne.

MARTIN. And Lady Letham, sir?

DAVENANT. She will ask for Mr Davenant.

MARTIN. You'll excuse me, sir, but you have tied your tie very badly.

DAVENANT. Yes, I have tied it rather badly. That drunken fellow coming in at the moment. (*Ties tie before the glass.*) I think that is better.

MARTIN. Yes, sir, that's quite right.

DAVENANT. Is there anything else?

MARTIN. No. (*A bell rings.*) The front-door bell, sir. (*Exit* MARTIN. *She returns a moment after, followed by* GABRIELLE.)

GABRIELLE. How do you do, Mr Davenant, and you see how running round I come to meet you eagerly; but this is not your writing. (*Hands him the letter.*)

DAVENANT (*takes letter and looks at it*). This letter is in Mr Davenant's writing.

GABRIELLE. Ach, let no more time be wasted putting jokes on each other, not just now. This morning I was all for making jokes, for I thought I was going to remain in England, and there would be plenty of time for reconciliation, plenty of time for laughing, and saying which had made the greatest fool of the other; but now it is all sad and gloomy.

DAVENANT. I really do not understand.

GABRIELLE. Oh yes, you do understand, and quite truly you do, Mr Davenant, so you must not tease me any more, nor must I tease you, Mr Davenant, for it is all too sad. But let that pass away. We will not talk of those things any more, for it would be useless, since I am going back to Austria.

DAVENANT. Going back to Austria! But when?

GABRIELLE. To-morrow or next day; and I've come here to-night because I could not go back to Austria without seeing the great author, Mr Davenant, whose books have been so much help to me at a time when my life has gone to wreckage. All this was spoken of lightly this morning, but my humour is not the same; it never is the same very long. But there has been great cause, which I will tell you about. But that will not be necessary, as perhaps you have heard the story already from him. Ach, I can tell by your face that you have. So it may be wrong of me to come here; but I could not go without seeing Mr Davenant as he is. For this morning you were not Mr Davenant, but merely Mr Davenant masquerading as – as your secretary; so if I had not come here to-night I should never have seen the real Mr Davenant. But now I have seen him and the room in which he wrote all those lovely books which – But we'll say no more about those books. Yet why not, for all the rest has finished. I am glad that it was here you wrote your books, and not in that horrid Claremont Villa, which I shall try to forget. But this room I shall remember. (*She walks round the room, looking at the pictures.*) You have some lovely pictures, and if I were not going away in a few minutes I'd ask you to explain them to me, for you explain pictures very well in your books. Your china I understand better; you have some lovely Dresden, but I do not want to talk about such things; and if I look at them it is only because they will help me to remember you better. And now, dear Mr Davenant, say: I forgive Gabrielle as Gabrielle forgives me, which is quite true.

DAVENANT. My dear Countess, you must not go like this. A foolish thought came into my head. One should not be judged by one's foolish thoughts. I don't know how it all happened that —

GABRIELLE. That you sent your secretary instead of coming yourself? Such a rude thing to do, and just at a time when I was saying every day: 'I'd die to know more about him'. And it is not better; it is worse since I have seen you. Yes, I think it is so.

DAVENANT. But, Countess, tell me. You cannot go away like this, for we have much to say to each other, so much that I hardly know where to begin or how to —

GABRIELLE. What, you, the great author, not to know how to begin a story! I can stay a little while longer to hear you try.

DAVENANT. What would you have me talk to you about?

GABRIELLE. About yourself, or I'll not stay another minute. I have been told that you go on writing from morning to night. Why do you do it? Really, I must scold you a little. I do not want you to fall ill. You may write four or five hours a day, but no more, and you must go for long walks. If I were living in this house I should send you out for two hours every day at least. This to me you must promise.

DAVENANT. Am I forgiven?

GABRIELLE. Yes, if you promise.

DAVENANT. I promise. How good you are. Mine was the original offence.

GABRIELLE. We will not talk about who began and who ended. I came here to-night, for I could not leave England with unfriendliness for the author of *Elizabeth Cooper*. I said in my letters, which you did not read, I will be in love with the author, not the man, a thing I did not mean at the time, but for the future I will think only of the author.

DAVENANT. My dear Countess, I should not like you to forget the man — not altogether. I cannot reconcile myself to becoming an intellectual abstraction, represented by seventeen volumes.

GABRIELLE. But they are such beautiful volumes. (*She turns to go.*)

DAVENANT. No, do not go. We must not part before we have laid aside the absurd disguises in which we have hidden ourselves, each from the other.

GABRIELLE. But I am speaking my heart open to you.

DAVENANT. A disguise is not rent and cast off in an hour. We must have patience. In a few minutes we shall be speaking out of our true selves. (*Detaining her.*) You have not told me yet when you discovered that I had sent my secretary –

GABRIELLE. Why do you want to know? Whether I took five minutes or one hour, what can it matter?

DAVENANT. A great deal, for the discovery in five minutes means one woman, and the discovery in an hour means another.

GABRIELLE. And which would you prefer me to be?

DAVENANT. You were returning to Vienna with the Baron von Allmen and two ladies, and it was in the train –

GABRIELLE. All that was my invention, part of the prank. But why do you make me talk of what will always be a very sad story to me?

DAVENANT. If you did not meet Sebastian in the train, he called on you, I suppose, one afternoon; and you were disappointed the moment he came into the room, for Sebastian did not correspond with the idea that you had formed of the man who had written *Elizabeth Cooper.* But the feeling of disappointment passed quickly into one of delight.

GABRIELLE. Now, you're making up a story, and I cannot wait to hear it. You will send it to me. (*Rises.*) It was fortunate for himself that he came to me before going to the theatre, for how could he be mistaken for the author of *Elizabeth Cooper*? No, never. My discovery saved him from disgrace, and the piece from being withdrawn, as it might have been. Ach! I wish you had seen our performance of *Elizabeth Cooper.* You missed a great deal, Mr Davenant, by not coming to Vienna.

DAVENANT. I did indeed. There is a puritan in the play –

GABRIELLE. We have no puritans in Vienna, and that is perhaps why we can act them so well. Why did you not come to Vienna to see your puritan? (*Sits.*)

DAVENANT. But you are not a puritan, Countess.

GABRIELLE. I'm talking now of your play. We should have sat in a box watching the performance, and afterwards we should have gone to supper at my cousin's, who has the *feu sacrè* and a lovely mouth.

DAVENANT. So the meeting in the train was merely one of your imaginations, Countess; and what about the banquet and the laurel crown?

GABRIELLE. All my imaginations on the battlements of the Castle of Heidelberg –

DAVENANT. And the old priest, was he, too, one of your inventions?

GABRIELLE. We were married on an island in the Danube by an old priest just as he told you.

DAVENANT. But he married you, I see, in his own name, and not in

166

mine.

GABRIELLE. Yes, in his own name. But that will make no difference, none whatever. I shall return to Austria, and my lawyers will tell me if I'm married. But let us not talk of these painful things, Mr Davenant, I beg of you, for, as I have said, I would leave Rockminster with one pleasant memory at least, and the time I have spent in this room, if you will not talk any more of unpleasant people and things, will be a pleasant memory in time to come. (*Rises.*)

DAVENANT (*rises*). No, you must not go. I would convince you that I meant only a little misunderstanding which would be cleared up in half-an-hour – in a day or two at most.

GABRIELLE. I, too, meant only a little harmless joke, and we have forgiven each other mutually, have we not? So why go back on that old story?

DAVENANT (*detaining her*). But I did not foresee that you would fall in love with him – how could I?

GABRIELLE. I do not wish to speak of him.

DAVENANT. Nor do I. It is true that I sent him to Vienna on a false errand, but he had no right to return to Rockminster and allow you – and encourage you, perhaps – to put a joke upon me. He is my cousin, and is many years younger.

GABRIELLE. (*with a change of tone*). Mr Davenant, you do not know me yet at all. How could you know me, for have we not come out of a masquerade, and not yet laid aside our clothes, as you have said? But if you should come to know me better, the first thing that you will learn about me is that I am not cruel – no, certainly I am not. Of course, I often offend people, sometimes even mortally; my temper is not very good, but when I think of it I have a great wish to be kind to everybody, even to him who sent my poems to Mrs Godby. So I beg you to believe me that the joke, the hoax, the humbug – What is a hoax, Mr Davenant?

DAVENANT. Much the same as humbug.

GABRIELLE. Must not be blamed to him, for the joke was mine, and was put on you in spite of all he could say. I would have my joke now; for at that time I was thinking of you as *un vieux farceur*, who would deserve to be hoaxed. But now I think quite differently. (*Looking round.*) If I were to live here I should move the sofa, for there is too much glare; and bowls of flowers I would have, and cushions. You have been in love many times, Mr Davenant – one can see that by this room, though there are too few cushions. How long have you been without cushions? Well, no matter. You must forgive

Sebastian. You two must not go on quarrelling about Gabrielle. No woman is worth that two such men as you should be quarrelling about her. You must promise, for the thought of it would make me very sad when I am far away in Vienna. You cannot refuse me what I ask.

DAVENANT. My dear Countess, you are asking me to promise to do something that you cannot do yourself.

GABRIELLE. But you have nothing to forgive him, only a prank; and he couldn't do else than as I told him. You two must go on writing heaps of books together, just as if Gabrielle had never written her letter, as if she had never crossed your lives.

DAVENANT. But if you had forgiven him you would not return to Vienna.

GABRIELLE. I forgive him for coming to see me as Lewis Davenant, but I cannot forgive him for sending my poems – But let us not go over the hateful story again.

DAVENANT. I understand, or I think I do. You are angry, for it seems to you but an accident that he didn't go to Southampton instead of Vienna.

GABRIELLE. Which might well have been. Tell me, isn't it so? I don't want to tease you. I only want to know.

DAVENANT. I should be a false friend if I failed to remind you that one woman inspires the poems that all women receive.

GABRIELLE. Laura inspired all Petrarch's sonnets, and they were circulated in manuscript.

DAVENANT. In print, but not in manuscript.

GABRIELLE. Then there was no print; but I will not argue with you, Mr Davenant. I am not in the humour to argue with anybody about such a thing as Petrarch and Sebastian.

DAVENANT. Quite true; let us not argue, but forgive him.

GABRIELLE. Not, that is not possible. There are things that cannot be forgiven. Were I to say I forgive him, my forgiveness would be merely words. It would not come from the heart. No; and now I must say good-bye. I really must go. (*She goes up stage, pauses a moment, and then returns.*) But, Mr Davenant, one thing more. To please your curiosity, I will tell you that when Sebastian came to see me I knew after the first five minutes that he was a friend of yours, your secretary, your cousin – anyway, not yourself. And now you will tell me something. Why did you not come to Vienna?

DAVENANT. I do not know myself.

GABRIELLE. That is a trick not to tell me that you are in love.

DAVENANT. No, I am not. You would know why I didn't go to Vienna!

It seems to me that I dreaded a hoax – that some of my friends here might have planned the letters.

GABRIELLE. What madness! My letters should have told you. But you didn't read them.

DAVENANT. If I had I should have gone.

GABRIELLE. But that was not the only reason for not going.

DAVENANT. There are always many reasons. Sebastian chided me for unwillingness to sacrifice a few pages of prose. But that was not the reason. I think the real reason was my incurable shyness ... hatred of the incongruous. I said if I were ten years younger I'd go.

GABRIELLE. Did I not say in my letters I did not like young men?

DAVENANT. You did. (*Detaining her.*) Many women write to authors about their books and ask for appointments, and if I have not accepted these invitations it is because I never could put the thought out of my mind that I should find a withered spinster waiting who would extend a sisterly hand to me, saying: 'I understand you, and you understand me; let us go under the willows and weep'.

GABRIELLE. But after looking at my miniature you needn't have feared to find a wrinkled face waiting for you.

DAVENANT. You forget that your miniature did not arrive till the last moment, after all arrangements had been made, and Sebastian was about to start.

GABRIELLE. No, I do not forget. But there were two miniatures, and you told me this morning that you had given the head and shoulders to him and kept the naughty miniature for yourself. And I must know at once if my naughty miniature, which is quite a disgrace, gave you much pleasure, Mr Davenant.

DAVENANT. It did indeed. Your miniature and your letters –

GABRIELLE. Ah, so you read my letters while – But what have you done with my miniature? You said this morning that it was not at Claremont Villa, so it must be here then. Let me see my miniature.

DAVENANT. Shall I show it to you?

GABRIELLE. Why not? You think I might be shocked; but one is not shocked at oneself; or do you think we should not look at the miniature together? Perhaps you are right; but fetch it all the same. (DAVENANT *goes over to bureau in the corner of the room and opens a drawer. He returns with the miniature.*)

GABRIELLE. So you keep it locked up faithfully. Come, dear Mr Davenant, and sit on the sofa beside me, and we will look at our miniature together. (*They sit.*) Well, you do not speak. It doesn't seem to you like me at all? Is that the reason of your silence?

DAVENANT. No, not exactly. You see, I know you only in a hat and feathers. If you will take off your hat –

GABRIELLE. I should have to take off more than my hat to look like a goddess. And now tell me, do you like goddesses or real women, Mr Davenant?

DAVENANT. If a man doesn't see the goddess in the woman, he does not love her.

GABRIELLE. But goddesses are so different in different countries. In our museums they are thin when they come from Italy, and fat when they arrive from Amsterdam. Do you like very young women – mere childs? I hope you do, for it was said that I looked like seventeen when sitting for that miniature.

DAVENANT. The artist who painted it had a great deal of talent. Who was he?

GABRIELLE. It was not a he; it was a she; nor would I sit to a man in veils. Now, Mr Davenant, if you go on looking at that miniature you will say something naughty. Give it to me. (*She puts the miniature into the bodice of her dress.*)

DAVENANT. You gave it to me. It is mine; and it is the only thing that I have to remind me of you.

GABRIELLE. Do you wish to be reminded of your cowardice? Men seldom do. (*Rises and turns towards the door.* DAVENANT *intercepts her.*)

DAVENANT. No, you must give me back my property. Nothing goes from this room that comes into it.

GABRIELLE. Your property, Mr Davenant? You speak to me as if I were a thief.

DAVENANT. Forgive me, but I must have my miniature.

GABRIELLE. You are thinking, not of me, but of your museum, for your house is like one. Is that so, Mr Davenant?

DAVENANT. To some extent, yes.

GABRIELLE. Well, then, come and walk round this room with me and show me your little museum.

DAVENANT. The house that might have been yours.

GABRIELLE. But you did not come to Vienna! Ah, here is a portrait of yourself, and very like you. I am very glad your hair is turning grey, and I am glad you have moustaches and not drooping ones. That would be dreadful, for you have a horse's face. My face is like a cat's.

DAVENANT (*still pursuing her*). You must give me my miniature.

GABRIELLE. But why are you so greedy for this miniature? For I am a goddess in it, and you do not want a goddess, Mr Davenant. You like natural things. I am freckled under the ear, where I always

170

freckle. See! (*She shows him her ear.*)

DAVENANT. The freckles make a beautiful neck still more desirable (*she draws away*) by their naturalness.

GABRIELLE. I would keep the miniature and have the painter add some freckles. Do goddesses freckle, Mr Davenant, or is it too cold up there for freckles?

DAVENANT. Gabrielle, listen. You did not write to Sebastian. You wrote to me. It was an accident that –

GABRIELLE. Ach! that horrid word – accident!

DAVENANT. The time has come to speak seriously. I would not play Sebastian false, but you do not love him, so you say. You are leaving him – returning to Vienna.

GABRIELLE. I did not say that I was returning to Vienna, not at once. I am going to Paris, to Dieppe, to Trouville, or some tiny little fishing village where I can bathe without being seen, which is what I like, for it gives me *des crampes* of every kind to think that somebody is watching me rise out of the seas in a sea-gown which is most unbecoming, exaggerating all one's little roundnesses.

DAVENANT. Which would not matter in your case, for you are as slight in nature as in the miniature which I must have.

GABRIELLE (*taking the miniature from her bosom, but holding it behind her back*). Now which would you prefer – to have the miniature to look at while I am away, or to come to see me when I return to Vienna?

DAVENANT. I may go abroad in the autumn, and we might meet in Venice.

GABRIELLE. It would be nice to meet you in Venice, and to sit in a gondola looking at the moon and listening to that noisy Italian music that would be dreadful elsewhere; but in Venice one likes it, and you could tell me your troubles holding my hand.

DAVENANT (*going to her*). Gabrielle, is this a promise?

GABRIELLE. Why should we not meet in Vienna? Everybody meets in Venice.

DAVENANT. But you said to hold your hand.

GABRIELLE. If I had not the miniature in my hand you might hold it now.

DAVENANT. Well, then, put back the miniature into your bodice. (*She puts the miniature back into her bodice.*)

GABRIELLE. Now you can hold my hand, Mr Davenant.

DAVENANT. Remember that I am but flesh and blood, and were I to go to Vienna I might ask you to love me.

GABRIELLE. Does one ask?

DAVENANT. I suppose not. (*He takes her in his arms.*)

GABRIELLE. We aren't in Vienna yet. (*He holds her.*) No, no, you must not kiss me.

DAVENANT. If you would not have me kiss you, why did you ask me to meet you in Vienna?

GABRIELLE. I do not know.

DAVENANT. A woman always knows. A man doesn't.

GABRIELLE. I swear, Mr Davenant, that I do not know why –

DAVENANT. Yes, you do. Why did you come here to-night?

GABRIELLE. I do not know – an impulse. I am full of impulses.

DAVENANT. Turn you head and let me kiss you.

GABRIELLE. No, not on the mouth. (*He kisses her.*) Had I known that you would kiss me by force I would not have come here.

DAVENANT. But you are not angry?

GABRIELLE. No, not angry.

DAVENANT. Worse still – disappointed?

GABRIELLE. A man is always wrong to kiss a woman against her will.

DAVENANT. Gabrielle, I had to kiss you.

GABRIELLE. Did you desire it so much as that?

DAVENANT. An obligation incurred to Sebastian.

GABRIELLE. To kiss me!

DAVENANT. Yes, for only through my kiss could the truth be made known to you.

GABRIELLE. What truth?

DAVENANT. That you came here in anger, with an idea in your mind of revenge. Sebastian sent your poems to Mrs Godby, and in somewhat vulgar parlance you came here determined to get even with him. But you couldn't, for you love your husband.

GABRIELLE. I think I hate you, Mr Davenant.

DAVENANT. But why should you hate me?

GABRIELLE. I do not like sly men.

DAVENANT. Sly?

GABRIELLE. Yes, sly, for you would have me believe that your kiss was only intended to prove that I still love Sebastian.

DAVENANT. If you didn't love Sebastian, you would have kissed me.

GABRIELLE. Do you think so? Tell me why you think so. Tell me, Mr Davenant, if it was only to wring the truth out of me that you kissed me, or are we still playing at comedy?

DAVENANT. In this world we are always playing a comedy of some sort, for nothing is quite true and nothing is altogether false. (*He rings the bell.*) (*Enter* MARTIN.)

DAVENANT. Will you tell Mr Dayne that I would like to speak to him?

GABRIELLE. So you think that I shall kiss and be friends again with my husband?

DAVENANT. I will not say I am sure, for one is sure of nothing.

GABRIELLE. And if I refuse, what then?

DAVENANT. You will lose an obedient lover, for when Sebastian returned here with Godby and I offered to relieve him of the tedium of telling you he was not the author of *Elizabeth Cooper,* he begged of me to tell you nothing.

GABRIELLE. That is a point in his favour; but why have you picked up that book, and why are you reading it? It isn't polite to read while you are talking to me.

DAVENANT. This book is an advance copy of his poems, and it is another point in his favour, for you will find all the poems dedicated to you. (*She takes the book of poems and looks through them.*) But one moment, Sebastian will be here in a few minutes. Give me my miniature.

GABRIELLE. I sent you this miniature before I married Sebastian, and I do not think you should have it.

DAVENANT. It seems to me that I have earned that miniature.

GABRIELLE. Well, perhaps you have, but let Sebastian never see it. (*She gives him the miniature.*) (*Enter* SEBASTIAN.)

DAVENANT. Sebastian, I have good news for you. The Countess is prepared to forgive you.

GABRIELLE. Is disposed to forgive him.

SEBASTIAN (*to* GABRIELLE). You see now that all I told you of my cousin is true. But I did not praise enough. He is a kind, a good and a true friend, and a great genius, for if he weren't he would never have persuaded you out of your cruel humour.

DAVENANT. Criticism and reproaches are from this moment forbidden, Sebastian.

SEBASTIAN I won't offend again, but how *did* you persuade her?

DAVENANT. I would not anticipate my old age, for in my old age I look forward to telling the story of the Countess's yielding to my persuasion when you both come from some distant country – Austria, perhaps Italy – bringing with you the children that I heard spoken of this morning, not forgetting the go-carts, the perambulator, the rocking-horses and the hoops – all the shows of their happiness.

GABRIELLE. And how would you like the children to be – two little girls, or two little boys? Two little girls, dear Mr Davenant; but I am not sure that myself and Sebastian would not prefer them mixed. But we will do all we can to oblige – shall we not, Sebastian? And now wilt thou be jealous if I kiss dear Mr Davenant for all he has done for us? (*Enter* MARTIN.)

MARTIN. Lady Letham, sir. (*Enter* LADY LETHAM.)

DAVENANT. How do you do, Lady Letham? Let me introduce you to the Countess von Hoenstadt and to her husband, Mr Sebastian Dayne, whom I think you have already met.

LADY LETHAM (*to* GABRIELLE). I am glad that Mr Dayne did not return from Germany empty-handed.

GABRIELLE. No, indeed he didn't, and I'm afraid that I've already proved myself somewhat of a handful. You do say somewhat of a handful in English, Lady Letham?

LADY LETHAM. We do. How well the Countess von Hoenstadt speaks English, Mr Dayne.

MARTIN. Dinner is served, sir.

DAVENANT (*giving* LADY LETHAM *his arm and turning to speak to* SEBASTIAN). If you choose to follow us, Lady Letham and I will be delighted to have your company; but it may be that you would prefer your company to ours, in which case you can take the Countess back to the 'Three Kings'; and after dinner you can catch the last train back to Claremont Villa and spend the rest of your honeymoon there, if you like, unless you would prefer to go farther afield. The Countess was speaking to me just now of Paris, Trouville and Etretat; but these things you must decide for yourself. Meanwhile the soup is getting cold. (*Exeunt* LADY LETHAM *and* DAVENANT.)

SEBASTIAN. Say which you would prefer, Gabrielle – to dine here or with me alone at the 'Three Kings'?

GABRIELLE. I have no thought for dinner just now. Let us sit for a while and talk. (*She goes towards the sofa and sits. He follows her.*) Read me your poems. (*Hands him the book.*)

SEBASTIAN. My book.

GABRIELLE. An advance copy. (*He begins to read.*)

END OF THE THIRD ACT

THE PASSING OF THE ESSENES

A DRAMA IN THREE ACTS

BY

GEORGE MOORE

CHARACTERS in the PLAY

JESUS of Nazareth

JACOB, a young shepherd

HAZAEL, President of the Essenes

MATHIAS
SADDOC
MANAHEM
CALEB
SHALLUM   Essene monks
ELEAZOR
ELIAKIM
BARTHOLEMEW
PAUL of TARSUS

SCENES

ACT I: Interior of the cenoby of the Essenes on a shelf of rock in the gorge of the brook Kerith. Evening.

ACT II: The same. Sunrise.

ACT III: The same. Later.

ACT I

SCENE: *The main hall of the cenoby of the Essenes, a rude, barn-like structure opening on to a balcony, on which there are seats. The* PRESIDENT'S *high-backed chair is on the right. Doors lead from the hall to the lecture-room and the cells.*
Enter JESUS, *with* JACOB, *a young shepherd. As they advance down the cave voices are heard.*

JACOB (*listening*). Were I out on the hills I'd say: Yoe bleateth after ram. Here my guess is that it is Mathias interpreting Scripture.
JESUS. Who then hath been talking to thee about Mathias, his voice and his doctrine?
JACOB Saddoc, whom I met the day I brought a message from thee to the President. He was sitting on the cliff's edge muttering: Heresies! Heresies! and so deep was he in his thoughts that a while went by before he understood my question enough to answer: Hazael is with the brethren, listening to Mathias proving the Scriptures to be parables; and having said as much he was off again. Adam and Eve, saith he, could not have been so foolish as to hide from God in a garden. Nobody hides from God.
JESUS. Saddoc and Mathias are of different minds about many things. Mathias, in truth, is hard to understand, and is a great trouble to Saddoc.
JACOB As this cavern will be to thee, Master; for it will breed a great longing in thee for the sky and the hills, the flock running merrily, following after the sound of the pipe, the sunny mornings on the hillsides and the oak wood where we have sat so often resting through the heats of midday. The drone from under yon door will set thee thinking of Eliab, who often soothed thee with sweet airs on the double flute, or of Bozrah, who ran his fingers over the strings of his harp to recall thee to us from the dim heart of the wood. But it was in answer, methinks, to Havilah's pipe that thou wouldst come to the rugged oak; he had a lonely ditty that fetched thee. Ah, Master, thou canst not forget, so why leave us?
JESUS. Thou'rt right, Jacob. I have lived too long on the hills to forget them. I shall not seek to forget, and not many days will pass over

177

without my coming to the hills to hearken to the sound of thy pipe. Mine I make over to thee.

JACOB. Thou must keep thy pipe, Master, to warn me of thy coming, and when I hear it I shall leap to my feet as the goat leaps at the sight of a quickening bough.

JESUS. I have taught thee much of my craft, Jacob.

JACOB. But Hazael will put questions to me that I cannot answer.

JESUS. Well, Hazael is without wit for sheep or goats.

JACOB. Hazael will say to thee: Jesus, thou must remain our shepherd till the next lambing season is over; and if he saith that he will say well.

JESUS. It is not long since he said to me: Jesus, there is grey in thy beard; how old art thou? And when I answered: Fifty-three, his head sank on his breast and he muttered: And I have heard thee always spoken of as the boy Jesus.

JACOB. He would like to have thee with him, but he must think of the flock, and he will ask if the dogs will follow me.

JESUS. Thema takes meat from thee, and after a two-days' fast Gorbotha will come to thy call, and when they have run down a wolf or a jackal for thee, they'll know thee for their master. Take heed of thy flock. Do well the work that God hath given thee to do, remembering always that though the distance be great from bad pasture to good, the journey from the bad to the good will profit thee, though the flock be weary before they attain it: but however weary, if the grass be good they will fall to nibbling. And now, Jacob, before we part, remember that when the lambs are folded with the yoes thou'lt put into their jaws a stick to keep them from sucking; and keep thine eyes upon the lamb I pointed out to thee, for he will come into a fine, broad-shouldered ram, strong across the loins and straight on his legs, the sort to get lambs that will do well on these hills; and thou'lt be wise to leave him for another hundred days on his dam. Shear him, for it will give him strength to take some wool from him, but take it not from his back, for he'll want the wool there to protect him from the sun. All the first year he will skip about the yoes and jump upon them, but it will be only play, for his time is not yet come. In two more years he will be at his height, serving ten yoes a day; but keep him not overlong, for thou must always have some new rams preparing, else the flock will decline. The ram that I chose for thy lesson to-night is old and must soon be replaced. He was a good ram in his time, but the white ram that came at my call is the best I have seen this many a year. The white ram is stronger than the black, though the black yoe will turn from him and seek a ram of her own colour. I have known a white ram so

178

ardent for a black yoe that he fought the black ram till their skulls cracked.

JACOB. But, Master – (*The door of the lecture-room opens and* MANAHEM *and* SADDOC *bear out* HAZAEL, *who has fainted. The* ESSENES *are clad in long white garments.*)

MANAHEM (*as they cross the stage to the balcony*). As soon as we get him into the air he will return to himself.

SADDOC. A little water! (*Exit* JESUS. *He returns with water,* SADDOC *motions the others aside and bathes* HAZAEL'S *temples.*)

HAZAEL. The heat overcame me. But I shall soon be well, and then thou shalt bear me back to hear –

SADDOC. Thou'lt do better to rest in the air of this balcony.

HAZAEL. It was not the length of Mathias's discourse, nor his eloquence, that caused my senses to swoon away, but my age, which will not permit me to listen long. Hearken, Saddoc and Manahem, I would be alone with Jesus, and do you return to the lecture-room at once, else our brother will be discouraged in his discourse. Hasten, lest ye miss any more of his arguments. (*The* ESSENES *are about to raise a protest, but at a sign from* HAZAEL *they go out.*) Who is this standing by thee, Jesus? Not one of the brethren, for if he wore a white robe I should see it.

JESUS. It is Jacob. I have brought him this evening to receive thy commands. To-night I remain with thee here.

HAZAEL. So thou biddest the hills farewell to-night?

JESUS. Why not to-night, since I am bringing thee a shepherd who will serve thee as well as I have served thee? Another may claim him whilst the winter lasts, for his fame is spreading.

HAZAEL. Thy master speaks well of thee, Jacob.

JACOB. He speaks too well of me sir. I had ill luck on the hills over against Cæsarea.

JESUS (*to* HAZAEL). He went thither in search of pasture, for tidings reached Kerith that rain had fallen in the west.

JACOB. I had no dogs, Master. Let Hazael know that my dogs were taken the night before by panthers.

JESUS. There is nothing so toothsome to a panther as a dog; he will risk his life fearlessly for one. And how many wolves were there, Jacob, in the pack that trailed thee?

JACOB. Ten or a dozen, and what defence would my poor dogs have been against a pack like that? 'Twas the fourth night, and I could not find the cavern I looked for and lay down in the open with my flock ... After the loss of my flock I lived as I could on the scraps the shepherds threw me. But they wearied of charity, and I'd be sitting

179

now with the lepers by the wayside above Jericho if Jesus had not given his lambs into my charge.

JESUS. Jacob lost faith in himself, as we all do at times.

JACOB. I am young, said I to myself, and can wait. Jesus, who knows more than all the other shepherds together, holds me to be no fool. I am young and can wait, and who knows, Jesus may tell me his cure for the scab, and by serving him I may get a puppy when Thema litters.

HAZAEL. Jacob, it is for thee to listen rather than to speak, and since Jesus believes that thou canst replace him, the flock from henceforth is in thy charge. (JESUS *goes up the stage with* JACOB.)

JESUS. Thou'lt come to fetch me in the morning; we'll count the sheep together. And take heart, Jacob, for I shall always be by in case of need.

JACOB. Am I to feed the dogs, Master?

JESUS. To-morrow they'll take food from thee at my bidding as before. (*Exit* JACOB.)

HAZAEL. I gave Caleb a letter this morning for thee, charging him to search the hills.

JESUS. After reading thy letter I held my peace with Jacob, and it was not till the last yoe was made clean for the winter that I said to him: I have come to the end of my life on the hills. He was frightened at the thought of leaving me before the lambing-time –

HAZAEL. And I am frightened at the thought of leaving thee before the springtime. I shall be sorry to leave thee, Jesus, for our lives have been twisted together, strands of the same rope. But it must be plain to thee that I am growing weaker; month by month, week by week, my strength is ebbing; I am going out. But for what reason should I lament that God hath not chosen to retain me for a few months longer, since my life cannot be prolonged for more than a few months? My eighty and odd years have left me with barely strength enough to sit in the doorway looking back on the way I have come. Every day the things of this world grow fainter and life becomes to me an unreal thing, and myself becomes unreal to those around me. Only for thee do I retain anything of my vanished self. So why should I remain? For thy sake, lest thou be lonely here? Well, that is reason enough, and I will bear the burden of life as well as I can for thy sake. A burden it is, and for a reason that thou mayst not divine, for thou art still a young man in my eyes, and, moreover, hast not lived under a roof year after year listening to learned interpretations of the Scriptures. Thou hast not guessed, nor wilt thou ever guess till age reveals it to thee, that as we grow old we do not love God as once we loved him. No one would have thought, not even thou, who art more conscious of God's presence than any one under this roof, I say not even thou wouldst have thought that as we approach death our love of God grows weaker, but this is so. In great age nothing seems to matter, and it is from this indifference that I wish to escape. Thou goest forth in the morning to lead thy flock in search of pasture, and God is nearer to us in the wilderness than he is among men.

JESUS. Art afraid that under this roof I, too, may cease to love God?

HAZAEL. Not cease to love God.

JESUS. Thou wouldst warn me that God is loved only on the hills under the sky?

HAZAEL. I am too weak to choose my thoughts or words, and many things pass out of my mind. Had I remembered I would not have spoken.

JESUS. But why not speak, Father? for I would be ready to resist the changes that may befall.

HAZAEL. Only this can I say with certainty, Jesus, that the sky will always be before thine eyes and the green fields under thy feet, yea, even whilst listening to Mathias.

JESUS. Thou, too, didst live once under the sky.

HAZAEL. In beforetimes the love of God was ardent in me, and whether walking by day or by night I was always watchful for the young man in whom I might discover an Essene for Kerith. But, Jesus, why this grief? Because I am going from thee? Dear friend, to come and go is the law of life, and perchance I shall be with thee longer than thou thinkest. Eighty and odd years may be lengthened into ninety; the patriarchs lived till a hundred and more years, and we believe that the soul outlives the body. Out of the chrysalis we escape from our corruptible bodies, and the beautiful butterfly flutters Godward. Grieve for me a little when I am gone, but grieve not before I go, for I would see thy face always happy, as I remember it in those years long ago in Nazareth. Jesus, Jesus, thou shouldst not weep like this! None should weep but for sin, and thy life is known to me from the day in Nazareth when we sat in the street together to the day that thou wentest to the Jordan to get baptism from John.

JESUS. A year of my life is unknown to thee, Hazael.

HAZAEL. We will not speak of it, nor of thy transgression of our rules, atoned for on the hills. Since God hath forgiven thee, why should we be laggards in forgiveness?

JESUS. I pray thee, say not another word, Hazael, for none is less worthy than I. The greatest sinner amongst us is sitting by thee, one that hath not dared to tell his secret to thee for twenty years or more.

HAZAEL. On thy return to us thou wouldst have told all that befell thee in Galilee, but neither I nor the brethren wished to hear thy story.

JESUS. John's doctrine of repentance entered into my life and I preached it, but little by little –

HAZAEL. Jesus, I beseech thee! Twenty years agone it was decided that we should not question thee. We were certain that thy hand had done no wrong and that no sinful thought ever entered thy mind.

JESUS. I lacked courage –

HAZAEL. No, Jesus, thy conscience deceives thee. Courage was not lacking. But we did not wish to hear thee, and thou, in thy great kindness, forbore for our sakes to speak.

JESUS. I said then that I could not come to live among you without confessing my sins, and went to the hills to lead my flock. And now that I have come again to live with you, the quiet and peace that I seek would be far away if –

HAZAEL. If thou didst not tell all the scruples that infect thee. But, Jesus, more than ever I beg that thou wilt not disturb the cenoby with confessions of past sins, tribulations and doubts. Silence is required of thee. Twenty years agone we were content with the Scriptures and with the rules of our Order. Questions were not rife. But ever since Mathias came from Egypt and read the Scriptures differently from Saddoc, finding allegories everywhere, all is changed. Some of our brethren, feeling that the solitude of Kerith was not enough, sought a deeper solitude in the clefts above us. Whatever may have befallen thee in Galilee, and afterwards in Jerusalem, would set the cenoby aflame with violent discussion were it disclosed now. Hatreds would spring up, and the desire to escape.

JESUS. Are there then brethren amongst us who would break their vows?

HAZAEL. I say naught against any brother, but there is disquiet. I had looked forward to a peaceful old age, with thee beside me. Shatter it not with disclosures, whatever they may be. (*Pause.*)

JESUS. I am too old to follow the flock any longer on the hills. I have done my best with it, and have given it in good condition to Jacob. There is reason in what thou sayest, Hazael. I would not disturb the peace of thy last years, and if I come to live with thee, and accept thy guidance, my first duty is obedience. (*The door of the lecture-room opens and the* ESSENES *come out singing:*)

In the Lord put I my trust:
How say ye to my soul, Flee
As a bird to your mountain?
For, lo, the wicked bend their

Bow, they make ready their arrow
Upon the string, that they may privily
Shoot at the upright in heart.
If the foundations be destroyed, what
Can the righteous do?
For the righteous Lord loveth
Righteousness; his countenance
Doth behold the upright.

JESUS. These words of the Psalmist were meant for me, and now that the brethren are here I may not speak. But to-morrow –

HAZAEL. There may be no to-morrow for me. (*To the* ESSENES.) Our brother Jesus hath given over the charge of our flocks to a young shepherd.

SADDOC. All the cells, Father, are filled.

HAZAEL. Jesus can sleep here on this bench. A mattress and a cloak will be enough for him who hath slept in caverns or in valleys on stones piled high to keep him above the floods. Manahem will get thee a mattress, Jesus; he knows where to find one. (*Exit* MANAHEM.) I am strong enough to walk alone, Saddoc. (*He disengages himself from* SADDOC'S *arm and walks with the* ESSENES *towards his cell, joining them in the psalm:*)
All the powers of the Lord
Bless ye the Lord; praise and
Exalt him above all for ever. (*Exeunt* HAZAEL *and the* ESSENES. SADDOC *remains with* JESUS.)

SADDOC. The brethren are weary of hearing Mathias prove that the Scriptures are but allegories, and for a long time have been talking of thee, saying: He'll come back with stories of the robbers he hath met and the wolves and the bears he hath escaped. True enough, there are some that would have thee stay on the hills, for thy Jacob, not being one of us, will claim one lamb out of every twenty, and these he may send to the temple for burnt-offerings, the which, as thou knowest, is forbidden by our laws. I have much more to tell, but here Manahem comes with a mattress for thee. (*Enter* MANAHEM *carrying a mattress.*)

MANAHEM. Wilt thou sleep, Jesus, within the cavern, or on the balcony under the sky?

JESUS. On the balcony, dear brother.

SADDOC (*helping* MANAHEM *to lay the mattress on the balcony*). On this bench he will lie comfortably under a covering, for though the evenings are still warm the nights are chilly. Fetch a warm covering, Manahem. (*Exit* MANAHEM. SADDOC *approaches* JESUS.) Since

183

Mathias came we have never had an easy day with our own thoughts. What dost thou think he was saying when we returned to the lecture-room?

JESUS. I cannot read the mind of Mathias, Saddoc.

SADDOC. That there are two beings in man, one that hath prudence and the other that exerts it; and he doth liken these two principles to a carbuncle and an emerald! (*Enter* MANAHEM *with a quilt.*)

MANAHEM. The warmest I could find, perhaps too warm.

JESUS (*feeling the quilt*). My thanks, brother, my thanks. (*He passes to the farther end of the balcony and leans on the rail.*) How still the night is, not a sound in it but the murmur of the brook flowing down the gorge to Jordan ... Ye have voices of wayfarers sometimes at your door asking for shelter and bread?

SADDOC. The dangers of the path save us from wayfarers.

MANAHEM. Once on a time a wayfarer dared to follow the path by night, and he lost his life over the cliffs in the brook.

JESUS. Come, Manahem, and tell me if thine eyes discern not a man in the path yonder.

MANAHEM. I see none.

JESUS. Look again, Manahem.

SADDOC (*going to the balcony*). Truly, our shepherd's eyes are better than ours. A man is on the path, trying to follow it, and if he be a man of flesh and blood like ourselves, he will topple.

MANAHEM. He hath not yet gone over into the brook, but keeps the path as if he knew it. He is maybe one of our dissident brothers come up from Jordan.

SADDOC. Now he is crossing the bridge, and now he begins the ascent. Let us pray that he may miss the path through the terraces.

JESUS. But thou wouldst not have him miss it, Saddoc? He shall have my mattress.

SADDOC. If not an evil spirit, of a certainty he is coming to ask for shelter for the night. And if not a demon, he may be a prophet or a robber; for once more the hills are filled with robbers.

JESUS. Or it may be the preacher of whom Jacob spoke to me this evening. He came up from Jordan with a story of a preacher that the multitude would not listen to and sought to drown in the river; and he told me how the rabble had followed the man over the hills with intent to kill him

MANAHEM. Some great and terrible heresy he must be preaching to stir them like that. Did Jacob bring news of his escape or death?

JESUS. He thought the prophet must have escaped into a cave, for he came upon the crowd going home like dogs from a hunt when they have lost their quarry.

SADDOC. A robber is at our door, for sure. He escaped the crowd and hath been hiding in a cave. Only a robber who knew the hills could have kept the path ...Now he sees us! He is no shepherd, but a robber. (*They wait for a few moments, and the knocking they expect comes at the door.*) Open not the door, Jesus! There are Sicarii who kill men in the daytime, mingling themselves among the multitude with daggers hidden in their garments, their mission being to stab those that disobey the law in any fraction. We are Essenes and may not send blood offerings to the temple. Open not the door! Sicarii or Zealots travel in search of heretics through the cities of Samaria and Judea. Open not the door! Men are for ever fooled, and will never cease to open their doors to those who stand in need of meat and drink. It will be safer, Jesus, to bid him away. Tell him rather that we'll let down a basket of meat and drink from the balcony to him.

JESUS. Art thou, Manahem, for turning this man from the door or letting him in?

MANAHEM. There is no need to be frightened. He is but a wanderer, Saddoc.

SADDOC. A wanderer he cannot be, for he hath followed the path through the darkness, a thing we could not do. Open not the door, I tell thee, else we all hang on crosses above the hills to-morrow. (*He goes to the door and listens.*)

MANAHEM. But, Saddoc, by our law we may not refuse bed and board to the poor.

JESUS. If we do not open he will leave our door, and that will be a greater misfortune than any he may bring us. Hearken, Saddoc!

SADDOC (*to* MANAHEM). He speaks fair enough. But we may plead that after sunset in the times we live in –

JESUS. Manahem, art thou with me or with Saddoc? We know that there is but one man, and we are more than a match for one. Put a sword in Saddoc's hand.

SADDOC. No, Manahem! I should feel like a fool with a sword in my hand. Since thou sayest, Jesus, there is but one man, and we are three, it might be unlucky to turn him from our door.

JESUS. May I then open to him? (JESUS *unbars the door, and* PAUL *staggers in, bald-headed, his turban having fallen in his flight. He is a powerful man of medium height, with broad shoulders, piercing black eyes, shaggy eyebrows, and a hooked nose. A black beard covers the lower part of his face. He stands like a hunted animal, breathing hard, looking from one to the other.*)

185

PAUL. May I rest a little while? If so, give me to drink before I sleep. No food, but drink. Why do ye not answer? Do ye fear me, mistaking me for a robber? Or have I wandered among robbers? Where am I? (*To* JESUS.) Hearken, I am but a wayfarer, and thou'rt a shepherd of the hills – I know thee by thy garb. Thou'lt not refuse me shelter?

JESUS (*to* SADDOC *and* MANAHEM). He shall have the mattress I was to sleep upon. (*To* PAUL). Thou shalt have food and a coverlet.

PAUL. No food, but a drink of water.

SADDOC. There is some yoes' milk on the shelf, Manahem. (MANAHEM *fetches the milk, which* PAUL *drinks greedily.*)

JESUS (*to* PAUL). I'll get thee a linen garment; sleep will come easier in it; and I'll bathe thy feet. (*Exit* JESUS.)

PAUL. A shepherd told me that after I had passed the bridge I'd find terraces leading upwards to this ledge of rock.

MANAHEM. We watched thee from the balcony. At every step we feared thou wouldst topple out of the path into the abyss.

SADDOC. If the shepherd hath told thee that we in this cavern are of the Essenes, and that no traveller was ever turned from our door, he hath told thee truly. But we would know whom we are guesting.

PAUL. I am Paul of Tarsus, a prisoner of the Romans –

SADDOC. A prisoner of the Romans! (*To* MANAHEM). Mayhap with soldiers at his heels! Let us put him beyond the door. Manahem, aid me! (SADDOC *tries to drag* PAUL *to his feet.* JESUS *enters, with a basin of water and a garment.*)

JESUS. Are we not forbidden by our rule to thrust a stranger from our door?

SADDOC. But he tells us he is a prisoner of the Romans.

JESUS. Even so, we cannot turn him away to fall into the abyss.

SADDOC. He kept to the path on his way hither and will doubtless return by it safely to the hills.

PAUL (*to* JESUS). I am not a criminal fleeing from the Romans, but a Roman citizen escaping from Jewish persecution.

SADDOC. Why, then, didst thou say thou wert a prisoner of the Romans?

PAUL. I am a prisoner of the Romans for a riot that began two years ago in Jerusalem, whither a great pressing of the spirit urged me, for I would not leave Asia before preaching once more in Jerusalem to the Jews, a stiff-necked, gainsaying race, but dear to me despite its stubbornness. But the people were stirred up against me, and would have stoned me had not the Roman guard come out to quell the uproar and borne me on their shoulders up the steps of the castle, whither the people thronged after me, rending their garments, throwing dust in the air, crying: Away with him for the scourging! As I was being bound I turned to the centurion and asked him if it were lawful to scourge a Roman citizen and he untried; whereupon they desisted, and I was sent to Cæsarea to be judged. And the Jews, still thirsting for my blood, sent elders from the temple to Festus, saying: We would question this man in Jerusalem on some points of the law; give him over to us. But I said to the noble Festus: These men are planning to kill me in an ambush; I appeal to Cæsar. And he answered me: Thou hast appealed to Cæsar, and to Cæsar thou shalt go. But the ship that was to take me to Rome was delayed, and a great pressing of the spirit came upon me to preach in Jericho, for I was loth to leave many Jews without knowledge of the Lord Jesus. And the noble Festus said to me: Go then to Jericho and preach thy doctrine, but I shall expect thee back within six days.

SADDOC. And how was thy doctrine received in Jericho?

PAUL. With stones, from which I escaped through the hills. But of all this I will tell ye to-morrow. Do ye tell me now of a young man, Timothy, who followed me along the cliff.

JESUS. Thou wast alone.

SADDOC (*whispering to* MANAHEM). He must have preached some terrible heresy for the Jews to seek his life with stones.

PAUL. Should Timothy have fallen into the hands of the Jews he is lost to me for ever.

JESUS. We know not of whom thou art speaking.

PAUL. Of Timothy, my son in the faith, who missed me where the hillside tumbles into shale and rubble and the road disappears. I must go in search of him.

JESUS. God hath upheld thee in a dangerous path for his purposes, and thou art welcome to remain with us for the night.

PAUL. Thy thought is that Timothy would be sought in vain in the darkness. (JESUS *unties* PAUL'S *sandals and bathes his feet.*)

SADDOC. Since thou art guesting among us we would hear more of the great pressing of the spirit that bade thee to Jericho.

PAUL. To preach the Lord Jesus, the Messiah promised to the Jews, who was raised from the dead. But the people would not listen.

MANAHEM. And why would they not listen? for 'tis not every day a tale is told of a man being raised from the dead.

PAUL. Stirred up by the priests the many sought to capture us; but we escaped into the hills and hid in a cave to which the spirit of the Lord directed us.

MANAHEM (*whispering to* SADDOC). Hark, an angel pointed out a cave to him!

SADDOC. Mayhap an angel did, but whether a good or an evil angel we know not. (JESUS *relieves* PAUL *of his garment and passes a white robe over his shoulders.*)

PAUL. Jericho would have done well to hearken to me, for have I not testified in many synagogues of the great light that blinded me on the road to Damascus, and the voice that cried to me out of the clouds: Saul, Saul, why persecutest thou me? (*Consciousness passes from* PAUL. *He falls back in the arms of* JESUS *and* SADDOC.)

SADDOC. Of what is he telling us?

JESUS. He hath fallen asleep. Help me to lift him to a couch on the balcony. (JESUS *and* SADDOC *carry* PAUL *to the balcony and lay him on one of the benches. They cover him with a quilt.* JESUS *lies down beside him on another bench.* SADDOC *returns to* MANAHEM.)

MANAHEM. Now, what did he say before he fell asleep?

SADDOC. He was telling us that on the road to Damascus a voice cried to him out of the clouds. (*They move a little nearer to* PAUL.) A heavy man to carry and to lift on to a couch.

MANAHEM. He spoke of many things besides Damascus.

SADDOC. He did; but words pass out of the mind quickly. I recall that the Jews drove him out of Jericho with stones, and that he lost his son in the faith, Timothy, on the hillside.

MANAHEM. His very words.

SADDOC. Had I had my wits about me I'd have asked him if his doctrine came out of the Scriptures.

MANAHEM. He was too weary to tell it plainly.

SADDOC. And we shall stumble when we try to tell it to the brethren. Let us go over it together.

MANAHEM. Mathias will put cunning questions to him. A rare occasion it will be for the Egyptian to entangle him and press him into evasions and contradictions.

SADDOC. Mathias will resolve the story of the voice speaking out of the clouds into allegory.

MANAHEM. In truth, whatever befell, his account of it is nowise clear.

SADDOC. He said the Lord Jesus was raised from the dead. Said he not so, Manahem?

MANAHEM. He said many things, speaking like a man in a dream.

SADDOC. Try to recall if he were stoned because of a heresy.

MANAHEM. I barely remember...My thoughts are dim and treacherous, but at daybreak the mind is clear. (*Exit* MANAHEM. SADDOC *returns to the balcony, looks anxiously at* PAUL *and goes out.*)

CURTAIN

ACT II

SCENE: *The same. Sunrise. When the curtain rises a shepherd's pipe is heard from afar. A slight interval, and the pipe is heard again, this time much nearer.* PAUL *and* JESUS *are asleep on benches on either side of the balcony. Neither awakes.*

JACOB *appears at the end of the gallery. He advances cautiously. He is about to play his pipe again with a view to awakening the sleepers. He hesitates, decides not to do so, and advances towards them. Touching* JESUS *with his pipe he awakens him.* JESUS *rises to his feet and signs to* JACOB *that he is not to speak.* JESUS *and* JACOB *come down the stage.*

JACOB. So the preacher found his way into the cenoby!

JESUS. A great knocking came at our door, and I gave him the bed that Manahem and Saddoc were making for me.

JACOB. But his fellow – where is he?

JESUS. He asked for his fellow, and would have gone in search of him. But he fell asleep in our arms whilst talking.

JACOB. At daybreak it was reported that the twain escaped through a swirl of water that no man would have dared his life into but to save it. On seeing them carried down to the sea, the people laughed and clapped their hands, saying: They will drink of bitterness before they drown, and if they drown not we shall take them in Moab. But they kept to the bank they plunged from, and belike a sudden flux in the current carried them up a shelving strand, whence they escaped into the hills.

JESUS. We can get this man to Cæsarea by crossways known only to us.

JACOB. We can indeed; and be sure I'll lead him to safety, Master.

JESUS. An evil blow might befall thee, or many stripes, or a stoning.

JACOB. I owe thee my life, and thine being worth twenty such lives as mine –

JESUS. I am but a shepherd on the hills of Kerith like thyself.

JACOB. Thou art above us, Master, and always in our thoughts, whether we speak of sheep or of the sick. Of what art thou thinking? I said yesterday to a man, and got from the him the story of the ram Cæsar, brought by thee from Cæsarea, the original Adam of the flock. And

189

when he heard from me that thou wert about to bid the hills farewell, he sighed and began the story of his wife, who was bed-rid for three years and would be so still if thou hadst not called to her from the doorway: Woman, rise and gown thyself! The sick ask for something thou hast touched – the laces from thy shoe, a strip from a veil thou hast worn. We cannot spare thee, Master.

JESUS. Come with me into the hills to warn the shepherds that should a strange man come to them asking for direction to Caesarea, they must guide him and give him bread and drink, and sandals, should he need them. (JESUS *and* JACOB *go up the stage, and* SADDOC *and* MANAHEM *enter, followed by* CALEB *carrying bread and a jug of milk.*)

JESUS (*to the* ESSENES). Our guest still sleeps. Do not awaken him, and when his eyes open tell him that I have gone in search of his fellow and will return to guide him to Cæsarea. (*Exeunt* JESUS *and* JACOB. *The* ESSENES *approach* PAUL.)

CALEB. He sleeps like one whom naught could awake but the trumpets of Judgment.

SADDOC. I would he were away. He hath had his rest, and I am mindful of the great danger it is to hide a man alike an enemy of the Jews and Romans. (PAUL *awakes, and seeing the three figures looks round with staring eyes, like one who believes himself to be the victim of an hallucination.*)

PAUL (*rising to his feet*). Who are ye? And where am I? Yonder is daylight ... I must escape!

MANAHEM. Hast forgotten knocking at our door last night?

PAUL. Last night I was swimming in Jordan and escaped through the hills ... I shall disentangle it all presently ... But Timothy, my son in the faith – where is he?

MANAHEM. The shepherd who slept by thee hath gone in search of thy fellow.

PAUL (*trying to recover himself*). When my eyes opened and I saw you in your white garments ...

CALEB. I bring thee bread and a jug of milk freshly drawn. (PAUL *drinks.*)

PAUL. My feet pain me.

MANAHEM. Jesus, our shepherd, bathed them. Hast forgotten?

PAUL. No. He gave me a garment, saying I would sleep easier in it. (*Exit* CALEB.)

MANAHEM. The rule of our Order is to succour the tired traveller.

PAUL. And assuredly I was one last night. (*He begins to eat the bread, and whilst he is eating* MATHIAS *enters, followed by* SHALLUM,

190

ELEAZOR, ELIAKIM, BARTHOLOMEW, *and* CALEB, *who carries a plate of lentils. Seeing that* PAUL *is eating* CALEB *whispers to* BARTHOLOMEW, *who goes out and returns with a small table, which he places before* PAUL.)

CALEB (*laying the plate on the table*). Lentils boiled in water is our fare, but our rule allows butter to our guests.

MATHIAS (*to* PAUL). Our President will be ready to speak with thee before midday and will press thee to remain with us till thou hast regained enough strength to continue thy journey. (*The* ESSENES *make a movement of withdrawal.*)

PAUL. A few hours' sleep is enough for a hardened wayfarer like me. Stay, noble Essenes, I thank you for the rest I have had, and for the delay that your President would press upon me; but I am under bond to return to Cæsarea to go on board the ship that will take me to Rome.

MANAHEM (*to* MATHIAS). Our guest hath appealed to Cæsar.

MATHIAS (*to* PAUL). Thou art then a rich man, who paid a great sum of money for thy citizenship?

PAUL. My citizenship was not purchased. I was born free.

MATHIAS. Yet thou art at enmity with Jews and Romans alike.

PAUL. A prisoner of the Romans for a riot in Jerusalem, and hated of the Jews for I preach a new dispensation, but an enemy of no man, rather the friend of all men.

CALEB. We would hear of this riot in Jerusalem.

MATHIAS. He hath come to rest, not to tell stories.

CALEB. But is he to leave us without knowledge of the Lord Jesus. Manahem and Saddoc had the story overnight. Are we not to hear it?

MATHIAS. What sayest thou, Saddoc?

SADDOC. That I'd liefer see the man eat his lentils than listen to him telling stories of the Lord Jesus.

CALEB. Paul is leaving us at midday, and we would not forgo the story he tells.

BARTHOLOMEW. Of the man raised from the dead.

MANAHEM. The first of all mankind to escape death.

MATHIAS. Elijah was spared death.

MANAHEM. A miracle – no man denies it; but a greater miracle was the raising of the Lord Jesus from the dead.

PAUL. God loves his creations – this earth and the men upon it, wherefore he sent his only begotten son to suffer death on the cross that all men might believe and be saved. And the Jews being a stiff-necked race, he decreed that the birth of the Lord Jesus should be as miraculous as his resurrection. He was born of a virgin.

191

MATHIAS. In the absence of our President –

PAUL (*rising to his feet*). I leave at midday, but I would not withhold from the Essene brotherhood the story of the Lord Jesus.

SHALLUM. We would hear it!

PAUL. Time, always on the march, will allow but a fragment –

SEVERAL ESSENES. Speak! Speak! (*The* ESSENES *fetch seats and range themselves round* PAUL, *who speaks from behind the table.*)

PAUL. Learn then that I am Paul of Tarsus, a Hebrew like yourselves, beforetimes a Pharisee standing by the law, obeying it and hating those who denied it or questioned it. Such a manner of man I was in the city of Tarsus, a tent-maker, clever at the loom and learned in the Scriptures.

MATHIAS. I would warn our President –

ELEAZOR (*detaining him*). Stay! Stay!

SADDOC. If thou leavest us, Mathias, who will trip up this wandering soothsayer when he reasons falsely?

ELIAKIM. If to listen to him be a breach of the law –

SADDOC. We were afraid to open the door to him –

PAUL. Mistaking me for a robber!

BARTHOLOMEW. On with the story!

ELEAZOR. We would hear it! We would hear it!

PAUL. One day there came to Tarsus tidings that a man was preaching in every town and village in Galilee that the end was come of the law given to Moses and the Prophets, and the promise given in its stead of eternal happiness for Jews and Gentiles alike. I was wroth indeed, and went about asking if there was nobody with authority to confute this man and cast him into prison, to bind him with chains, and if needs be, to flog him with rods. Further news of the man Jesus came to Tarsus, of the Apostles he had gathered round him, and of the crowds that accepted his promises of the new dispensation that God had vouchsafed to his people. My rage increased, and then the news came that the man Jesus had been seized by order of the High Priest and crucified. More than that I knew not, and urged by a great pressing of the spirit I left Tarsus, and in the streets of Jerusalem beheld the first martyr, Stephen, stoned by the populace, a sight that gave me great joy. One heretic the less! I said, and went to the High Priest to ask for letters that would give me the right to arrest all ill thinkers and lead them back in chains to Jerusalem. But when we came in view of Damascus, and saw the roofs between the trees, I heard a voice crying to me: Saul, Saul, why persecutest thou me? It is hard for thee to kick against the pricks. And trembling I fell forward, my face upon the ground. The

192

voice continued: I am Jesus whom thou persecutest. Arise and go into the city, and it shall be told to thee what thou must do. My followers, who were but stricken and not blinded as I was, took me by the arm and led me into Damascus, where I abode as a blind man till Ananias laid his hands upon me and the scales fell from my eyes and I cried out for baptism; and having received baptism, which is spiritual strength, and taken food, which is bodily, I went up to the synagogue to preach the passing of the old world, till the Jews of the city rose up against me and would have killed me if I had not escaped them, let down from the wall in a basket.

SHALLUM. From a window?

PAUL. From a window, in drenching rain and in darkness, carried many times by the wind against the wall. But I escaped from Damascus and went into Arabia to take counsel with myself, for I could not doubt that the Lord Jesus, speaking out of the clouds, had appointed me his Apostle and established my authority above that of Peter or John or James, or any of the twelve who walked with him in Galilee. All the same, I could not forget Stephen, whose death I had witnessed in the streets of Jerusalem, and my words: One heretic the less! and I was tortured by a memory of my journey to Damascus, whither I had gone to persecute the Saints. But my doubts were assuaged by the Lord Jesus, and I learned that the words spoken to me out of the clouds were not intended for me alone, but for all the world.

CALEB. Did the Lord Jesus speak to thee again out of the clouds?

MATHIAS. There are few clouds in Arabia, Caleb.

PAUL. God liveth above the clouds, wherefore he speaks out of them. My doctrine was not born of the imaginations of my heart, but given unto me by the Lord Jesus in Arabia. From Arabia I went up to Jerusalem to speak with them that were in the city when the Lord was crucified, and it was Barnabas who brought me to Peter, saying that albeit I had persecuted, I was now zealous in the faith and had preached in many synagogues that Christ Jesus had died and been raised from the dead. Paul, said Barnabas, hath come from Arabia to hear the story of the Lord Jesus from thee, and Peter answered: That story I will tell willingly to whosoever asketh it of me, for it is a story of exceeding worth to men. And he told that one day, distracted with grief, his wife being nigh to death, he rushed out of the house to bring a physician, and meeting with a man coming up from the lake, and mistaking him for a physician, his grief being such that he had no eyes for his torn garment, he said: Come thou to my house; impose thy hands and bid my wife rise from her bed and walk. I will do this, Jesus answered, but he charged Peter not to believe all he heard about him, nor to speak of what might happen in his house; and he had barely spoken these words when Peter said: Here! throwing open the door for him. A miracle it was, as great as any, for at the imposition of his hands and the words he uttered, Peter's wife rose from her bed as she was bidden to do, and coming over to Peter she asked: How shall we reward him? and he answered her: So torn is his garment that it trails about his feet as he walks, tripping him; if I be fortunate with the fish to-night I will buy him a new garment. She said: Meanwhile I will mend his cloak for him; and she sat down to stitch the torn parts together. Afterwards he abode with them. For the truth of the story I tell, Peter said to me, my good friend Barnabas will avouch, and shouldst thou wish to have further testimony, come with me to Galilee and I'll show thee the bed on which he lay, the table at which he sat, and the plate from which he ate his meat. In my boat I will take thee over the sea of Galilee and show thee the spot where he quieted the waves that were threatening to drown us, and where we took the biggest draught of fishes ever known in those parts. Come, stranger, I trust thee. But I said: Peter, why should I go up to Galilee? At this question he stood abashed, saying: I thought that thou wouldst hear all I could tell thee of the Master. All thou canst tell me of his resurrection from the dead I will hear willingly, I answered him, and from thee sooner than from another, for thou wert in Jerusalem at the time. My reply troubled him, and wondering at his trouble, which seemed to me to be without cause, I waited till he was out of hearing to ask Barnabas to explain it to me; and his answer was that Peter was a timid man and shy, always infirm in his faith, as the Master himself knew well, for on the night before the crucifixion Jesus said to Peter: Before the cock crows thou shalt deny me thrice. And it was so; Peter denied, and then rued his denial. The same Peter to-day, Barnabas said, that the Master judged rightly; he hath changed in nothing. And this judgment of Peter that I received from Barnabas was confirmed afterwards when on our return from Cyprus, whither we had gone to preach, we went up to Antioch, a city dear to me, for it was there that the word Christian was spoken for the first time. My return was fortunate, for there I met Barnabas, whom I rejoiced to meet again after these many years. All memory of our dissensions was forgotten; we had much to tell each other of our travels and the conversions we had made, and our joy was increased by Peter, who appeared amongst us, bringing a brother with him, Silas, who must have been grieved, though he said nothing to me of it. He must have seen that the law to which he was attached was forgotten at Antioch, not by us only, but by his new leader, Peter, who mixed like ourselves with the Gentiles and did not refuse to eat with them. One day we came out of a house heated with argument, and as we loitered by the pavement's edge we came upon Peter in a public inn eating and drinking with the uncircumcised; whereupon the men of Jerusalem said: We see now what thou art, Peter, a Jew that eats with Gentiles and of unclean meats. Peter did not withstand them and say, as he should have done: How is it that you call them that God hath made unclean? but excused himself and withdrew, and was followed by Barnabas and Silas.

An angry soul I have been since God first separated me from my mother's womb, gaining something on one side and losing on another. But we make not ourselves; God makes us; and there is a jealousy still within me. I know it, and have suffered from it, and never did it cause me greater suffering than in those days in Antioch. My jealousy was like a hungry animal, gnawing at my ribs, till unable to bear it any long, and seeing in visions all that I had raised pulled down, I started with Titus and travelled all over Galatia and Phrygia to Bithynia, founding churches everywhere I went, and everywhere persecuted by the Jews. But my life hath never been my concern but God's, a thing upheld by God for so many years that I shun danger no longer, and now it hath even come to me that I am lonely in security, withdrawn from God in houses, and safe in his arms when clinging to a spar in the dark sea. God and our Lord Jesus Christ, his beloved son, have walked on either side of me in mountain passes where robbers lie in wait. We are nearer to God in hunger and thirst than when the mouth is full, in fatigue rather than in rest, and to know oneself to be God's servant is good cheer for the traveller, better than the lights of an inn, for false brethren may await him in the inn, some that will hale him before rulers; but if he know he is God's servant he will be secure in his own heart, where alone security abides. Shipwrecked I was many times, stoned at Lystra, escaping death by feigning it, followed wherever I went by persecution from the Jews, determined to undo my work; but undeterred by stones and threats and stripes – forty save one – I returned to Lystra and preached there again, and in Perga and Attalia. From thence we returned to Antioch, and there was great rejoicing in Saigon Street when we told of the churches we had founded in Galatia, how we flung open the door of truth to the Pagans and many passed through. But what is my life to you? As I have said, it hath never been my concern, wherefore it can be no concern of yours, noble Essenes. Time never lags; I see the sand running through the glass as I speak. Not much more is left, only enough for me to tell that I would have ye meet my friends and disciples and learn from them that the revelation of the Lord Jesus of himself on the road to Damascus was not the only one. He hath appeared to his disciples many times. Witnesses abound ... (*He staggers into* MANAHEM'S *arms.*) Only a faintness ... it will pass.

MANAHEM. A cup of water! (*One of the* ESSENES *goes out and returns with a cup of water.* MANAHEM *holds it to* PAUL'S *lips.*)

PAUL. Many are the revelations, but Jesus of Nazareth is the greatest and the last.

MATHIAS (*looking round*). So ye would exchange the study of the Scriptures for a gospel that a misadventure on the hills hath cast among you!

PAUL. My sickness is not that which overthrew me on the road to Damascus, but a faintness ... air ... lead me to the balcony. (*The* ESSENES *crowd round* PAUL *and move towards the balcony, leaving* MATHIAS *and* SADDOC *in the middle of the stage.*)

MATHIAS. I will set a noose for him, and thou shalt see him run into it.

SADDOC. Like a foolish rabbit. And though he never comes to kick in it, I shall abide in Kerith till God calls me unto himself, the same in the end as in the beginning.

BARTHOLOMEW (*coming from the balcony*). The schism widens every minute, and I would ask if Hazael should not be warned that his authority is needed here.

MATHIAS. He should indeed! (BARTHOLOMEW *makes a movement towards the inner cavern.*) Stay, Bartholomew. Art thou with us, Saddoc and I, or with Paul?

BARTHOLOMEW. I fear to break my views, Mathias, but still greater is my fear to abide in Kerith. (*Exit* BARTHOLOMEW.)

MATHIAS. I offer thee friendship, Saddoc, and shall not desert Kerith though the brethren leave us.

SADDOC. Thou'lt weary in Kerith without brethren to instruct in the Scriptures, and in the end wilt return to thine own Egypt. But the Lord and the Scriptures are on our side, and in the debate, thy wit, Mathias – (MATHIAS *is about to call to the* ESSENES, *but* SADDOC *stops him.*) Bartholomew hath gone to warn Hazael, and I would hear Paul confuted and overthrown in his presence.

MATHIAS. His defeat would be greater truly, but at any moment Jesus may return from the hills to guide him to Cæsarea. We may not delay. And there are other excuses for our haste. Hazael may be too feeble this morning to give his mind to the arguments that will be settled, for Paul is a keen debater.

MANAHEM (*from the balcony*). And this wonderful passing of the old world was wrought by the coming of the Messiah promised beforetime, a child born of a virgin's womb!

MATHIAS (*raising his voice*). I know of no such prediction, Manahem. The word in Isaiah is not virgin but girl, who shall conceive and bear a son and shall call his name Immanuel. In thine eagerness to accept Paul's gospel thou hast forgotten the Scriptures.

SHALLUM (*from the balcony*). The prophecy in Deuteronomy is fulfilled in the Lord Jesus.

MATHIAS. I would answer thee, Shallum, out of Deuteronomy: The prophet that shall presume to speak a word in my name which I have not commanded him to speak, or that shall speak in the name of other Gods, even that prophet shall die. (PAUL *and the* ESSENES *come down the stage.*)

SHALLUM (*to* ELIAKIM). It was an act of God that separated Paul from his companion, Timothy.

ELIAKIM. And upheld him in the dangers of the path.

CALEB. Soon Jesus will return from the hills to lead him to Cæsarea, wherefore let the stranger give us instruction.

PAUL. Before I leave you I would have you learn that there is but one mediator between God and man, the Lord Jesus, and that you are free men now, the curse of the law lifted from you.

SADDOC (*aside to* MATHIAS). The curse of the law! When he says such things it is like running a knife into me!

MATHIAS. Hush! (*To* PAUL.) The law was given to us by God.

PAUL. And hath been repealed by God, who sent his only begotten son with the joyful tidings that there is salvation for all, Jews and Gentiles alike.

MATHIAS. Thou hast fared up and down Asia for twenty years, founding churches, persecuted by the Jews and making converts among the Gentiles, which is strange – unless indeed thou wouldst maintain that the study of the Scriptures and the laws that God gave to Moses have rendered the Jews less able to receive the truth than those who worship idols.

PAUL. The conversion of the Jews was confided to Peter, that of the Gentiles to me.

MATHIAS. Already a division among you! To enlighten us thou'lt tell why the conversion of the Jews was confided to Peter?

PAUL. For that Peter and Barnabas accept circumcision. I told them at Antioch that the Gentiles would not accept circumcision, and put it to them: Can it be that God sent down his beloved son to die on the

197

cross and be raised from the dead for no greater end than that the Jews should remain Jews and the Gentiles idolaters?

MATHIAS. Thou speakest Greek of a sort, Paul, and art specious in argument despite the rudeness of thy language.

PAUL. My language serves me well enough. My mission is among the poor and ignorant rather than among the rich.

MATHIAS. So the Christians began among the poor and uninstructed?

PAUL. Thou wouldst not have had them begin among the wise and learned, among the Jews of Alexandria?

MATHIAS. Truly not. But a Jew of Alexandria would put to thee some simple questions which thou wouldst be troubled to answer plainly.

PAUL. Put them.

MATHIAS. A dangerous doctrine is implicit in thy gospel, Paul – that whosoever hath faith may sin and sin again, and come into salvation despite his sins. (PAUL *begins to interrupt*.) Bear with me a little while. The promise made to Moses counts for nothing?

PAUL. It counted for a great deal when we were as children lost in a desert and the law was our guide. We are no longer children, but heirs to the kingdom of heaven, Jews and Gentiles alike.

MATHIAS. The promise made to Moses was then a duplicity? (*Again* PAUL *tries to interrupt*.) Trouble not to explain, for I will pass over this matter and will ask thee instead how we may come into the faith.

PAUL. Through grace.

MATHIAS. But how comes grace? Whence comes it?

PAUL. Grace is a gift from God, which he gives or withholds.

MATHIAS. At his pleasure?

PAUL. Doth the vase ask the potter: Why hast thou made me thus? Hath not the potter power over the clay to make from the same lump two vases for noble and ignoble use? (*A murmur of approval is heard among the* ESSENES.)

MATHIAS. Hath it then come to pass that I discern a heed in the countenances around me for a potter God, a maker of things according to pattern? (*To* PAUL.) The Christ that possesses thee, Paul, is but the Logos, the principle that mediates between the supreme God and the world formed out of matter, which hath no being of its own, for being is not in that mere potency of all things alike, which thou callest power, but in divine reason.

PAUL. Thou'rt nearer to Christ than thou knowest, nearer than any of the Greeks I heard in Athens.

MATHIAS. I gather from thy Greek that thy stay in Athens was not long, and from thence I would have had thee go to Alexandria, my city, to learn philosophy from the masters. Philo would have persuaded thee into a purer conception of God than a mere potter.

PAUL. Neither life nor death nor angels can separate me from the love of our Lord Jesus Christ. (*Rising from his seat* MATHIAS *passes on to the balcony and leans on the rail. The babble of voices ceases when he holds up his hand.*)

MATHIAS. Jesus's feet are already on the last terraces, and in a moment he'll be knocking at our door. (*The door is opened by an* ESSENE.)

PAUL. He brings news of Timothy! (JESUS *enters with a wallet over his shoulders, carrying another in his hand.* PAUL *rushes towards him.*) Before all else, thy news of Timothy!

JESUS. Soon after he missed thee a shepherd put him on the way to Cæsarea.

PAUL (*aside*). For the safety of Timothy, my beloved son in the faith, I give thanks to thee, O Lord.

JESUS. Thou'lt have three days in which to thank God for the safety of Timothy. (*He hangs the wallet over* PAUL'S *shoulder.*) Cæsarea is a three-days' journey and thou'rt a tired man.

PAUL. Tired in mind rather than in body.

JESUS. I had looked forward to rousing thee myself when I returned from the hills, but I find thee disputing with the Essenes. (*To the* ESSENES.) An evil trick ye have played upon me, brethren, making it doubtful if I shall get our guest to Cæsarea in three days.

PAUL. Blame not the brethren. For remembering that I was leaving Asia for ever I could not keep back the story of him crucified –

SADDOC. Begin it not again for the sake of Jesus, lest in the telling of it the hour of departure slips by unperceived by him.

JESUS. So the Lord Jesus was on the cross?

SADDOC (*to* PAUL). A story hath often been told in the hills – sometimes it is forgotten, sometimes it is in everybody's mouth – that Jesus, the great shepherd, was put on the cross by some Roman Governor in Jerusalem. He will tell it to thee on the way to Cæsarea.

PAUL (*struggling against the sickness that is rising in him*). So thou wert crucified, shepherd of the Judean hills? And how didst thou escape from the cross?

JESUS. I was raised from the tomb.

SADDOC. The hour of thy departure is nigh, Paul, but we will send Jacob to Cæsarea –

PAUL. With news that I have worn out my strength in argument with the Essenes?

SADDOC (*laying his hand on* PAUL'S *arm*). If I read thy face aright, the sickness is rising in thee.

199

PAUL. A sickness of the flesh, no more. A man is as strong as the soul within him. Loose me, Saddoc, loose me! (*To* JESUS.) Didst say thou wert raised from the dead by the power of the Father?

JESUS. I said I was raised from the tomb.

PAUL. He is possessed of an evil spirit! A madman! A madman! (PAUL *breaks away from* SADDOC *and rushes out of the cavern.* SHALLUM, CALEB, ELEAZOR, ELIAKIM, *go on to the balcony to watch him descend the terraces.* JESUS *and* MANAHEM *remain with* SADDOC *and* MATHIAS.)

JESUS. He said: Possessed of an evil spirit. But I am a shepherd of the hills, no more, without knowledge of him or of the dissensions he hath brought into our company.

MANAHEM. Thy words may have frightened him.

JESUS. My words were simple. As I remember them they were: I was on the cross and was raised from the tomb. And at these words his face changed as I have seen men's faces change at the approach of the sickness.

MANAHEM. The sickness rises in a man like a wind in the air. But why did he cry: A madman! A madman! Was he possessed of a bodily or a spiritual terror?

JESUS. I must warn Hazael that our guest hath left us. (JESUS *goes into the inner cavern and* MANAHEM *joins the* ESSENES *on the balcony.*)

MATHIAS. (*to* SADDOC). Hast a reason in mind for his flight?

SADDOC. His anxiety to arrive in Cæsarea according to his bond.

MATHIAS. On hearing Jesus say he was raised from the tomb Paul's disturbed brain might have begun to doubt the death and resurrection that he hath preached for the last twenty years, and in his desperation at seeing his whole life crushed like an empty eggshell underfoot strange words would come to him, and why not the words he spoke?

SADDOC. A subtle divination, Mathias – true or false, I know not which, but one that we shall be able to turn to our advantage if ...

MATHIAS. Explain thy hesitation, Saddoc.

SADDOC. My thoughts were that if Paul should return to us after the seizure –

MATHIAS. Why should he return? He will continue his journey to Cæsarea. We are rid of him for ever.

SADDOC. Wherefore thy heart is moved with pity for a man that can no longer injure us.

MATHIAS. I am moved with pity at the thought of a man who sees his whole life crushed, as I have said, like an empty eggshell. Many men have suffered this crucifixion, and I pity them all for reasons well

200

known to myself. (*Enter* HAZAEL, *leaning on* JESUS'S *arm, followed by* BARTHOLOMEW.)

HAZAEL. I have come to hear of the flight of our guest, dissensions having arisen among you. It is unfortunate –

MANAHEM. (*from the balcony*). He hath fallen on the pathway beyond the bridge, stricken!

SHALLUM (*from the balcony*). Close by the brink, and should he stir he will fall into the brook!

HAZAEL. Four of our company must go to his help with a litter.

MANAHEM. A change of bearers will be needed, for the ascent is steep, and no four men will endure it for more than two or three terraces.

HAZAEL. Thou, Manahem, and Shallum, Eleazor, Eliakim, will bear him easily across the bridge, and Bartholomew and Caleb will lend their shoulders when needed.

JESUS. I opened the door to him last night and would go to his help.

HAZAEL. I cannot spare thee, Jesus.

MANAHEM. Jacob, our shepherd, is by Paul at this moment. He leans over him, lifts him – dead man or living man I cannot say.

HAZAEL. Jacob will give his help, too, and if further help be needed he'll know where to look for it. (*The* ESSENES *come from the balcony and* HAZAEL *addresses them.*) Put all your thoughts into the saving of this man. Forget your differences, remembering that our first duty as Essenes is to succour the sick and wounded. I pray you to be Essenes and nothing else. Whatever may happen afterwards is in the mind of God. (*The* ESSENES *go out.* HAZAEL *and* JESUS *enter the inner cavern.* MATHIAS *and* SADDOC *remain.*)

CURTAIN

ACT III

SCENE: *The same. Later. When the curtain rises Mathias and Saddoc are discovered sitting at a table talking.*

MATHIAS. Thinkest Saddoc, that by now they have reached the bridge-head?

SADDOC. Not yet. Methinks they should now be about half-way down the terraces.

MATHIAS. Thy guesses are not enough, Saddoc. I need thine eyes. Tell me, is Jacob still striving to get Paul to his feet? (SADDOC *rises from .the table, and going to the balcony looks over the rail.*)

SADDOC. Paul wrestles with Jacob on the path. One or the other will fall over the brink, mayhap both, and our trouble will be over.

MATHIAS. None of our brotherhood may hope for any man's death.

SADDOC (*coming from the balcony*). Nay, I entertained no hope of his death, but at thy request went to the balcony to report what mine eyes should see. I was one of the brotherhood before thou wert, Mathias, and know the rules of Order. (*He sits at the table.*)

MATHIAS. Saddoc, put off thy despondency. Thy wishes may be gratified yet. They are, if I read thee correctly, that Paul may be able to continue his journey and perchance find shepherds to guide him to Cæsarea, where he'll take ship. (*Pause.*) Forgive me, Saddoc, if I seemed to instruct thee. 'Twas a chance word, no more. Forget it, and return to the balcony and tell me if the litter-bearers are at the bridge-head.

SADDOC. I can tell thee without going to the balcony that they are still among the terraces. But to please thee I will report what I see. (*He goes to the balcony.*) I see Paul lying on the path by the cliff's edge quite still, and Jacob standing by. . . . Now the litter emerges from the pepper-trees . . . Soon he'll be laid out on this very balcony, his new followers in attendance on him, listening with exalted eyes and suspended breath. His sickness will serve his heresy well!

MATHIAS. The time hath come for us to lay our heads together and discover how we may save the brethren from this interloper, this false Jew, this heretic. Were Jesus of Nazareth not amongst us we should be without the proof that cannot be denied. His hands and feet are tokens that Paul preaches a dream. (*Pause.*)

SADDOC. The plan is well laid, but ...

MATHIAS. But what, Saddoc?

SADDOC. A man's faith is subject to his desires, and should thy plan fail and the brethren depart, there will be none left of the ancient Order of the Essenes, but Hazael, Jesus, thyself and I.

MATHIAS. There'll be always broken bones among the shepherds for thee to join together, but for me there will be naught in Kerith.

SADDOC. Thou'lt return to Alexandria, whence thou camest.

MATHIAS. There is no return for me to Alexandria.

SADDOC. Why not, Mathias? (*A gesture from* MATHIAS *makes plain to him that he must put no further questions.*) Whilst I cure the sick among the hills thou'lt sit by the brook interpreting the Scriptures to Brother Jedaiah. In his cleft up yonder he must regret sometimes the noise that seemed too much for him when he was with us here.

MATHIAS. I have heard naught of him for long.

SADDOC. For three days he did not let down his basket for food, and we thought him dead or dying, and I went up to succour him and found him weak but still living. He had fallen and lamed himself, and when I had mended his leg, and he could get about, he was again happy in his solitude and willing to continue in it.

MATHIAS. And this is the man whom thou proposest to me as a listener! His thoughts are in himself, never outside of himself, just as this Paul hath no thought for himself but for mankind, hurrying from city to city and preaching his doctrine of the resurrection. (*Pause.*)

SADDOC. Of what art thou thinking, Mathias? Of a new plan to defeat Paul and to save Kerith?

MATHIAS. No. I was thinking of what my life will be in Kerith if the brethren leave us to follow Paul.

SADDOC. There is another future for thee, Mathias – to write a book, for there is much wisdom in thee.

MATHIAS. It may be that wisdom still lingers in me, but the power to write a book is no longer mine.

SADDOC. Often we have wondered at the fortune that brought thee hither.

MATHIAS. And still greater would be your wonder were I to tell how it came to pass that I left Alexandria at the height of my fame, when the city was babbling of me and of my book, portions of which I had begun to read at my lectures. At first it pleased me to think modestly and to speak modestly of myself, but as time went on and the throng of them that came to hear me was so great that many were turned away, it seemed to me that all that men wished to know unfolded itself as I wrote, and I thought of myself as one born to write this book. I knew not whether it would bring joy and encouragement to all men; I write not as Paul speaks. The book had life within itself, and every night when I laid down the pen I believed that all I had written had existed in the mind of God from all eternity. I looked upon myself as an instrument in the hands of God as much as Paul doth himself. But much remained to be set down in writing; what is not written perishes, and death watches for every man. In the dead of night my pen would pause, stayed by the fear lest I might not wake up in the morning to continue my book – men die often in their sleep. And there was another fear; I bethought myself how even the wise have been beguiled by the pleasures of this world, the pleasures of women, and I became watchful over myself, frightened lest I might fall into the pit that other men had fallen into. Soberly as I live, I said to myself, I may fall from this life of moderation and chastity; philosophy may no longer be enough. The flesh may overpower the mind in me as it hath in other men. For the sake of my book I must make myself safe against danger. This thought became fixed; I could not escape from it; and there were wandering spirits, all determined on my overthrow. A voice spake within me: There is but one way; sacrifice thy manhood. I had seen youths in the temple of Ashtoreth sacrifice their manhood with sharp shells. I did likewise ...

SADDOC. And having rid thyself of these beguilements, did thy book prosper?

MATHIAS (*starting to his feet*). Why torment me with questions?

SADDOC. Thy choice, Mathias, was to open thy heart to me, and being a physician, a healer -

MATHIAS. We cannot separate the body from the soul without loss to one or the other. As I lay rejoicing in the thought that I could now write what would outlast time itself, I felt suddenly – a spasm of thought it was – that my book no longer lived from itself, and when I went to it words failed me, or was there no thought to sustain the words? My thought dissolved in images and I wrote on, believing I had accomplished something, but when I returned to what I had written there were on the page only words, nothing of what I would have written. And after vain efforts of many months I said: The spirit will never again awaken in me; I am dead; and going to a friend I told him my story. He reminded me how I had spoken the day before in the school, how all had listened entranced to my eloquence, and I answered: Only eloquence remains, mists of words seemingly beautiful in themselves but which have no substance.

Here is my manuscript, I continued; do with it what thou wilt, but let no man know that I have given it. Next day I departed for Lower Egypt, where as thou knowest there are Essenes; but the heat of their rocky solitudes was too great for my health, and looking northward I came to Kerith. Such is my story, Saddoc, and I would ask what conclusion thou drawest from it.

SADDOC. Thou shalt die here in Kerith, and be buried under the rocks within hearing of the brook's threnody. Hearken to it, Mathias! It goes by whispering some great secret plainly enough.

MATHIAS. But if we ask ourselves what the brook is saying we get no answer. We hear only water going by ... There comes a trampling of feet!

SADDOC. The litter-bearers are coming up the last terrace. (*They listen for a moment. Enter the litter-bearers with* PAUL.)

DIFFERENT ESSENES. Not here ... No, not there ... On the balcony, where the air is fresher. (*The* ESSENES *carry Paul to the balcony and lay him on a bench amid a murmur of voices.*)

SADDOC (*to* BARTHOLOMEW). Hath he spoken?

BARTHOLOMEW. He murmured and raved incontinently as we came up the terraces.

SADDOC. Do thou go and fetch a basin of water and some cloths. (*Exit* BARTHOLOMEW. *A pause.* PAUL *rouses a little.*)

CALEB (*to* PAUL). On seeing thee fall we ran without stopping till we came to the bridge.

MANAHEM (*mopping his brow*). As nimbly as we might with the litter. The descent is only a thought easier than the ascent.

ELIAKIM. 'Twas a stiff climb truly.

CALEB (*to* PAUL). To ensure thine ease we changed bearers at every terrace.

MANAHEM. My shoulder saith not so, Caleb. I bore him for three without a change.

SHALLUM. And I still feel his weight after one!

MANAHEM. And my shoulder was again under the litter when we set him down here. (SADDOC *goes to* PAUL *and feels his pulse.* BARTHOLOMEW *enters with a basin of water and a cloth, which he hands to* SADDOC.)

SADDOC. In a few minutes he'll be himself again. (*He bathes* PAUL'S *temples.*)

MATHIAS. Ready to begin the journey to Cæsarea?

SADDOC. Hush! Speak not of Cæsarea. He may awaken at the word, and I would have him sleep a while longer. (*Enter* HAZAEL *supported by* JESUS. SADDOC *goes forward to meet them.*) A man may rise from these fits and continue his work without knowledge of what hath befallen him, or he may lie helpless for a day, or even two.

HAZAEL (*looking towards the balcony*). If he awaken now, will he be able for the journey?

MATHIAS. In case of a lesser seizure, his guide will know where to find him shelter.

HAZAEL. Go, Eleazor, and bid Jacob hold himself in readiness. (*Exit* ELEAZOR.)

SADDOC. Thou dost well to choose Jacob, Hazael. 'Twere hard for thee that Jesus should leave thee on the day after his return.

HAZAEL. Speak not of myself. It is our brotherhood that is divided between me and yon man who lieth stricken in sickness.

MATHIAS. If we would save Kerith we must cast out Paul.

SADDOC. Let me speak now, Hazael, no longer as a physician. It is not meet that Paul should leave us until he and all the brethren have heard from Jesus the story of his crucifixion.

HAZAEL. Our rule disfavours any inquisition into the past life of one of our brethren, but be it now as ye will. Speak truly, Jesus, if thou wouldst help us in our strait.

MATHIAS, SADDOC AND THE OTHERS. Speak, Jesus!

JESUS. I had a purpose to speak when I returned hither yesterevening, and I sought counsel concerning it with Hazael. I could not remain, I told him, without revealing how I came to break my vows. He urged that there is much disquiet in Kerith, that old stories would only add to the confusion, and begged that I should be silent. And unable to withstand his pleading, I said: Be it so. But since these words were spoken a man hath come amongst us with a story that Jesus of Nazareth was raised from the dead by the power of the Father and spoke to him out of the clouds, and if it may allay the perplexities that have arisen thereby in our community I will now declare that I myself was born in Nazareth and followed Hazael to Kerith. How it came that I left him I need not delay to tell, save only this, that I received baptism from John, and like him preached the gospel of repentance. My preaching was received with joy and acclaim along the shores of the lake by the fishermen and by many from Tiberias, and miracles were performed by me, for at that time the power of God wrought in me – there is no power in the world but God's. I speak not now vaingloriously, but confess to you that at that time I was puffed up with pride and arrogance. I forgot God and went down to Jerusalem expecting a great welcome. On an ass richly caparisoned I rode into the city, the people strewing palms before me and crying Hosannas, and when some reproved them for so doing, I said: If they did not proclaim me the stones themselves would do so. (*The* ESSENES *murmur amongst themselves.*) Unwilling that your eyes should look upon a blasphemer you cover your faces with your hands, and you would seal your ears if you could against the story I am telling ... In Jerusalem I said I could destroy the temple and build it up again in three days, and my words coming to the ears of the High Priest, Caiaphas, he sent his servants in search of me. I was taken in a garden whither I had gone to pray and was brought before the High Priest, who questioned me and tore his hair and cried; A blasphemer! Pilate was my judge, and the punishment he meted out to me was a scourging and the carrying of my cross to Golgotha. On it I hung till I passed into a swoon, and being deemed dead at the end of the third hour, my body was given to Joseph of Arimathea for burial. (PAUL, *rousing, listens intently.*) He laid me in the tomb that he had had carved for himself, and as he was about to close it I stirred in my grave-clothes, and seeing I was not dead he carried me to his house, where I remained till my wounds were cured. When I was able to move about I worked in the olive garden, carrying faggots and pruning the trees, my wits happily away, till the smell of a camel-driver recalled the hills, and henceforth I could wonder only if my flock was thriving or wasting under Brother Amos's care. (*At this moment his eyes fall on* PAUL.) See, Paul listens. His wits are returning to him.

MATHIAS. He hath missed nothing.

PAUL. A strange story indeed, and well worth the hearing, so truthfully is it told.

MATHIAS. As well worth the hearing as the voice that spoke to thee out of the clouds, Paul, and should a memory of that voice still haunt in thee, we shall be glad to hear if thou canst distinguish a sameness in the two voices.

PAUL. Thy words enter my ears, Mathias, but for what thou intendest –

SADDOC. Brethren, crowd not about him. Let him enjoy the air of the balcony till he is rested and his mind composed.

MANAHEM. We would hear what he hath to say ere he leaves us at midday.

SADDOC. He dozes, and must not be awakened. Mayhap sleep will bring him into his full mind, and then you can put questions to him.

MANAHEM. Thou shouldst have been with us, Mathias, when he spake to us on the balcony. His words fixed themselves in the memory of his hearers for ever.

MATHIAS. I would hear the words that are fixed in thy memory for ever, Manahem.

MANAHEM. Not in my memory alone, but perchance in the memory of all men. Even thou wouldst have been exalted hadst thou heard him speak. (*Murmuring to himself.*) When I was a child I spoke as a child, I understood as a child, I thought as a child; but when I became a man I put away childish things.

PAUL (*rousing*). Brethren, I hear your voices ... Saddoc and Manahem were in dispute, and then my wit slumbered. But now it wakes, and I remember that my day among you is shortening. Question me.

MATHIAS. We disputed which was the true Jesus, he whom thou teachest or the Jesus that heretofore hath led our flocks home. So alike are their stories that we are perplexed. Our brother Jesus preached in Galilee and was crucified in Jerusalem twenty years agone, and it was at that time that thy Jesus of Nazareth spoke to thee out of the clouds. Wherefore either a great miracle or a great deception is wrapped up in thy teaching, and we would hear from thee, who hast seen and heard both the dead and the quick, which we should follow.

PAUL. Thou wast a listener when I told my story, how after three years spent in Arabia I went up to Jerusalem and spoke with Peter, the Lord's Apostle, and with James, the brother of the Lord. Wherefore I guess thee to be a caviller, one who would take advantage of my plight. But I would not have thy questions refused an answer. A long journey awaits me –

MATHIAS. A single question and its answer will free us from doubt. Which Jesus is the Messiah promised to the Jews?

PAUL. The Lord Jesus Christ, who sits in heaven by the side of the Father. Jesus, thy shepherd, liveth before me in the flesh.

MATHIAS. Before thy seizure he was declared to be possessed of an evil spirit. A madman! was thy cry. We would hear if thou holdest by these words. (*Turning to the* ESSENES.) When the mind darkens in sickness the truth slips out.

PAUL. To hide my sickness from you I ran away. All else is forgotten.

MATHIAS. We have the witness of our brother's hands and feet.

PAUL (*rising with an effort*). I have no need to look into his hands and feet for the scars of his crucifixion. He was on the cross, I deny it not, like many another, and escaped death as some have done. The man liveth for examination. Look into his eyes; touch his hands and face. (*Suddenly becoming calm.*) Thou art a philosopher from Alexandria, Mathias, and judgest all things by the light of reason; wherefore examine the story with which thou wouldst confute me, and tell me if it be within the purposes and devices of the Father that his son should be crucified and raised from the dead for no further end than to lead flocks from pasture to pasture, keeping the great truth buried in his breast that there is salvation for all. Thou wouldst have done well to have put these question to thyself before coming to me for answers.

MATHIAS. Nay, look thou into the shepherd's hands and feet and thou'lt read testimony that he was on the cross.

PAUL. As to that, have not my words been clear?

HAZAEL. Jesus, I would hear thee speak. Hast thou naught to say in this dispute?

JESUS. Perchance Paul knoweth of another Jesus, the Christ –

PAUL. Yea, him that was raised from the dead and will remain till the last man perishes, to be united then to the Father which is in heaven, and henceforth there will be but one God.

JESUS. It may be that my name hath been mingled with these happenings, whatsoever they were. I know not. Nor do I doubt that a voice spoke to Paul out of the skies. He that walks with God will hear his voice. To some it is a thunderbolt from the heavens, to some it is a voice that speaks from within, but every man that prayeth well may hear the voice of the Father. He that hath ears to hear will hear. It may be, as I have said, that my name hath crept into these reports, and that my sufferings, which were great, have been used by God for his own glory. (*He smiles.*) Paul, I would not rob thee of my namesake!

MATHIAS. That is well spoken, Jesus! Wisdom hath uttered a voice even among the Gentiles, to Socrates, to Pythagoras. Nay, I myself, did I not once hear a voice?

PAUL. Thou speakest, Mathias, after the wisdom of Egypt, in empty phrases, to withdraw the thoughts of the brethren from the miracle of the resurrection. The Greeks seek after wisdom, but the need of all peoples is a miracle. They hearkened unto me in Athens till I began to speak of the resurrection, whereupon they jeered, crying out that no man was ever raised from the dead. And I returned to Asia cast down by the thought of the great numbers that would die without knowledge of the Lord Jesus, however long I might live, however far I might travel. O, my Lord Jesus, I cried, I would hold myself accursed for the sake of my brethren, my kinsmen according to the flesh; and remembering that I was within twenty leagues of Jericho, I went to the noble Festus to ask for six days' absence from Cæsarea to preach in Jericho. The journey to Jericho is now over, and my feet are already on the way to Rome. Three days hence I shall be in Cæsarea, in a month in Rome, preaching my gospel without fear of persecution by the Jews.

SHALLUM. And after Rome?

209

PAUL. Spain.

MANAHEM. And after Spain thou'lt return to Asia to take account of our stewardship.

ELIAKIM. Whilst thou art absent in Rome and in Spain we shall found many churches, and a great welcome will be given to thee on thy return. In my thoughts I can see the converts crowding round, welcoming the Apostle of the Gentiles.

MANAHEM. The seed hath been sown.

PAUL. But he who hath sown will not garner.

MANAHEM. Thou wilt not die in Spain.

PAUL. How knowest thou? My sleep is often broken by a dream in which I behold myself striking in haste across a rocky plain towards mountains which lie afar off. As my strength departs the Lord Jesus comes to my help, and I cry: Give me strength to reach the village beyond the mountains and to preach thy resurrection, and salvation through thee, for, my Lord Jesus, they are guiltless − thy name hath never reached their ears; it is but just that they should hear it. The world perishes year by year; in a few it will be gone. My dear Lord Jesus, thy servant comes to thee at the end of a long day, weary of the world but refreshed by sight of thee, and still ardent to bring the innocent of law and sin to salvation. Bend down, Lord Jesus, till I see thee, whom I have seen so often in sleeping, in waking, in perils in the sea, in deserts −

MATHIAS. Belike it will be another shepherd lad, Paul, bending over thee, to give thee to drink from his gourd − (*Enter* ELEAZOR, *followed by* JACOB *carrying two wallets.* HAZAEL *and* JESUS *retire into the inner cavern.*)

JACOB. (*to* PAUL). Master, art thou ready? When Eleazor brought me now Hazael's message, bidding me guide thee to Cæsarea: It cannot be, I said, that he can start without another night's rest!

PAUL. Do always as thou art bidden to do, Jacob.

JACOB. Here then is thy wallet, with food for three days. (*To* SADDOC.) Hath he strength for so long a journey?

SADDOC. No other ill but weariness can I find in him, a profound weariness.

JACOB. We shall sleep in caves on soft sand. If go he must we should go now.

PAUL. My promise is given or I would remain with you a little longer, for much hath been left unsaid that should have been said. I would speak to you of good will to one's neighbour, of affection one to another, and of many other things. But Jacob's eyes are upon me. (*He turns to go.*) Farewell, brethren. Stop on the roads now and then

210

to speak of me. Think of me in Italy, and afterwards in Spain by the great sea that no man knows the end of. Each man here hath a trade and he will live by it, accepting bread from no man but living by the work of his hands, as I have lived. Think of all that is lovely, of all that is pure, of things that are kind, of things that are good. Avoid the blasphemous and the evil-living –

JACOB. Paul –

PAUL. Good-bye, brethren, whom I shall never see again in the flesh, mayhap, but whom I shall always see with the eyes of the spirit. I salute you all, even Saddoc and Mathias, who would have caused division between us. I bear no grudge to them. The truth will be revealed to them by the Lord Jesus himself in good time. I thank you for the food I have had and the bed I have slept in ... My spirit is bowed down, but go I must. Even Timothy I cannot bring with me. He returns to Derbe, to his mother, to preach the gospel to the idolaters of that city, and you, Manahem, Bartholomew, Shallum, Eliakim, Eleazor, Caleb, will preach in Macedonia, Thessalonica, Galatia. In Corinth you will meet Aquila and Priscilla, faithful servants whom ye will greet in friendship and with a holy kiss. There is Apollos, too, and many another. Their names crowd upon me, but of what avail were it to speak them now? They would pass out of your memory. I will write to you from Rome. (PAUL *goes out, followed by* JACOB. SADDOC *and* MATHIAS *remain apart, and the* ESSENES, *with the exception of* MANAHEM, *crowd on to the balcony.*)

SHALLUM. He strides away like a shepherd, and last night was the first for many nights that he slept in a bed.

ELIAKIM. Already we are forgotten.

BARTHOLOMEW. Not forgotten. We shall be with him in his prayers, and he'll be with us in ours. (*Exeunt* SADDOC *and* MATHIAS.)

ELEAZOR. Come to the balcony, Manahem, if thou wouldst see him for the last time.

MANAHEM (*crossing to the balcony and speaking with his hand on* SHALLUM'S *shoulder*). At every stride he grows smaller in our eyes and greater in our hearts.

SHALLUM. After Rome he will take ship for Spain.

MANAHEM. But not to die. He will return to us, and a joyful day it will be when he visits the churches we have founded and sees the converts we bring to him.

SHALLUM. Thou speakest well, Manahem. Henceforth we are no longer Essenes but Christians, and the doctrine we preach shall be the doctrine we have received from Paul.

211

ELIAKIM. His eyes were upon me when he spoke of Corinth, and his voice was addressed to me when he said: Aquila and Priscilla you will meet in Corinth, and they will instruct you more fully than I can before my departure.

ELEAZOR. I heard him say none of these things to thee, Eliakim. Methought when he spoke of Corinth that his eyes were upon me.

MANAHEM. Remember his words, that there should be no envyings amongst us. (*Pause.*) He hath passed under the overhanging rock.

CALEB. Yes; but we can overtake him if we hasten.

MANAHEM. Then let us hasten, for the instructions he hath given us are not sufficient. Dissensions may arise amongst us. Let us hasten. We shall overtake him before he hath reached the level road. (*The* ESSENES *go out hurriedly. Enter* JESUS, *leading* HAZAEL.)

JESUS. Here is thy chair.

HAZAEL. Are the brethren all gone?

JESUS. Be thou seated and I will go to the balcony and make count of them as they descend the terraces. (*He goes on to the balcony and looks over the rail.*)

HAZAEL. How many of our brethren follow Paul?

JESUS. Saddoc and Mathias are not among them.

HAZAEL. Then we shall be four in Kerith.

JESUS. (*crossing to the other side of the balcony*). Saddoc and Mathias are in the path down which I came last night with Jacob. Walking studiously, they consider how the brotherhood of the Essenes may be saved.

HAZAEL. Thinkest, Jesus, that the brethren can be persuaded to return to Kerith?

JESUS. In three days Paul will be on board a Roman ship.

HAZAEL. But his Apostles will remain in Asia. (*Footsteps are heard outside. Enter* MATHIAS *and* SADDOC.)

MATHIAS. In a few minutes the brethren will overtake the new prophet.

SADDOC. And before they reach Cæsarea we shall have already made a laughing-stock of Paul's doctrine in Jerusalem.

HAZAEL. And how may ye accomplish this?

MATHIAS. If Jesus will come with us it will be easy. (*Turning to* JESUS.) Have no fear, Jesus, for thyself. Thy reception will be a great one. The past will be undone, and the High Priest will send servants to Rome to confute Paul in thy name.

JESUS. I stumbled once in the belief that we who did not make the world can remake it, but I have learnt since that the world is ever in the hands of God. He is moulding it always, without our help and warily.

MATHIAS. Thou art not with us, then?

JESUS. I am neither with you nor against you. (*Exeunt* MATHIAS *and* SADDOC.) They go in such haste to confound the errors of men that Brother Jedaiah's basket of food is forgotten. I will take it to him. (*He picks up the basket.*) Mayhap they will learn in time that it is better to love the good than to hate the wicked. (JESUS *goes out.* HAZAEL *falls on his knees and prays.*)

CURTAIN

THE HEATHER FIELD

A PLAY IN THREE ACTS
BY
EDWARD MARTYN

DRAMATIS PERSONAE

BARRY USSHER, a landowner, student, philosopher, &c.
LORD SHRULE, a neighbouring landowner.
LADY SHRULE (LILIAN), his wife.
CARDEN TYRRELL.
MRS GRACE TYRRELL (born Desmond), his wife.
KIT, their son, nine years old.
MILES TYRRELL, scholar of Trinity College, Dublin,
and brother of Carden.
DOCTOR DOWLING, DOCTOR ROCHE, physicians.

The action takes place about the year 1890 in CARDEN TYRRELL's
house on the West coast of Ireland.

ACT I

SCENE:– CARDEN TYRRELL'S library. On the right a door leads to the dining-room and rest of house. On the left is a large empty fire-place. At back through openglass folding-doors a small garden is visible, below which the Atlantic Ocean, flanked by a mountain at left, stretches out to the horizon. Between fire-place and folding-doors stands a writing-table with chairs on either side. At the opposite part of the room near folding-doors is a large sofa. Books in shelves line all walls. In front at the right is another table covered with papers, magazines, &c., which are likewise thrown negligently over other chairs in the room. It is a bright forenoon in the Autumn.

MILES TYRRELL, a young light-haired man of about nineteen, dressed in a blue serge suit, is seated at the writing-table in deep study with several books around him. After a pause he looks up wearily, then again bends over his books.

BARRY USSHER, a lean man of about two and thirty, of medium height, with dark hair, a short pointed beard, and dressed in a riding-costume of sombre grey, enters from garden at back.

MILES (*starting*). Ah, Barry.

USSHER. (*throwing his hat and hunting-whip on the sofa*). Hallo, Miles, good morning. I see you are determined to win that gold medal at Trinity – and become one day Lord Chancellor of Ireland too, I'll be bound.

MILES (*with a faint smile*). Lord Chancellor, indeed! I shall be lucky if I can pass my examination and then find just so many briefs as will afford me a living.

USSHER. Why are you so despondent? You have ability.

MILES. Perhaps – if there was an opportunity of displaying it. Oh, this is no place for work.

USSHER. I know what you mean. But why not study in your room upstairs?

MILES. I might do that. Still it is not so much the interruptions. It is the knowledge of what goes on, perpetually.

USSHER. Are things as bad as ever?

MILES. Yes—my brother and his wife cannot agree.

USSHER. How sad it is.

MILES. Oh, if only I had a quiet house to study in like yours. You live there like a sage absorbed in your books and ideas.

USSHER. I fear I also find difficulties in cultivating the tastes that are congenial to me.

MILES. Why ?

USSHER. You see, Miles, an unfortunate landowner must devote all his attention to keeping a little of his belongings together in these bad times.

MILES. As if you were affected by bad times—you, with that fine place here joining us, and with your unencumbered estate, and no one depending upon you. You're a lucky fellow. No wonder the luck of Barry Ussher is a by-word with the country people.

USSHER. They know nothing about it.

MILES. Well, in any case you seem able to live as you please. You have always means to travel, and never want for anything.

USSHER. So that is your idea of luck, Miles?

MILES. Well, somewhat I fancy. Isn't it yours?

USSHER. I don't think these things make much difference either way.

MILES. Oh, come, Barry, you can't expect me to believe that.

USSHER. Yes, I mean that what we have on one side is taken away from the other; so the world's lots are more fairly divided than you imagine. Our natures remain much the same at their root. There is always the original pain.

MILES. I suppose you cynical philosophers must invent some grievance from lack of real troubles.

USSHER. No, Miles.

MILES. Well, if you only knew how my brother envies your good fortune.

USSHER. There are others Carden Tyrrell might envy, but he need not envy me. By the way, where is he?

MILES. He is out – I suppose in the heather field.

USSHER. Oh – (*After a short pause*) He has finished all his work there, hasn't he?

MILES. Yes, the young grass is coming up beautifully now. Do you want to see him at once? I can send for him. In any case he is sure to be back soon.

USSHER. That will do. I am in no great hurry.

MILES. You have some business with him?

USSHER. Well, yes. It is about this very subject of land reclamation. I hear he is about to raise another large loan from Government, in order to extend these operations of his.

MILES. Really?

218

USSHER. So they told me yesterday in Dublin at the Board of Works.

MILES. When Grace hears this, there will be more troubles and disputes.

USSHER. Most likely. What a pity your sister-in-law defeats all her objects by her manner towards Carden.

MILES. Oh indeed, she is very impatient with him. Yet she is good enough in her way too.

USSHER. Precisely; and would probably have made an excellent wife for almost any other man; but for your brother – well, it might have been better if he had never thought of marriage at all.

MILES. What? Surely he might have found some one to suit him. Why should you say such a thing?

USSHER. (*with a frightened look*). Why?

MILES. Yes, Barry. But what is the matter with you?

USSHER. (*quickly recovering himself*). Oh, nothing, Miles – nothing. I merely meant to say that it would be very difficult for anyone to suit Carden. He is a person so much of himself, you know.

MILES. Ah, it is certainly a great misfortune he ever met Grace. And their estrangement is so extraordinary for he once used to be so fond of her.

USSHER. Yes, they generally begin that way. I remember just before he became engaged he told me that he thought till then he should never marry, but that at last he had found real happiness. They all say that, you know.

MILES. You may very well philosophise over what is past, Barry. But why did you not then try to dissuade him?

USSHER. Of course I tried to dissuade him then. I did my best.

MILES. Oh, you did, did you?

USSHER. Yes, of course. I warned him against the danger of marrying a girl with whom he was only acquainted so short a time. I entreated him to wait a while at all events, as he was then only twenty-one and she something younger. But all to no purpose. Ah, if he had waited, he could not have failed to discover that she was only marrying him for his means and position, and that she did not in the least care for him. Besides I was certain from the first that he had no real affection or respect for her.

MILES. Indeed? What made you so certain of that, Barry?

USSHER. Well, you see, Carden and I had been intimate so long. We had been brought up together in fact, so that I fancy I understand him better than anyone. The sudden overturning of all his ideas at that time seemed to me strange and unnatural. He was like one bewitched. A man's whole nature somehow does not change in a moment. You were too young, Miles, to know him in those days; but

219

he was so ideal, so imaginative, as engaging as some beautiful child who saw nothing real in the world outside his own fairy dreams.

MILES (*with a baffled look*). I have memories of those days!

USSHER. They are vivid with me. Oh, he always did *so* fascinate and interest me. What poetry he put into those days of my youth – the days that are dead. (*Pause.*) Then to see him suddenly changed, grown even prosy under the power of her influence, it made it impossible for me to consider this attachment of his genuine or likely to endure. And has not the result proved that I was right?

MILES. I fear I must admit, Barry, that you were, alas, a reliable prophet.

USSHER. Oh, I foresaw all. I knew this change could not last. The old, wild nature had to break out again when the novelty was over. It was a misfortune since he was married, but it was inevitable. There are some dispositions too eerie, too ethereal, too untamable for good, steady, domestic cultivation, and if so domesticated they avenge themselves in after time. Ah, foolishly his wife and her friends thought they were going to change Carden to their model of a young man, but the latent, untamable nature was not to be subdued. Its first sign of revolt against suppression was when he began this vast work in the heather field.

MILES (*with a puzzled look*). Barry, I – I do not understand.

USSHER. Miles, you must admit it was rather an extravagant work. He has sunk a fortune of borrowed capital in the reclamation of that mountain. Look at all the men he employed to root up rocks, and the steam ploughs, too, that have been working during these last years.

MILES. But surely he will obtain a large rent for the rich grass he has made to grow there. That ought to more than compensate for his outlay.

USSHER. Meanwhile interest is accruing. The grass has not grown sufficiently for letting as yet. Then payment of rent cannot follow till long after, always supposing that it ever produces much rent.

MILES (*surprised*). Why do you say that? Is not the land good now.

USSHER. Ah, Miles, do you not know that the soil in such places is very wild and untamable? If heather lands are brought into cultivation for domestic use, they must be watched, they must have generous and loving treatment, else their old wild nature may avenge itself. (*He averts his look.*)

MILES (*with mingled wonder and uneasiness*). Avenge itself? How, Barry?

USSHER. Why, the wild heather may break out upon them soon again.

MILES. Oh – (*Then eagerly*) But don't you think Carden has given the best of treatment to the heather field?

220

USSHER. (*slowly and gently*). I do not know whether his treatment was sufficiently kind, as farmers say here in West Ireland. Somehow he seemed too impatient for the change. He was hardly considerate enough, perhaps, in the accomplishment of his will.

MILES (*with dejection*). You evidently think there is something unsatisfactory in the business.

USSHER. Let us hope for the best, Miles. In any case we ought to try and prevent him from embarking in further schemes.

MILES. Do, Barry. If there is one person in the world he will listen to, it is you. Besides you will remove a fresh cause of quarrels with Grace: and who knows but you may be able to do more afterwards. Stop – I see him coming now through the garden. (CARDEN TYRRELL, *a rather powerfully built man of one and thirty, with light hair, spare growth of beard, unsteady eyes, very large forehead, and lower part of face small, dressed negligently in a dark suit, enters from the back.*)

TYRRELL (*smiling*). Oh, how goes it with you, Barry? You have not favoured us with visits much of late. What have you been doing?

USSHER. Well, I have been to Dublin for one thing.

TYRRELL. So I heard. But is it true you are reducing all your rents?

USSHER. Yes, I *have* been reducing them somewhat.

TYRRELL. My goodness. I suppose you will end by making the tenants a present of your property. You call me a dreamer, but it seems that I am the practical man.

USSHER (*laughing*). Oh, that does not follow at all. I consider it wiser to give a little in time, than later on to have perhaps more wrung from me by the Land Commission.

TYRRELL. But one should never depreciate the value of one's property. I am afraid, Barry, you are mismanaging your affairs. Have you begun yet to reclaim that bog outside your demesne, as I advised?

USSHER. No, Carden.

TYRRELL. There, you see. Well, a fortune is to be made by such work. You would be much better employed at it than at reducing your rents. But, my dear old Barry, there is no use in arguing with you, when you are once set upon a thing. I suppose it is because you knew I would not approve of what you are doing that you have not been to see me for so long.

USSHER. Always suspicious, Carden. But, may I ask why you never come to see me?

TYRRELL. You forget all I have undertaken – all my responsibilities. I have little time.

USSHER. And one would think my time was of no value. Perhaps,

Carden, the real reason is that I might possibly not appreciate some of your undertakings and responsibilities.

TYRRELL. (*with a swift shy glance*). Why should you think so?

USSHER (*smiling*). Oh, I don't know. I was only wondering.

TYRRELL. But why should that prevent me from going to you?

USSHER. Precisely, why indeed? I should never have thought of it, if you had not first suggested the thought.

TYRRELL. Well, you have no reason to think anything of the kind. Just as if I could be occupied in the way you imagine.

USSHER. It seems odd that you should, Carden.

TYRRELL. Yet you have an idea all the same, that I could.

USSHER. Well, to tell you the truth, I heard yesterday that you were contemplating what seems to me certainly most rash.

TYRRELL. Oh, you did, did you? Let us hear what seems to you most rash.

USSHER. It is true, is it not, that you are about to borrow another large sum of money for new land improvements?

TYRRELL. (*somewhat confused*). Yes – it is true – well?

USSHER. Well – don't you think you had better not?

TYRRELL. Why not?

USSHER. Don't you think you have done enough work – for the present, at all events? Would it not be better to wait for a time and see whether what you have already accomplished is going to be successful ?

MILES. Yes, Carden, don't you think you ought to wait for a while longer?

TYRRELL. Wait? Why wait, when I know the work must be successful – nay, is already successful?

USSHER. You can scarcely yet be sure of that, Carden.

TYRRELL. Why not?

USSHER (*rather confused*). Oh, the nature – (*He hesitates.*)

MILES. You can scarcely yet be sure of what the land is capable, you know.

TYRRELL. Can I not see what grass it has produced.

USSHER. Yes, but will that continue?

TYRRELL (*scornfully*). Will that continue? Who ever heard so absurd a question. As well ask will the air continue to bear up the birds? Will its myriad life continue to pant underneath the sea? Come – my old friend, my brother – I will not have you talk in this discouraging way and make such insinuations, as if you were indeed nothing more than mere country neighbours, who cannot understand my ideas. No, you must believe in me, and inspire me with heart.

MILES. We do believe in you, Carden – but –

USSHER. We only suggest prudence.

MILES. Be prudent, Carden.

TYRRELL. Oh, but when you understand the matter, you will see how prudent I have been. For it was absolutely necessary to obtain this further loan unless the value of the previous one was to be destroyed.

USSHER. I do not follow you. Will you explain?

TYRRELL. Well, you see, the drainage of the heather field has practically swamped the lands below it; so I now must necessarily drain the water off from them right down to the sea. When I have finished all that grand ramification of drains, I shall have created a whole vast tract of fertile pasture which will double the value of my property. What do you think of that? Why, I believe all you people imagine that I am working in the dark, that I do not know what I am about. But 1 tell you I have excellent reasons for everything I undertake.

USSHER. Yes, Carden, of course – but you have borrowed a vast sum of money. Take care that the interest you will have to pay the Board of Works does not exceed your income.

TYRRELL. There is no danger, Barry. Have I not told you that my income must be greatly increased?

USSHER. You have indeed. I can only hope most sincerely that it will be so.

TYRRELL. But you still seem to doubt it all the same. (USSHER *is silent*). Oh, come, Barry, this is unfriendly of you. Barry, you are a prophet of evil. Heaven grant that your doubts may be vain else – Oh, I should be the most miserable of men. But they are vain – they are, they are – even despite your other memorable prophecy that, alas, has come too true. Ah, do you remember your warning to me ten years ago?

USSHER. You mean just before your marriage? Yes.

TYRRELL. (*gloomily*). I wonder had that anything to do with its unhappiness. I wonder if these doubts now will bring misfortune on my present undertakings.

USSHER (*in a frightened voice*). Carden, for pity's sake stop. Don't speak like that. Forget any doubts I may have now expressed. Forget them – forget them. I was wrong ever to have interfered with my advice. Never will I do so again. No – I have not the right. See, Carden, for all I know you may succeed now. I heartily hope you will. You are determined to, and discouragement might only caust you to fail. No – you must not have a second misfortune to cast at me. Good-bye. (*He prepares to go.*)

223

MILES. Oh, Barry, do not leave us in this way. Think –

TYRRELL. Oh, I am sorry you should take anything I said in that light. I did not mean, Barry, really to –

USSHER. NO, Carden, forgive me, but I was for the moment unnerved by the thought that you should attribute to me any of your ill luck. No – I hope you will always find me a help to you instead, whenever you may require me.

TYRRELL. Ah, now you are like yourself again – the Barry of other days. I knew you would understand me when I explained everything to you.

USSHER. I hope, Carden, at least I may never be to you the cause of ill luck. (*Exit at back.*)

TYRRELL. Dear old Barry, it makes him positively angry to see me improving my property, because he has not the enterprise to improve his own. But I think I have convinced him that he was mistaken in his estimate of my work.

MILES. You certainly frightened him, Carden. I have never seen him as he was just now.

TYRRELL. Oh, I really did not mean what I said. He only annoyed me by his stupid doubting.

MILES. Still – as a matter of fact long ago he tried to dissuade you from marrying Grace – isn't that so?

TYRRELL. Yes. He was full of doubts and objections then as now – only then he was right. But now – ha, ha – well, I know he is altogether wrong.

MILES. Why do you say you know, Carden? Why are you so certain now?

TYRRELL. Because I see so clearly before me.

MILES. That at least is a comfort. But perhaps he might be wrong in the other matter too. Don't you think it would be well also if you would determine to belie his doubts of long ago as well as of to-day?

TYRRELL. What do you mean?

MILES. Why, Carden, to try and prove that after all he was wrong when he advised you not to marry Grace.

TYRRELL. (*with a sigh*). Ah – impossible.

MILES. Don't say that, Carden.

TYRRELL: Oh, Miles, you do not understand.

MILES. But have you never tried?

TYRRELL. Tried –?

MILES. Yes, tried. You know there is nothing really wrong about her.

TYRRELL. Nothing, nothing – and everything. The same thing that is wrong about me. That is how it is between us.

MILES. But might you not try to fall in just a little with her ways? She is good after all.

TYRRELL. My dear Miles you don't know what you are talking about. Of course she is good enough. I know that perfectly well. But she has no sense of compromise – no consideration for me at all. She always despised me.

MILES. Oh, Carden, no –

TYRRELL. Oh, but yes. That is why she is so indignant I should take an interest in anything except herself. She would shape my life altogether after her own standard and that of Lady Shrule. I have often given in before, but the result was she became more and more exacting, until at last I found matters quite intolerable. Oh, it is useless to deny that here at least Barry's warnings have come true.

MILES. How extraordinary that you should have changed so towards her – you who once were so devoted.

TYRRELL. Ah, Miles, I have simply found her to be absolutely different from what I once imagined her. I was very young then, very inexperienced. I longed for sympathy, and thought it was easy to find. I idealised women in those days. I believed that they were idealists. Ah, that was my fatal error.

MILES. But surely you don't mean to deny that some are?

TYRRELL. I don't believe any are, really. They may be on an average more fanciful than man, but your true idealist can only be a man. Alas! had I known that then, my fate would have been very different. I thought others were easy to find, in whom I could confide as in Barry.

MILES. Do you consider him an idealist?

TYRRELL. I should think so indeed – a true idealist – only he is in a way so drilled and careful, that he will never let himself go. But he is such a friend, and understands everything. No, I never knew isolation when we were together in our youth. Isolation only began with my marriage which led me out into a lonely world. Oh, it was a great misfortune. And I have no one to blame but myself.

MILES. And yet – and yet were you really so much to blame? She was so beautiful.

TYRRELL. Ah, you have said it. There you have found the cause of all the trouble. But Barry would never have wavered.

MILES. Oh, he is a hardened philosopher whom no beauty could soften.

TYRRELL. That is because, unlike most people, he can see the truly beautiful, and so is heedless of shams.

MILES. Shams? And you can speak like that of her beauty. How I remember her on your wedding-day when as her little page I held

225

her train? I was only nine years old then, and thought she was some tall white fairy that had come to live with us. Oh, Carden, think of that time. Its memory might banish much bitterness.

TYRRELL. Too late, too late. You are still very young, Miles. I have outgrown the capability of such sentiment.

MILES. But you have not outgrown the great kindness of your nature. No, that I could never believe. Ought it not in these difficulties to help you? Why, see how good you are always to me.

TYRRELL. Ah, yes, that is different, Miles.

MILES. And Kit, too – are you not most affectionate and kind to him?

TYRRELL. My poor little son, of course – how could I be otherwise to him? He is really so lovable and such a companion to me. For just now he is wonderfully like what you were, Miles, when you acted as that pretty page. His age besides is the same as yours was then; so that the very sight of him calls back to me the days of my youth. Oh, that happy time before my fatal mistake! Miles, *do* you remember that time?

MILES. Remember? How well I remember!

TYRRELL. I suppose I had troubles then, as now; but memory has idealised those past scenes, till only their beauty remains, wafted back to me like an aroma from some lost paradise. I feel I shall never know the joy of those days again.

MILES. You must not think such things, Carden. Days as good as these will, I am sure, return.

TYRRELL. Ah no, Miles – their poetry, never – the hope that shines like a spring-day sun upon our youth! It warms us with such life. It inspires us to attempt so many deeds. With what expectations we travel. What materials we are to make out of it all. Do you remember when we went abroad together?

MILES. (*joyfully*). Oh, yes, of course I do, Carden.

TYRRELL. Well, it seems funny that I should have taken you with me then on travels you were too young to appreciate: but I could not bear to leave you who had no protector save me after our father died.

MILES. You kind brother.

TYRRELL. Yes, I carried you off, my little Miles, as you were then.

MILES. And how I enjoyed myself.

TYRRELL. What fairie towns we came to – Boppart on the Rhine with its quaint old houses. Then we sailed our boat through the hills to Lorlei, and watched where the river nymphs used long ago to glide, laughing, through the gold-lit depths of the stream.

MILES. Yes, and you told me the legend of their gold – how it was robbed and restored and still guarded by them.

TYRRELL. I did; and you, little practical man that you were, you bent down to the water expecting to see the glitter of the Rhine Gold!

MILES (*laughing*). The marvellous seemed real in those days.

TYRRELL. Ah, those bright happy days ! And do you remember that Sunday morning in Cologne Cathedral when all the boys sang Palestrina so divinely?

MILES. I remember we stood by great iron gates. I looked up in your face and wondered why it shone through its tears.

TYRRELL. How pure the silver voice chords soared to the vaults of stone! Pure as our joy in those days. Fit music for those bright young days.

MILES. Yes, everything seemed joyful then.

TYRRELL. Oh, what brave times we used to have together. You know we were always such friends.

MILES (*with emotion*). Indeed we always were, Carden. There is no one in the whole world I love as well as you. You have ever been the best of brothers to me.

TYRRELL. (*goes over mysteriously to* MILES). Then you think, Miles, you will always help me ?

MILES. (*surprised*). Why, Carden, of course -

TYRRELL (*with anxious intensity*). You will not leave me, if – if ever I should stand helpless and alone, will you Miles?

MILES. Good gracious, no. But what makes you imagine such a thing?

TYRRELL. Well, somehow I feel that persons and objects are receding from me and becoming more unreal in these later times. (*Crosses over to sofa at right and kneeling on it with one knee, gazes out at the mountain.*) Do you know, Miles, I often think that my life of pain and unrest here is only a dream after all.

MILES. And like a dream this suffering will pass away, Carden, let us hope never to return.

TYRRELL (*sadly*). No, oh no. It would be too much to expect that. A dream – a bad dream (*as if suddenly illumined*), yet with intervals too of wakefulness now and then.

MILES (*approaching him*). Of wakefulness? What do you mean? When are those intervals?

TYRRELL. When I am out in the heather field.

MILES. The heather field?

TYRRELL (*with enthusiasm*). Yes – the great mountain field out there (*points out at back*), that it was my ideal to bring to fruitfulness. There I awaken to true life indeed, as I stand looking over the Atlantic; and sea winds sweep against my feet the young grass in its matchless Irish green that gleams a golden green in the Autumn sun

227

to-day. There I am haunted by those departed joys of my youth –
again and again.

MILES (*with a puzzled look*). There? But why there, Carden. Why there
more than anywhere else?

TYRRELL. Oh you matter-of-fact Miles – still the same as the little wise
Miles of long ago, who used to ask such quaint questions. How
different we are? Yet how delightful I always find you. 'Why there?'
you ask. Ha, ha!

MILES (*a little disconcerted*). Evidently you consider it a superfluous
question. But I think I may very reasonably ask it all the same.

TYRRELL. Well, then, because there after years of joyless stagnation I
find myself again in an ideal domain – away from fretful
surroundings – alone! Except for little Kit who loves the mountain
and its wild flowers. You know, Miles, how like I have said he now
looks to what you were in the old days? At moments, indeed, I can
hardly believe it is he and not you. So his presence there is no
hindrance to that evocation of the past. No; he serves rather to
quicken the magic of the heather field.

MILES (*with sudden, emotion*). Oh, to think I could ever have been so
much to you. How good you always were to me, Carden.

TYRRELL. I could not help it. You belonged to the beauty of that time.

MILES. All this sounds like the marvellous tales you used to tell me
when I was a child. I see your imagination is the same as ever.

TYRRELL. And you call what I tell you only imagination.

MILES. Well, Carden – but what else.

TYRRELL. (*resignedly*). Ah, I suppose I cannot help you. You too are
like Barry who said the same thing when I once told him of the
voices –

MILES. (*with vague alarm*). Voices, Carden? Why – what now are these?

TYRRELL. Out there – over the mountain. Oh, the vivid brightness of
those voices, as they float back from the past on each changing
breeze!

MILES (*anxiously*). You only heard the wind whistle along the coast.
Don't heed it any more, Carden.

TYRRELL. Why should I not heed such celestial song?

MILES. A dream phantom of the desolate mountain.

TYRRELL. No; it is only your words I hear as in a troubled dream.

MILES (*gently*). Carden, it is deceiving you – this wonderful
imagination.

TYRRELL. What? – imagination again?

MILES. Of course.

TYRRELL (*patiently*). Ah well, I cannot convince you, Miles. But what does it matter? You are delightfully sympathetic to me all the same. I feel this opening of my soul to you has even done me good. Yes, it does me good to be listened to occasionally. It leaves a great peace after it; and I have not felt so peaceful as now for many a day. Indeed, if this could last, it would be almost like the old time again. (MRS GRACE TYRRELL, *a rather tall, thin woman of about thirty but looking younger, with a pale face, brown hair and an undefinable attractiveness in her outward manner and movements enters by door at right. She is dressed plainly, but with exceeding neatness. TYRRELL takes a large book from the shelves at back of sofa on which he then sits and turns over the leaves, suppressing a look of annoyance).*

MILES (*going towards her politely*). I suppose you have been out on your rounds this morning as usual, Grace?

GRACE. Yes, as usual. Have you been here since breakfast?

MILES. Yes.

GRACE. Studying, I suppose.

MILES. Not much.

GRACE. Why?

MILES. Oh, Barry Ussher was here, and then Carden and I have been talking.

GRACE. And so your morning was wasted, Miles?

MILES. Oh, not wasted, Grace.

GRACE. I think it would have been more profitably employed in working for your examinations than in talking to your brother.

MILES. I am not at all so certain you are right.

GRACE. You must admit you have plenty of time for talking without allowing it to interfere with your studies.

TYRRELL (*looking up from his book*). It is so hard for us, Miles, is it not, when we are together, to refrain?

GRACE. What you two can have to say perpetually to each other puzzles me. You never visit anywhere nor seem to know what is going on in the neighbourhood.

TYRRELL. If we did, I am certain we shouldn't trouble to speak about it.

GRACE. Oh, indeed.

TYRRELL. No; the subjects that mutually interest us are far different. Among other things, we were talking before you came in over our journey long ago on the Continent. (*Then as if carried away by the subject of the moment*) Look, in this architectural book there are plates representing some buildings we saw then. Here is a Romanesque house at Boppart on the Rhine. It is a unique specimen of domestic architecture in that period. And here – this is the bishop's house at Würzburg. How beautifully the oriel is poised there at the angle, like a hooded falcon on its perch; what a genius these medieval architects had for soothing with picturesque ideality the restless suffering spirit of their time. To gaze on their work makes one forget oneself and everything else –

GRACE (*who the while has been looking about her with an impatient and wearied expression*). Goodness me, what a litter the room is in with all these books and papers.

TYRRELL (*with a momentary look of humiliation*). Oh!

GRACE. What brought me here, by the way, was to tell you that I must have it thoroughly dusted and tidied at once, as the Shrules come to lunch to-morrow.

TYRRELL. Yes, but what have they got to do with my room?

GRACE. We shall want it to sit in. I could not think of letting anyone see it in its present state.

TYRRELL (*fretfully*). Can't you leave my room alone?

GRACE. There! as usual, you are disagreeable when your wife wants anything.

TYRRELL. No; but I have a quantity of important papers that it would give me endless trouble at present to sort, and put away.

MILES. Oh, why cause him all this inconvenience, Grace? Will not the drawing-room suit you just as well?

GRACE. Lord Shrule has had an attack of gout and does not like going upstairs –

MILES. Then bring them here. But you need not upset the room. Everyone knows it's a work-room.

GRACE. I could not think of allowing any strangers to see it in this state.

MILES. I wonder how you can attach so much importance –

GRACE (*coldly*). That will do, Miles. As usual you don't know what you are talking about.

MILES. Hei-ho. (*He begins to gather his books together on the writing-table.*)

TYRRELL. You are not going, Miles, are you?

MILES. I think I shall try if I can read in the summerhouse outside. (*Exit at back, carrying with him his books.*)

GRACE (*quietly*). Well, I suppose you had better put away all these old papers at once, and let the housemaid come in.

TYRRELL. Impossible. – I am too busy.

GRACE. That's what you always say. You imagine yourself the busiest man in the world; and as a matter of fact you have nothing to do.

TYRRELL. Nothing to do?

GRACE (*calmly*). What have you to do?

TYRRELL (*checking his irritation*). Very well, we won't discuss that old subject. Anyhow I require my papers, as a man comes to see me tomorrow on business connected with them.

GRACE. Who is this man?

TYRRELL. The drainage inspector of the Board of Works.

GRACE. Indeed! Why, I thought he had finished everything here long ago.

TYRRELL. Oh, so he has.

GRACE. Well, what is he coming for now?

TYRRELL. (*vaguely*). Oh – you see – it would take too long to explain just at present. Besides you might not understand.

GRACE. (*with a penetrating look*). You know I would understand well enough. But you never were a person to be relied upon! You are now trying to hide something from me. Come, it is as good to tell it to me at once.

TYRRELL (*bridling up*). I am not trying to hide anything from you. I don't care whether you know it or not.

GRACE. Well, then, why is this man coming?

TYRRELL. He is to lay out some drains in the valley beneath the heather field.

GRACE (*astounded*). What? – You don't mean to say you are going to drain all that immense tract of land too?

TYRRELL. Yes. It is necessary now after the other work. So I am going to obtain a new loan from Government to carry it out.

GRACE. A new loan! We shall certainly be ruined this time.

TYRRELL. No – no – Why, can you not see the enormous improvement this work must be to the estate?

GRACE. Oh, that is what you are always saying; and the estate for some years past has been steadily growing worse and worse, uutil now we are almost reduced to difficulties.

TYRRELL. You are quite mistaken. I tell you we are on the eve of seeing our income doubled. Just consider the rent that must soon be produced by the heather field.

GRACE (*with a gesture of impatience*). The heather field. Up to this, indeed, it has been nothing but a gigantic loss. And who knows but it may never be anything else? My goodness, can you not wait to see if it will be a success before you swamp the estate with this new debt?

TYRRELL. No – no – every delay is a loss of profit. You do not understand.

GRACE. Oh, I am tired of your always telling me that I do not

231

understand. I understand perfectly that you are bringing us to beggary.

TYRRELL. Well – it is certainly amazing that you should think so. But then, you know, you are never open to reason – never in sympathy with my ideas.

GRACE. How on earth can I be, when like everyone else I believe you to be utterly mistaken in what you are doing?

TYRRELL. I do not mean what I am doing at present – but the whole tenor of my life and ideas. You have never understood them.

GRACE (*sharply*). Look here, it's beginning to irritate me this talk about my not understanding. So I see – you think yourself the great incomprehensible, ha, ha. Well, you are quite mistaken. Everyone understands you. So do I, absolutely. For in spite of all your efforts to be singular, you are a very ordinary person, in whom there is nothing particular to understand.

TYRRELL (*helplessly*). What on earth do you mean by always harping on my efforts to be singular? Heaven knows I cannot see how I try to be so.

GRACE (*with a little laugh, as she taps her foot on the floor*). I suppose you are now habituated to the effort.

TYRRELL (*looking at her with a sort of wonder*). Oh, how impossible it is for you ever to know how I have suffered – how I have aspired!

GRACE (*impatiently*). Really, it becomes too provoking when you begin talking about these imaginary sufferings and aspirations of yours. What on earth have you to suffer? You are in good health are you not? Were you not more than fortunate to have married as you did? Have you not independent means? What then can a man like you aspire more to? It is true, of course, that you have crippled your resources by mismanagement and extravagance. But, if you will now be led by me, and put this new scheme of drainage out of your head, and if we are economical for a while, the property must recover. Then you can have absolutely nothing to trouble you.

TYRRELL. Oh, this matter-of-fact way you have of looking at things! This simple barren prose of your mind ! It is that, that is driving me mad.

GRACE. Driving you mad – (*Pause, during which they look at each other.*)

TYRRELL. Well, I suppose you think I am so. (*He waits for her answer.*) What an absurd idea This is another means of annoying me.

GRACE. I must defend myself.

TYRRELL. What do you mean ?

GRACE. Seeing you are so bent on ruining our child and me, I can only think one thing.

TYRRELL. That I am mad?

GRACE (*without answering him walking to back*).

TYRRELL. Grace.

GRACE (*turning*). Well – what is it?

TYRRELL. Do you mean this?

GRACE. (*still walking to back*). What did I say?

TYRRELL. You said – I mean you insinuated that – I am mad.

GRACE (*Does not answer.*)

TYRRELL. You do not mean this. Take back what you have said.

GRACE (*turning suddenly*). I cannot. (*She still walks to back.*)

TYRRELL. Before you go take back your words. You don't know how they frighten me. Again I beseech you to take back those words. You do not believe what you say.

GRACE. I do believe them. I believe you to be mad. (*Exit at back*).

TYRRELL. (*laughing nervously*). Oh – ha— mad. How can she say such a thing? Mad – who is saner than I am? Ha – ha – I suppose people of her type think everyone who differs from them, mad. How curious! Ah, we have not a single sympathy. That is what it is. (*With a look of terror*) Merciful heaven, is it possible, though, she may be right? Can there possibly be a doubt as to which is the reality and which is the dream? Oh, horror – horror! (*He sinks upon the sofa and covers his face with his hands.*) (MILES TYRRELL, *carrying his books as before, enters at back.*)

MILES. It is rather chilly reading out of doors. As I saw Grace just go through the garden, I may perhaps again have this place to myself. (*Perceiving* TYRRELL.) Oh, you here still. Why, Carden, what is the matter with you?

TYRRELL (*rising, approaches in a dazed manner, and seems involuntarily to feel his way with his hands*). Nothing – only that persons and things now more than ever seem strangely to recede from me and become more unreal. But you – *you*, Miles, said you would never leave me (*glances around with a shudder*) if ever I should stand helpless and alone. Oh, Miles, my brother – (*He hides his face on* MILES' *shoulder.*)

MILES. Carden – (*The books fall from his arms on the floor.*)

END OF ACT I

ACT II

SCENE: *The same as last, except that the room is tidied, the window doors at back are closed, vases of flowers stand on the tables from which the papers, &c., have been removed and replaced by sundry drawing-room ornaments. It is the afternoon of the following day.*

MRS GRACE TYRRELL *opens the door at right for* LADY SHRULE, *a plain, fashionable looking woman of about five-and-thirty, in a riding habit and straw hat which fit her to perfection. She enters somewhat jauntily.*

GRACE *(following her)*. I thought we might as well sit here after lunch instead of in the drawing-room. I know Lord Shrule is not very fond of going upstairs.

LADY SHRULE. No; my husband, dear old man, finds it trying after his attack of gout. Well, upon my word, Grace, this is quite a pretty room. What a pity not to turn all these frowzy books out of it.

GRACE *(sighing)*. Oh, of course, it ought to be a drawing-room.

LADY SHRULE. Then why don't you make it one?

GRACE. My goodness, Lilian, you know I can do nothing in this house.

LADY SHRULE. I know you have a wretched time of it, dear, with that husband of yours. Still I cannot help thinking that if, at the beginning, you had really tried, you might have made him more amenable.

GRACE. That sounds very easy. You have no idea what he is.

LADY SHRULE. Oh, nonsense, Grace. Most men have notions before they marry: but they are soon brought to their senses, if their wives are clever. And you are clever: so that is why I say you cannot have tried.

GRACE. I have tried everything, Lilian, although you won't believe it.

LADY SHRULE. What – everything?

GRACE. Yes.

LADY SHRULE. There is one thing I am sure you have never tried.

GRACE *(eagerly)*. What is that?

LADY SHRULE. Flattery.

GRACE. Lilian, don't be silly. As if there was anything I could flatter him about.

234

LADY SHRULE. Well, you know, in spite of all, people *do* say he is clever.

GRACE (*impatiently*). I must say I have never found him so.

LADY SHRULE. I confess I never have either. But then I don't see very much of him. To tell you the truth he always seemed to me odd and ridiculous: for he never cared for society, never went to races, dances, or tennis parties, you know, like other people. Still it might be worth your while to do as I advised. You can hardly imagine what effect it has even on the most unpromising men.

GRACE. That may be, that may be, when they are really superior to one; but to flatter him – ugh – never (*half to herself as she turns away*). Besides it is impossible after yesterday.

LADY SHRULE. (*pricking up her ears*). Yesterday? What happened yesterday, Grace? (GRACE *is silent.*)

LADY SHRULE. (*goes up to her*). What is the matter, dear?

GRACE (*petulantly*). Oh, nothing, Lilian. I did not mean you to hear.

LADY SHRULE. Oh, but there *is* something, Grace. I see it by your troubled look. He must have done something dreadful yesterday. Perhaps I might be of help to you. What was it?

GRACE. Well this. Yesterday I discovered that he has embarked on a new folly which must end in our ruin; and when I tried to remonstrate with him he would not listen to a word I said. Just think, he – he –

LADY SHRULE. He must be a great savage. But what else can you expect from the life he leads?

GRACE. Quite true. You are perfectly right, Lilian.

LADY SHRULE. What is this new folly you say he has embarked on, Grace?

GRACE. Oh, a monstrous plan of draining another immense morass. As if our means were not already sufficiently crippled by his extravagance in this way.

LADY SHRULE. I should think so, indeed. What a misfortune for you that you ever married him.

GRACE. Yes – what a misfortune!

LADY SHRULE. I have always wondered why you did, Grace. You know you never cared for him. How, indeed, could any girl care for such a man – least of all the Grace Desmond I remember in those days, when we used to meet at every party and ball in the county.

GRACE. Yes, yes, Lilian, I know that. But you see he was a good match at the time; and I thought I would be able to make him sensible, and to lead him; – for he *was* so much in love with me.

LADY SHRULE. Was he ever really, do you think?

235

GRACE. Oh, I think so: he must have been at first; for then it seemed to me that I used to monopolise all his attention.

LADY SHRULE. How came he to change? Some other woman, I suppose –

GRACE. No – no. There is no one else. I am sure of that. I have watched him closely now for some years.

LADY SHRULE. Nonsense, dear – just as if *you* could watch him. I tell you it is impossible that a man can exist without loving some woman.

GRACE. Yes – I know we women all think so. But this is quite a case in itself. He is such a queer creature. You cannot imagine how strange his ideas are. (*With a certain relief and confidence.*) Oh, no – there is no one else; and it is very wicked of you, Lilian, to suggest such a thing.

LADY SHRULE. (*a little nettled*). How then, do you account for his behaviour?

GRACE. I cannot think, for I have always been most amiable to him and patient with his eccentricities, which are dreadfully irritating. Gracious, I remember when he first began to weary me with his strange ideas that I could not make head or tail of. (So you may be sure, dear, they were sheer nonsense.) It was then, when I tried to draw him from such folly, and to centre his interest upon myself, that I noticed a curious change in him. It seemed all at once that I became as nothing to him – that what he loved was something mysterious – beyond me.

LADY SHRULE. Ah, he never loved you, Grace. I am certain, now, he never did.

GRACE. Oh, yes, he must have at first. You should have seen how I made him do almost anything for me. Why, he settled down, entertained, shot, even farmed. Imagine that for him.

LADY SHRULE. (*composedly*). Well – what was the result? What about the farming, for instance?

GRACE (*crestfallen*). Indeed – the only result of the farming has been – the heather field.

LADY SHRULE. Ah, Grace, for all you made him do, you were not able to make him give up the heather field – my poor Grace!

GRACE. (*with violent emotion*). Oh, that folly! That abominable work! With the beginning of it I noticed his first change towards me.

LADY SHRULE. He never loved you, Grace. He is a terrible man. These Tyrrells were always a queer lot. You know the father was very eccentric; and the mother – well, Shrule tells me she went quite out of her mind before she died, at the birth of the young brother. What kind is he, by the way? He is very good-looking, don't you think?

GRACE. Oh, Miles is all right. He is a harmless creature, – wonderfully clever at college, I hear. He is certainly amiable, but vexes me occasionally with his foolish admiration for my husband.

LADY SHRULE. Yes, I can imagine how annoying that must be.

GRACE. Yes, and to have that fellow Ussher, too, dropping in to complete the mutual admiration society! Oh, I always disliked him.

LADY SHRULE. I don't think much of him either, with his sad, lonely way of living there in that great place of his. I believe he has it filled with such strange things.

GRACE. Yes, books and hideous pictures. I have not been there for years. I avoid him as much as possible; for he was always my enemy, and does his best to destroy whatever influence I might have with my husband.

LADY SHRULE. My poor Grace, what a strange crew you have fallen among! This dreadful husband! So at last he is going selfishly to sacrifice you for the gratification of his theories and whims.

GRACE (*with determination*). He shall not sacrifice me, Lilian. I am certain of that now.

LADY SHRULE. Why, dear, what are you thinking of?

GRACE. All those facts you have mentioned about the Tyrrells only confirm a suspicion that has haunted me for some time.

LADY SHRULE. (*with increasing curiosity*). What suspicion, Grace?

GRACE. That my husband is not in his right senses.

LADY SHRULE. Do you mean you think him mad?

GRACE. Yes – mad.

LADY SHRULE. Oh!

GRACE. Yes, Lilian; I feel there can be no doubt about it now. You know his monstrous extravagance, his wild manner of talking – and then what you tell me about his father and mother. – Oh, he must certainly be mad.

LADY SHRULE. I suppose you are right.

GRACE. Of course – that is what it is – poor man! Measures ought therefore to be taken at once to prevent him from ruining his family.

LADY SHRULE. What measures can you take, Grace?

GRACE. I don't see why I should not commence a legal suit to deprive him of control over the property.

LADY SHRULE. But that would mean placing him under restraint, wouldn't it?

GRACE. I suppose so, if necessary. All I know is that I am determined to prevent this new burden from being put on the estate.

LADY SHRULE. Wouldn't it be well, Grace, if you were first to have medical advice as to the state of your husband's mind?

GRACE. I have already thought of that, Lilian. I have been in communication with Doctor Dowling and Doctor Roche.

LADY SHRULE. What – really?

GRACE. Yes. I believe two doctors are required, are they not, in cases of this sort?

LADY SHRULE. I don't know: but we can ask Shrule.

GRACE. Of course: he is sure to know, How lucky I have you both here.

LADY SHRULE. When do you think of sending for the doctors?

GRACE. Well, Lilian, the sooner the better, if this government loan is to be stopped. (*Hesitating*) Well, the fact is I – I have sent for them to-day.

LADY SHRULE. To-day?

GRACE. Yes. Was I not right?

LADY SHRULE. But your husband suspects nothing of this?

GRACE. Good heavens, no! Neither do the doctors as yet. No – I have sent for them upon the plea of their holding a consultation about Kit. As Doctor Roche has been attending him lately off and on for little attacks of feverishness and nausea, their visit will not look in any way suspicious. I will then take care they have conversation with my husband. You see?

LADY SHRULE. What energy and resource you have, dear, to be sure.

GRACE. Ah, when a woman is reduced to such desperate straits as I am at present, it sharpens her wits. But the doctors may arrive now at any moment, and as I must see and prepare them beforehand for this task, let us go out to the end of the shrubbery where we can meet them on their way.

LADY SHRULE. Very well – and you can bring Shrule to join in our consultation afterwards, when he comes from the dining-room.

GRACE. What a comfort, Lilian, to have you both to consult. (*Vehemently*) You must help me. I tell you I must succeed in this undertaking. It means the very existence of my child and me. (CARDEN TYRRELL *enters hastily at the back*.)

TYRRELL. Oh, have you finished lunch so soon? How do you do, Lady Shrule? (*They shake hands*). I hope you will excuse my absence. I was very busy all the morning with the Board of Works inspector.

LADY SHRULE. Oh, not at all. Have you finished your business?

TYRRELL. No – but I expect to by to-night. The inspector has gone in before me to lunch – so, with your permission, I will leave you to look after him.

LADY SHRULE. Of course, Mr Tyrrell – we will excuse you. Grace and I were just about to take a stroll around the garden. You will find

Shrule in the dining-room. (*Exeunt* LADY SHRULE *and* MRS GRACE TYRRELL *at back.* CARDEN TYRRELL *gazes after them as they disappear in the garden, then goes to writing table where he searches for something which he cannot find, while he grumbles indistinctly. He looks around the room with an expression of annoyance at its altered condition, then exit by door at right. Enter at back* BARRY USSHER *and* KIT TYRRELL, *a rather wild though pensive-looking boy with short, fair hair, and dressed in a sailor suit. He has a daisy chain swung across his shoulder, and holds a bunch of wild flowers in his hand.*)

KIT (*dragging* USSHER *by the sleeve*). Come in, Barry, come in. I missed you yesterday. Have you brought me anything this time?

USSHER. I am afraid nothing this time, Kit. You see, when I left home I did not intend to come here; but on the road I met by chance Doctor Roche, who told me he had been sent for by your mother. So I thought I would just turn in, and see if anything was the matter. There is no one ill is there?

KIT. No, of course not. They are only bringing him to bother me again. I have nothing the matter with me; and still he is always saying I must not eat this and I must not eat that.

USSHER. What a nasty old fellow!

KIT. Yes – isn't he horrid? He says, too, I mustn't lie on the grass. I suppose he'll soon want to prevent me hunting for wild flowers.

USSHER. That *would* be a privation, Kit. You love them so much, don't you? What nice ones you have brought in to-day. Where did you get them – so late, too, in the year?

KIT. Oh, you can't think how I had to search for them here and there through the long grass in the heather field. It is the only place now where any wild flowers are left. How I love being there with father.

USSHER. So you, Kit, have also caught the sickness of the heather field.

KIT. What is this sickness you are all saying I have ? I tell you I am quite well. (*With impatience*) Oh, how I wish I were a man.

USSHER. Alas, are you not much better as you are? Why do you want to be a man?

KIT. Because then they could not prevent me doing what I like. I should be a sailor and find out what is beyond that great sea father and I are always looking at from the heather field.

USSHER. Be a sailor, Kit, and give up the wild flowers?

KIT. Oh, I forgot. But should I have to, do you think?

USSHER. I fear you could not gather flowers on the sea, except, perhaps, a few poor crushed ones, torn from its depths by the storms.

KIT. Then there *are* some, after all?

USSHER. Yes – down under the sea grow numberless fair flowers whose leaves close softly around many a poor sailor.

KIT (*dreamily*). What beautiful flowers!

USSHER. I hope you will never be such a sailor, Kit. No, you are far better as you are! Do not wish to be a man.

KIT. Why, Barry?

USSHER. Because you understand so many things now you never could then. How much nicer to be always a little wildflower elf! In the lives of dream children such as you it is beautiful to think of a heather field.

KIT. Oh, but can they prevent me from going there?

USSHER. They cannot. I will see that old Roche attempts no such tyranny.

KIT. Oh, thank you, Barry. How good you always are! (LORD SHRULE, *an elderly benevolent-looking man dressed in a somewhat old-fashioned riding costume,* MILES TYRRELL, *and* CARDEN TYRRELL *enter by the door at right.*)

LORD SHRULE. Now that the inspector has gone out again to his work, I must say, my dear Carden, I am astounded at hearing of this new expenditure you contemplate. I did not like to speak before him – Ah, Ussher, how do you do? (*To* KIT) And how is my little man?

KIT (*holding out his hand*). Very well, thanks.

LORD SHRULE. That's right, that's right. I was saying, my dear Carden, your fresh project of expenditure fills me with amazement. Have you heard about it, Ussher?

USSHER. I have indeed.

LORD SHRULE. Well, does it not seem to you extremely imprudent – nay, reckless?

USSHER. Oh, you must not ask me, Lord Shrule. Carden seems determined. And, after all, he is the best judge of his own affairs.

TYRRELL. Yes, Barry, that is just it.

LORD SHRULE. Come, come, Carden, you will not mind the advice of an old man who has a long experience in the management of land. Your father and I were always fast friends, and I naturally take a great interest in you and your family.

TYRRELL. I know you have always been very kind, Lord Shrule. Forgive me if I have spoken hastily. I did not mean –

LORD SHRULE. Of course not, my dear Carden. I quite understand you. I fear indeed you must think it rather impertinent of your friends to interfere in your business. But then, as I have said, I consider myself privileged.

TYRRELL. You may be quite sure, Lord Shrule, I could not take anything from you except in good part.

LORD SHRULE. I thought so. Well, let me implore of you, if only for the sake of your family, to desist. This is certainly the wildest scheme I ever heard of, and couldn't pay, even if the drainage were to turn out a success.

TYRRELL. But you forget it is necessary now that the drainage of the heather field falls into this land. I *must* make a cutting for the water to get to the sea. And then, what is easier than to reclaim the land through which this cutting goes ?

LORD SHRULE. My dear Carden, don't mind the cutting – don't mind the heather field. What you have only got to think of is to cease altogether from loading your estate with an ever-growing burden of debt. For goodness' sake leave these works alone. If you continue them you will simply beggar yourself.

TYRRELL (*uneasily*). I do not see that at all. The work will be very remunerative. It will double the value of the estate.

LORD SHRULE. Oh, Carden, listen to me. I know well the nature of such works as you are carrying on. I have tried them myself – on a far smaller scale, of course. They never repay their expenditure.

TYRRELL. That is a mere assertion unsupported by argument. On the other hand, I have excellent reasons why I should believe that what I am about to undertake must have the best results. Look at the rich pasture now in the heather field. And am I to suppose that I shall not have the same in the valley when it is reclaimed? Until you can prove logically that I am mistaken, I must continue those works, which I clearly see are so profitable. Am I not right, Barry?

USSHER. I have said I shall never again discourage you, Carden.

LORD SHRULE. Ussher, upon my word I thought you knew better. But I suppose it is useless remonstrating on these experiments, which amount with him to absolute mania. (MRS GRACE TYRRELL *enters at back.*)

GRACE (*after bowing to* USSHER). Oh, Lord Shrule, we have been waiting for you in the garden. Won't you come? I want to show you my little greenhouse. The plants you gave me are doing so well in it.

LORD SHRULE. I am delighted to hear you say so, Mrs Tyrrell. Let us go and see them. But I hope you will not make me walk much, as I have barely recovered from that last attack of gout, and can only get about as yet quietly on my pony. Let me see, I left my hat in the hall.

GRACE. We can go through there, just as well. (*Exeunt* LORD SHRULE *and* MRS GRACE TYRRELL *by door at right.*)

TYRRELL. It is really too bad that I should be molested thus perpetually with unsolicited advice. All my acquaintances seem to consider it incumbent upon them to interfere in and direct my affairs just like their own. One would think I had no right to do anything. That old fellow, you know, means well; but it is very annoying to be taken to task by a person who has really no right to meddle. Ha! – it is too absurd indeed that I should have to defend what I have a perfect right to do.

MILES. I know it must be very trying, Carden.

TYRRELL. I should think so, indeed. And I am not going to stand it any longer. I will live my life as I want, and will take dictation from nobody.

USSHER. But you must expect to be criticised, Carden. That is the penalty, you know, for attempting to do anything.

TYRRELL. Oh, I don't mind any amount of outside criticism – nor even the strictures of friends like Lord Shrule, as long as their remarks are not to my face. No, it is other criticism – nearer – that leaves a sting.

MILES. Well, Carden, I am sure Barry and I are not in the habit of finding fault with you. At least we never mean to.

USSHER. Of that, at all events, I am certain.

TYRRELL. No – not you two, kindest and best. It is even nearer home – this criticism and opposition – this hearing perpetually amidst the strain of labour, bitter and disheartening words. That is what is so unbearable.

MILES. Be patient with her, Carden. Grace cannot as yet understand. This is a period of trial. One day you will see her loyally helping and inspiring you.

TYRRELL (*impatiently*). Inspiring me! I wish, Miles, you would not use a sublime word in a vulgar sense. When you have more experience you will find that instead of inspiring they more often prevent us from doing anything.

MILES. Oh, Carden – how unlike you! That is more the style of the cynic philosopher, there – Barry. See how he is smiling. I am sure he regrets he missed saying such a thing himself instead.

USSHER. Well, really, Miles –

TYRRELL (*laughing*). Oh, you dear Miles. You were always the most wonderful body in the world for dispelling bitterness and gloom with that beautiful light you seem to carry about you! (*Hopefully*) Well, two friends such as you ought to compensate me for what I have to bear from others. Bah, I will not mind them. I will be merry while I work; and my work will be incessant, leaving no time for brooding over unpleasant things. And both of you will always be present with me, if difficulties should arise. Yes, with you I know

242

I cannot suffer defeat from the rest. (*Enter at back* MRS GRACE TYRRELL, DOCTOR DOWLING, *a thick-set man of about forty, dressed in a tweed suit, and* DOCTOR ROCHE, *an elderly, lean and somewhat prim man, wearing spectacles and black clothes. Looking a little ill at ease, the Doctors exchange salutations with* TYRRELL, MILES, USSHER, AND KIT.)

KIT. Mother!

GRACE. Yes, my dear?

KIT. Who is that with Doctor Roche?

GRACE. Doctor Dowling.

KIT. Is he coming to see me too?

GRACE. Just to look at you, Kit. That's all.

KIT. But I have nothing the matter with me, mother.

GRACE. Never mind – neither will hurt you – only save you from possible peril – oh, my own sweet boy. (*She kisses him.*)

TYRRELL. (*To* GRACE). You cannot think there was cause for summoning these two physicians.

GRACE (*vaguely*). Cause? – well – I was a little anxious on the child's account, and thought it best they should consult about him. But I expected to find you alone. (*She glances at* USSHER).

USSHER (*taking the hint*). Carden, I must go. I hope there is nothing really the matter with Kit. He doesn't look as if there was.

KIT. Oh, Barry, don't go. You know you promised –

USSHER. Hush, Kit.

TYRRELL. Yes, stay where you are, Barry. There is no reason for making such a mystery of this business. Besides, I must soon go out to the inspector, and we can walk together. (*To* GRACE) By the way, what has become of the Shrules?

GRACE (*uneasily*). Oh, Lord Shrule had to return home suddenly about some matter of importance. They both desired me to say 'good-bye' to you.

TYRRELL. So much the better. – Well, doctors, I certainly cannot understand the necessity of this consultation. The boy seems to me perfectly well.

GRACE. No, I assure you, Doctor Dowling, he is not so. He is often ill from eating all sorts of unwholesome sweets. How do you find him looking to-day, Doctor Roche?

ROCHE. He appears healthier, on the whole, I think, Mrs Tyrrell. (*To* KIT) Come here, and let me look well at you, my little man. There, put out your tongue.

KIT. Ah, I suppose, Barry, I must now expect the worst.

USSHER. Never fear, Kit. They don't look as if they meant to do much

243

to you.

GRACE (*suspiciously*). I am afraid, Mr Ussher, you spoil him as much as his father, and I shall get no good of him while you are here. You and Miles ought to take a walk. It would be so nice on this fine day, wouldn't it? But won't you return to dinner? Do return to dinner, Mr Ussher.

USSHER. No, thank you, Mrs Tyrrell, I regret I cannot. I shall be going now in a minute with Carden. Kit must not expect any countenance from me.

KIT. But I thought you said you would not let Doctor Roche –

USSHER. Now, Kit, you must do as you are told. Have I not said you needn't fear? (THE DOCTORS *look at* KIT, *feel his pulse, talk together, &c.*)

USSHER (*aside to* MILES). Your sister-in-law seems particularly anxious to get rid of us.

MILES (*aside to* USSHER, *with an enquiring look*). Do you really think so? I wonder why?

USSHER (*aside to* MILES). I am not certain yet.

TYRRELL. How needless this consultation is, to be sure. There is nothing the matter with the boy.

GRACE. You do well to say so – you, who are the chief cause of his illness.

TYRRELL. I, the cause?

GRACE. Of course you are. He is sick at night after those long days when you keep him out fasting on the mountain, and then feed him with sweets at dinner afterwards. This must all cease.

KIT. Oh, mother, do not prevent me from going to the heather field. I don't want these sweets – I was only sick once.

GRACE. Can you not see, Kit, that I am only acting for your good? (*Sadly*) It is I who fight for his interests, and he leaves me for his father.

TYRRELL. Only sick once, and all this fuss for that! Never mind, Kit, you shall not be prevented. I will take care in future that you get plenty to eat and at proper times. So there will be no danger of sickness again.

KIT. Then you will not let anyone prevent me from going with you, father?

TYRRELL. Ah, you see, Kit, I never could get on without you in the heather field. We should feel so lonely – both of us, shouldn't we? (GRACE *looks significantly at the* DOCTORS, *who now begin to observe* TYRRELL *closely.*)

KIT. Yes, father, dear.

USSHER (*aside to* MILES). The doctors seem strangely in-attentive now to Kit and his ailments.

MILES (*aside to* USSHER, *with a puzzled expression*). So it seems. What do you think they mean?

USSHER (*aside to* MILES). Wait. I have an uncomfortable suspicion. It is well we stayed here.

GRACE. Alas, the child's health must be sacrificed like everything else, I suppose.

TYRRELL. How sacrificed?

GRACE. Oh, to add zest to your infatuation for that mountain.

TYRRELL. Nothing of the kind. If I had known he had ever been ill, I would have taken every precaution, in spite of my infatuation as you choose to call the interest I take in my work.

DOWLING. Is that your land work, Mr Tyrrell?

TYRRELL. Yes.

DOWLING. You are an extensive reclaimer of waste land?

TYRRELL. Yes; I fancy there are few in Ireland more extensive.

ROCHE. You are certainly most enterprising.

TYRRELL. Ay – it is a grand work.

DOWLING. And you believe in the possibility of its paying?

TYRRELL. Of course. Wait till you see the profits I shall make. With these I shall extend my works; and with the further profits I shall embark on such a scale of business as in time will enable me to start a company for buying up and reclaiming or reafforesting every inch of waste land in Ireland.

USSHER. That is truly a gigantic scheme, Carden. Look here, I must really be going; and your inspector, too, must be waiting for you. Let us be off. Come along.

TYRRELL. Oh, wait a moment, Barry. I want to explain. I will go with you directly. (*To the* DOCTORS) With the far-reaching usefulness of my projects I must become a real benefactor to the country, and in a time, too, when so many quack remedies in the way of legislation are being offered to the public.

ROCHE. True, true. How very interesting.

DOWLING. Upon my word, most interesting.

TYRRELL. Oh, the work is a glorious one. There is something creative about it – this changing the face of a whole country! None of the humdrum, barn-door work of ordinary farming, with its sordid accompaniment of the cattle fair! When from the ideal world of my books those people forced me to such a business, I was bound to find the extreme of its idealisation.

DOWLING (*aside to* DOCTOR ROCHE). What the dickens does he mean by that?

ROCHE. You mean you have idealised farming, Mr Tyrrell?

TYRRELL. Of course, what else? Do you think I could go on doing the dull drudgery they forced upon me? No – I considered how I could elevate it. I pondered and pondered and never rested, until at last there came to me the master-thought of the heather-field.

ROCHE (*slowly nodding assent*). Oh, – indeed. Dear me.

TYRRELL (*with evident pleasure at the surprise he is creating*). Yes; was it not a discovery? And what contentment it brought after the previous life-drudgery. I felt like returning to my youth's ideals in that free mountain air. Oh! there is magic in those mountain breezes!

DOWLING. All I know, sir, is, that the Faculty consider sea air blowing over a mountain bog to be the finest remedy in the world for bile or dyspepsia. (*He looks around him facetiously.*)

TYRRELL (*with an exression of disgust*). So that is the only thought suggested to you by the ethereal mountain breeze! There are some people who can never recognize a beautiful meaning in anything.

DOWLING. Maybe so, Mr Tyrrell. (*As if struck with an idea*). Do you find any meaning yourself, though, in this mountain air?

TYRRELL (*disdainfully*). Do I? Why, of course I do. I find in it a medium between the beauty of the past and myself.

DOWLING. Indeed.

TYRRELL. Yes; nature's ethereal phonograph, as it might be, treasuring for my delight past ecstasies of sound. I hear in its waves those voices floating back to me from –

USSHER (*with alarm, aside to* MILES). You must take your brother away at once.

DOWLING. What is that you are saying, Mr Tyrrell?

ROCHE. Voices – you don't mean to say you hear voices?

TYRRELL. I do mean to say it.

DOWLING. Whose voices do you hear?

TYRRELL. Choristers singing of youth in an eternal sunrise!

ROCHE. But you must know that this is all imagination.

TYRRELL (*irritably*). Imagination – always imagination. How wearisome that word sounds to me. I tell you there is no such thing as imagination.

DOWLING. That is a bold statement, sir.

TYRRELL. No – you either perceive or you don't perceive. Therefore it vexes me, when I perceive anything, to be told that it is only imagination.

GRACE. Wouldn't it be more accurate, then, to call it hallucination?

246

TYRRELL (*hastily to her*). That's always how you enter into the spirit of my ideas.

DOWLING. You can hardly expect her to agree with them.

TYRRELL (*resignedly*). No – I suppose there must always be distortion of my meaning.

DOWLING. Then would you mind explaining your meaning?

ROCHE. You told us you hear voices?

TYRRELL. Yes, of course.

ROCHE. Do you ever remember anything they say?

TYRRELL (*thinking*). Yes.

DOWLING. Well, would you let us know?

TYRRELL. They keep telling me I am not what I am.

ROCHE. How very strange!

DOWLING. Humph! do they say anything else, sir?

TYRRELL. They often call me back to my real life.

ROCHE. What do you mean by your real life?

TYRRELL. That life before I wandered into this dream.

DOWLING. And so you think you are only dreaming now?

TYRRELL. How can you tell that *you* also are not now in a dream?

USSHER. Answer that, if you are able, doctor.

DOWLING. A man ought to know very well whether he is asleep or awake.

TYRRELL. That is just it; and I know I am in a dream.

USSHER (*impatiently*). Really, Carden, I don't see what you gain by discussing your ideas with people who can neither understand nor sympathize with them. Come, come away. I cannot wait any longer.

TYRRELL (*rather dejected*). Yes, Barry, I suppose you are right. It was stupid of me. Let us go out. Good evening, doctors.

USSHER (*to* TYRRELL). You walk on with Miles and Kit. I just remember I have something to consult Doctor Roche about.

MILES. Come, Carden. (*Exeunt at back* CARDEN, MILES, *and* KIT TYRRELL.)

USSHER (*very gravely*). Doctor Dowling and Doctor Roche, you were sent for by Mrs Tyrrell to-day to consult on a matter altogether different from the health of the little boy.

GRACE (*defiantly*). Well, then, and if they were!

USSHER. Your husband fortunately suspects nothing; and I have warned Miles against saying anything to enlighten him.

GRACE. If you consider me in your power, you are greatly mistaken.

USSHER (*austerely*). I consider nothing of the sort, Mrs Tyrrell. You have strangely misunderstood me.

GRACE. I don't know. Anyhow, I have nothing to fear from you. The opinions of Doctor Dowling and Doctor Roche will ensure the success of the measures I have decided upon for the security of the child's interests and mine.

USSHER. You seem very sure as to the conclusions these gentlemen are to arrive at.

GRACE. Well, they know all about my poor husband's reckless expenditure, his inability to act like other people, his futile disputes with the tenantry, and to-day they have seen how he has conducted himself, and have heard him speak. I hardly think they can have any doubt as to the condition of his mind. What do you say, Doctor Dowling and Doctor Roche?

DOWLING. I am of opinion, ma'am, it is a case of dementia – but curable with proper treatment.

USSHER. Indeed. And what are your reasons for considering it dementia?

DOWLING. The general tenor, Mr Ussher, of the patient's behaviour; his reckless expenditure of his means, as Mrs Tyrrell says; his queer deranged enthusiasm; and, above all, his talk about hearing voices. There is no more common sign of insanity than for persons to believe that they hear voices.

ROCHE. Quite so. That is by far the most serious symptom in the case.

USSHER. But surely you must see that a highly-gifted man like Carden Tyrrell is not to be judged by your everyday rules. These voices you speak of he heard long ago in happier days. They are only memories made vivid by the force of imagination. Why, he told you as much. Did he not?

DOWLING. That was not the impression conveyed to me.

USSHER. Doctor Roche, you cannot agree with this, I am sure.

ROCHE. Well, really, Mr Ussher, I fear I must – that is to say, with certain reservations. Our responsibility in certifying to madness is no doubt grave; but then, on the other hand, we would incur a graver responsibility if, by our indulgence, the patient afterwards were to harm himself or anyone else.

GRACE If he is not restrained he will surely bring the child and me to irreparable ruin. You see he has almost done so already. Oh, think of that, Doctor Roche. You know he is not fit to have the control of anything.

ROCHE. I know there might be some doubt as to the question of madness, if we had nothing more to go upon than these extravagant land improvements of his.

USSHER. (*eagerly*). Yes.

ROCHE. But then I am confronted by this unpleasant symptom of his hearing voices that have no existence – a most common sign, as you say rightly, Dowling, of insanity.

USSHER. Did not Joan of Arc declare she heard voices calling on her to accomplish a work which proved to be one of the most wonderful and practical in history ? Was not Socrates firmly convinced that he was in the habit of receiving admonitions from his daemon? I might quote you several other instances of celebrated personages whose imaginations led them to believe they heard voices. Yet no one has ever thought of calling them insane. Come now, Doctor Roche, a man of your experience and culture must admit the truth of what I say.

ROCHE. Ah, Mr Ussher, I fear all forms of madness might be explained away by your arguments.

GRACE. Of course, Doctor Roche. Pray don't listen to him.

ROCHE. But, at the same time, Mrs Tyrrell, I am bound to admit that madness partakes more of an infirmity whereby the natural sequence of ideas is disconnected.

USSHER. Quite so, quite so. If you talk with a lunatic you find that you can never keep him to any consecutive line of thought. He is perpetually off here, off there, on some new and irrelevant tangent. You can never obtain a direct answer to a question. His mental process resembles a chain, at intervals unlinked. These are the real symptoms of that pitiful and uninteresting malady. Are they not?

ROCHE. Yes, Mr Ussher, on the whole you are fairly right.

USSHER. Very well then, are any such symptoms discoverable in Carden Tyrrell? Who is more clearly consecutive in his ideas than he? Discuss any question with him – politics or books – what you will – I am bound he acquits himself ably.

GRACE. And land improvement too, Mr Ussher, you forget that.

DOWLING. There you just have it, ma'am.

USSHER. His reasons for making these improvements are quite consecutive and rational. (DOCTOR DOWLING *and* GRACE *laugh*.) Oh, but I assure you they are so. His work may or may not be practical. Who knows? Personally I agree with you in thinking it is not. Still, that is no plea for trying to deprive him of his liberty and rights. If it were, I fear that many, and those too in responsible positions, might have their freedom of action endangered. It is only common-place and unimaginative people who consider the poetic and original temperament to be a mark of madness.

ROCHE. There is a great deal in what you say, Mr Ussher. I –

GRACE (*alarmed*). Doctor Roche, you cannot be serious. You are not giving in to such arguments?

ROCHE. (*apologetically*). No – no, Mrs Tyrrell. I merely admit their truth in a general way. That is all.

USSHER. You are far too clever a man, Doctor, not to see their truth. Then again, think of the gravity and danger of what you propose doing. You know, of course, gentlemen, that you will be asked to confirm on oath before a Commission of Lunacy the opinion you now so rashly form of my friend.

DOWLING. I'm quite prepared, Sir, to swear before any Commission.

USSHER. That may be, Doctor Dowling. However, Doctor Roche, the matter doubtless appears in another light to you. You may be quite certain that when Carden Tyrrell is forewarned, he will be particularly careful not to compromise himself at his private examination by the Commission, who will then, of course, ridicule the idea of preventing him from managing his estate. The defeated parties afterwards will be open to an action by their victim for damages, of which action the law costs, whether he succeeds or not, are sure to be considerable on all sides. When this conspiracy –

GRACE. Mr Ussher, you forget yourself. How dare you –?

USSHER. Yes, Mrs Tyrrell, it is an unpleasant word, but excusable in my resentment of this cruel injustice to my old and best friend. You may be sure, too, it is the word the world will use. Why did the Shrules leave here so suddenly to-day?

GRACE (*haughtily*). You have already heard the reason.

USSHER. I am bound to accept it. But I cannot help thinking that Lord Shrule invented his excuse.

GRACE. I think we have heard quite enough from you, Mr Ussher. You are not likely to intimidate us by your threats. (*To the* DOCTORS) Isn't that so?

DOWLING. Oh, I am prepared to stand by my opinion, ma'am.

GRACE. And you, Doctor Roche –?

ROCHE. (*nervously*). Well, you see, Mrs Tyrrell, I never held so decided an opinion of the case as my friend Doctor Dowling. I think – for the present – that is to say – perhaps –

GRACE. For the present? Surely, you must know that if we do not act at once we shall be too late to prevent the raising of this ruinous loan.

ROCHE. Ah, yes, yes, but I am afraid I cannot make up my mind about the patient as yet. I could not undertake to swear on oath that he is now insane.

GRACE. It is quite clear that you are intimidated, Doctor Roche.

ROCHE. (*indignantly*). I allow no one to intimidate me, Mrs Tyrrell.

GRACE. And you will leave the child and me to be ruined?

ROCHE. What can I do? Have I not told you my difficulties?

GRACE. Oh, Doctor Roche, we are in your hands. Our fate lies upon your decision. I implore of you not to fail us.

ROCHE. (*very confused*). You must excuse me, Mrs Tyrrell; but on consideration I would not venture to grant your request. I have an appointment just now. Pray excuse me. Good afternoon, Mrs Tyrrell. Good afternoon, good afternoon. (*Exit bowing to all, at back.*)

DOWLING. Well, I suppose after this I am not much use here, so I may as well also be on my way. I am sorry, ma'am, the Doctor was persuaded to change his mind; but he is a nervous, timid man. To me the case seems a pretty clear one. However, perhaps it is better to do nothing just at present. (*He bows, and exit by door at back.*)

GRACE (*to* USSHER, *with suppressed anger*). I suppose you are prepared to bear the responsibility you have incurred.

USSHER. Yes – I am prepared to bear it. But did you fully consider the responsibility you were so eager to take upon yourself, Mrs Tyrrell? I can only hope that you had not considered the question.

GRACE. I do not understand you.

USSHER. I am sorry for it. Is it then so light a matter to imprison a man, – and above all such a man as your husband? It would practically mean his death. To take him away from all that he loves, – his free life on the mountains, his intimate delight in nature, his interests and occupations, without which life would become for him meaningless – can you not understand the cruelty of this?

GRACE. I have no wish to be cruel. I must only protect myself.

USSHER. Yes – but it seems to me in attempting this protection you are very inexorable – very cruel. And the worst of it is, you appear not to realise the cruelty which you are so ready to inflict. Have you forgotten that he is your husband, that he once loved you very dearly? Have you forgotten everything except yourself?

GRACE. I have not forgotten my child –

USSHER. You are, of course, bound to think of him, but not, I am sure, to the detriment of your husband. Carden has his rights as well as Kit. Is the father to be wholly sacrificed for the child? (*Pause.*) But, Mrs Tyrrell, were you only thinking of your child?

GRACE. What do you mean?

USSHER. Was there not another reason besides the child which caused you to be so resolute? That personal dislike – Remember you and Carden have not been living very amicably for some time.

GRACE. Oh – you consider that ill-feeling has actuated me in this matter?

USSHER. I don't say so – I only suggest the probability. Are you sure that it is not so?

GRACE (*indignantly*). What a base insinuation. No – I am sure it is not so – of course it is not so. I may no longer care for my husband. Perhaps I never cared much for him. But I know that now I am only thinking of my child. It was for little Kit's sake that I wished –

USSHER. Yes – to imprison his father in a madhouse.

GRACE. I was willing to accept the responsibility. Are you still willing to accept yours? It is a heavy one. There was a chance of saving our fortune; and you have wrecked it. What will you now do to save the child and me from this madman who is devouring our substance?

USSHER. Hush – hush. For heaven's sake do not talk in this manner.

GRACE. Oh, why did you do me this cruel wrong today?

USSHER. I only prevented your doing a cruel wrong.

GRACE. You have done us all a cruel wrong.

USSHER. No – I feel I have done you all a good deed to-day.

GRACE (*scornfully*). A good deed truly – a deed giving power to carry out those projects which are our ruin!

USSHER. Who can tell but that his projects may succeed? Be patient. Be gentle with him. I believe you might win him yet by gentleness from very great extravagance. Try.

GRACE. (*gloomily*). Too late.

USSHER. Why too late?

GRACE. It was too late from the moment his thoughts first turned to the heather field.

USSHER (*starts and looks at her for a moment with vague alarm. Then says very gently*) There is no reason why he should ever learn the part you have played against him to-day. Henceforth you will be different to him, will you not?

GRACE (*gazing steadfastly before her*). Too late –

USSHER. Ah – well – (*Exit quietly at back.*) (*Pause. There is a noise as of some one approaching.* GRACE *looks out at back, then recedes to door at right.* CARDEN TYRRELL *enters hurriedly, carrying a sheet of the ordnance map, which he lays upon the writing-table at left and studies, unaware of his wife's presence. She watches him with an expression of gathering anger, then exit sobbing by door at right. He starts and turns to see her just disappear, then sighing he shrugs his shoulders, and resumes his eager study of the map.*)

END OF ACT II

ACT III

The same as last, only that the place, by the absence of all drawing-room ornaments, has assumed once more its aspect of a library. A fire of fresh ashwood in the large fireplace burns cheerfully, while sunlight streams in through the window-doors at back. A sheet of the ordnance map lies on writing table. Several months have passed; and it is now Spring.

KIT TYRRELL *runs in by door at right carrying a child's kite, which he examines as he kneels down in front of the fire. Measuring out the string at arm's length, he appears dissatisfied. Then, as if suddenly remembering, he runs over to the book-case at back, and climbing up on its ledge he takes from behind the books on an upper row a mass of cord. He returns, and disentangling it ties its end to the cord attached to the kite, which he then carries to the window-doors at back. These he opens, and stands in a flood of sunlight. Outside is heard the singing of birds.*

CARDEN TYRRELL, *somewhat aged and careworn, enters by door at right.*

TYRRELL (*half to himself as he watches* KIT). Oh, memories –

KIT (*after a short pause, perceiving* TYRRELL *and running to him*). Father.

TYRRELL. The little birds are singing in the sunlight to my little bird. Where are you going, Kit?

KIT. I am going to fly the kite. Oh, come out, father, with me to the heather field. There is sure to be a splendid breeze there to-day.

TYRRELL (*sadly*). Ah, the heather field. No, Kit, I cannot.

KIT. You have not been there for such a long time. Why can't you come?

TYRRELL. I can't; it is unbearable to be always followed and watched – and in that place above all others.

KIT. But, father, why don't you tell those policemen to go away?

TYRRELL. I have done so over and over again. They will not go.

KIT. But why must they watch you, father, dear?

KIT (*looks at* KIT *for a moment, then in an unsteady voice as he turns away*). Do not ask me, boy. You would not understand.

253

THE HEATHER FIELD – ACT III

KIT (*catching* TYRRELL *by the arm*). Really? Yet Barry says that I understand so many things better than if I were a man.

TYRRELL (*thoughtfully*). He is right. Only those who become as you are, can know the rarest joys of life.

KIT. Then why do you think, father, I would not understand the reason they are watching you.

TYRRELL. Because – because it would appear – well, something incredible to you. There, do not ask, boy. (*He flings himself moodily into the chair on the outside of the writing table. A short pause.*)

KIT (*coming near*). Father, dear, you are not angry with me?

TYRRELL. No, Kit. Only a bit worried by things in general.

KIT. I am sorry if I have ever worried you. I will try not to do it again. I love you. Oh, you don't know how I love you, father.

TYRRELL (*throwing his arms around* KIT). My darling, you have never worried me. I could not live without you.

KIT. (*hiding his face on* TYRRELL'S *neck*). Oh, father, father!

TYRRELL. Yes, Kit, you are the little elf that calls up for me the magic of the heather field. Henceforth we must never be divided – you and I.

KIT. Never, oh never, father dear. You don't know how lonely I feel away from you. I have not been to the heather field for ever so long. It seemed such a sad place when you were not there.

TYRRELL. Even in spite of its wild flowers, Kit? It is time for them now to be coming out again.

KIT. Yes, the heather field will be beginning to look lovely now.

TYRRELL. How I wish I were free to walk among its flowers on this soft spring day.

KIT. Poor father! – but would you like me to fetch you some of them. Shall I go?

TYRRELL. Yes, do, Kit. I should like some flowers from the heather field. (BARRY USSHER *enters at back.*)

KIT. Oh, there's Barry.

TYRRELL. What – Barry! It is an event when I see anyone now.

USSHER. As if it were not your own doing.

TYRRELL (*somewhat ruffled*). You may say what you like for all I care.

USSHER (*shrugging his shoulders*). Heigh-ho! Well, Kit, are you glad the winter is over?

KIT. Oh, yes, how horrid and dark it was.

USSHER. I wonder how you ever managed to exist through it. And you never got the pony, after all?

KIT. No – you see when father promised me one he thought he could afford it. But now he cannot, until he lets the heather field. I must wait a while longer. Is not that so, father?

TYRRELL. Yes, Kit, we must wait.

KIT. You know, Barry, I could not think of worrying him any more about the pony.

USSHER. You good little son, there is no need to wait any longer. I have just brought you such a nice pony.

TYRRELL. What is this, Barry? what is this!

KIT. Oh, where is he, Barry?

USSHER. Out in the yard waiting for you – bridle, saddle and all.

KIT. Oh, thank you, Barry. Father, is he not nice and kind?

TYRRELL. (*looking at* USSHER). Yes, always the kind friend – always the same.

KIT. Father, I shall ride the pony off to the heather-field at once, and get you those flowers. (*Exit at back.*)

USSHER. How happy the little fellow is.

TYRRELL. You have indeed made him so by your kindness, Barry.

USSHER. Bah – a selfish kindness at most. I tell you, I have not felt for a long time such real happiness as just now when I saw myself looked at like some good spirit by that little face.

TYRRELL. And to think that you who are so lucky, to whom most things come so easily, should say this! Why, even I, with all my troubles, could hardly speak more despondingly. What would you do if you were imprisoned as I am here since those evictions?

USSHER. Your health will be ruined by your obstinacy.

TYRRELL. What can I do ? The police have orders never to lose sight of me if I go out. They say I should be shot at otherwise.

USSHER. Ha!

TYRRELL. And you know I never could bear to be followed by a guard. It makes me feel like a criminal. I would much rather stay indoors.

USSHER (*after thinking for a moment*). Look here, Carden, you ought to leave this place for a while. We will go together. We will travel.

TYRRELL. Impossible, the drainage of the valley could never go on in my absence.

USSHER. Why not? You haven't been near it for ever so long.

TYRRELL. Oh, that doesn't matter in the least. I can direct it just as well from this room. There on the writing table is my map with all the drains marked upon it. The superintendent comes to me at stated intervals, reports the progress of each man's work, and takes the fresh orders which I give him from the map. I assure you it gives me greater pleasure to conduct operations in this way scientifically, than if I were to go on the ground. One can imagine oneself in such a situation, like Moltke fighting battles from his study.

255

USSHER (*gives a quick look at* TYRRELL. *Then after a short pause* –)
Well, if you won't leave here, at all events try and settle with those
peasants, so that you may dispense with police and be able to go
about again.

TYRRELL. Settle? How could I settle with them? The only settlement
they would hear of I could never grant. Oh no – a nice ending,
indeed, that would be to our battle!

USSHER. Is there no compromise you will come to?

TYRRELL. I will reinstate the evicted, if they pay in full their rents and
the costs I have incurred on their account.

USSHER. Oh, that is no compromise at all.

TYRRELL. Well, it is as much as I can agree to. I told these people when
they struck, that I could not afford to give abatements on rents which
had already been reduced so much by the Land Commission, and I
can less afford to give any now with pressing mortgagees who have
not been paid for so long.

USSHER. But would it not be better to get some rent for that land instead
of leaving it idle? Others, you know, will not dare to take it from
you.

TYRRELL. I cannot help that. I must work it myself.

USSHER. Meanwhile how are you going to pay the mortgagees their
interest?

TYRRELL. Oh, there is the great difficulty. The chief mortgagee is most
pressing, and threatens to foreclose immediately. I have implored
of him again and again to wait until I can let the heather field, but
in vain. Miles, whom I expect home this evening, was to have made
a final appeal to him in Dublin last night. I can only hope for a
favourable result.

USSHER. I think you had better come to terms with those tenants,
Carden.

TYRRELL. I shall never give in to them. I shall never voluntarily reduce
the value of my property. Besides, if the worst should come, I have
always the great resource.

USSHER. What is that?

TYRRELL. The heather field!

USSHER. Carden, take care. It is a dangerous thing – trusting to only one
resource.

TYRRELL (*a little irritated*). What do you mean? Are you too going to
join the enemy?

USSHER (*uneasily*) No, no, Carden, you do not understand me; but –

TYRRELL. But what?

USSHER. Oh, I should so like to see you on good terms with your people again. I am sure the remembrance of all that friendship with them in the past must make this quarrel unbearable to you.

TYRRELL. Yes, indeed that is true.

USSHER. And this continual watch upon your movements too must be dreadful.

TYRRELL. Dreadful, it is gradually wearing me out. I know I cannot stand it much longer. And most of the long dreary winter I had no one about me whom I could confide in or consult; for Miles has been away at College as you know.

USSHER. Yes, carrying everything before him. I see he has won a scholarship. He is sure of his gold medal now.

TYRRELL. Miles is of the stuff to succeed. I am so fond of Miles. He was always such good company.

USSHER. Of course, a most charming boy. I am glad he is to be at home to-day.

TYRRELL. Indeed his companionship will make a great difference to me, now that I can never get about.

USSHER (*anxiously*). Oh, but Carden, you cannot continue in this way. You have always been used to so free a life in the open air. I say this imprisonment will kill you. Already I see a very marked change in your appearance.

TYRRELL (*doggedly*). I cannot help it. My past demands that I must suffer. (*With a sigh, he passes to right of doors at back, where he looks out in a reverie.*)

USSHER (*watching him*). For heaven's sake, Carden, do not be so fatally unreasonable.

TYRRELL (*after a pause, still looking in the same direction*). No – I am not so; you think those remedies you suggest would avail to relieve me – but they would not.

USSHER. Why not?

TYRRELL. You ask – you who are such a philosopher? Can you not understand that the only remedy for me must be something that has no relation whatever with those circumstances that may affect me ill or otherwise?

USSHER. You mean that improvement of circumstances has little to do with bringing contentment.

TYRRELL. I mean that the only remedy must be something which would make me forgetful that I am myself. (*Mysteriously*) Barry, would you believe it, often in moments of darkest anxiety I am arrested by the sight of some flower or leaf or some tiny nook in the garden out there. And oh – I become then at once so peaceful that I care not what may happen to me – I think it is only when we turn to them in our misery that we can really see the exquisite beauty of these things.

USSHER. Ah, Carden, nature is a marvellous sedative. How infinite her ingeniousness amidst all our pains and fears.

TYRRELL. Yes – and just this moment when I looked upon the ocean there and the land awakening with such freshness from its winter sleep, I felt something that no improvement of circumstances could bring. (*Then with a strange enthusiasm*) Oh, to feel that despite all suffering one has the firmament, the earth, the sea! What more can one really require from the world?

USSHER. Ay – true enough 'For all things were made from these,' to quote the great mediaeval philosopher. Nevertheless I think I might bring you another and very real sort of relief from this present trouble, if you would but allow me.

TYRRELL. And what if you might? It would only be succeeded by some further trouble. That is the only sort of relief you could ever bring. Ah, there is a trouble past all your remedies.

USSHER. Alas, I fear there are many. How could I pretend otherwise? But will you tell me this particular one?

TYRRELL. I wonder will you understand.

USSHER. Why not, Carden?

TYRRELL. Well then, have you ever seen on earth something beautiful beyond earth – that great beauty which appears in divers ways? And then have you known what it is to go back to the world again?

USSHER (*sadly*). I know, I know – the pain of loss.

TYRRELL. Is it not misery? But you have seen the great beauty have you not? Oh, that immortal beauty – so far away – always so far away.

USSHER. Yes – yes, our ideal of beauty that for ever haunts and eludes us through life. (*With a movement of resignation*) But let us not speak of it any more.

TYRRELL. Why, Barry?

USSHER. Because, as you say, it makes one so miserable in the world, and it is such a hopeless phantom after all.

TYRRELL. How can you say so? You who know that it is alone the reality in the world.

USSHER (*cautiously*). Hush, Carden, I do not know.

TYRRELL. (*laughing bitterly*). There – just like you, Barry, careful never to let yourself go.

USSHER. No – no, Carden, but you brood too much on these thoughts. You are overworked – you ought really to come away from here. Do let us travel somewhere together for a change.

TYRRELL. Ah, not now – at some future time, perhaps – but not now.

258

My difficulties are gathering before me. I must stand and hew them from my path. (GRACE TYRRELL *enters hurriedly and excitedly by door at right.*)

GRACE (*pauses when she sees* USSHER, *then to* TYRRELL). Oh, but I suppose as you have no secrets from him –

TYRRELL (*starting*). Well, what is the matter?

GRACE (*holding out a paper*). A dreadful-looking man has just handed me this.

TYRRELL. Let me see (*takes paper*). Ah –

GRACE. I have so often asked you for money to pay this person.

TYRRELL. I am very sorry. I had nothing to give you.

GRACE. Alas, you always had plenty to squander on that mountain.

TYRRELL. That was Government money, and it could not honestly be expended except on the object for which it was advanced.

GRACE. I am afraid I must have some of it now. I cannot be left in this condition.

TYRRELL. Indeed you shall not have one penny of it.

GRACE. What – you mean to leave me under the stigma of such an insult?

TYRRELL (*impatiently*). There is no particular urgency. I will see if I can possibly meet this writ by some money of my own. (*With a painful distracted look*) Oh this worry – this worry. (*Exit by door at right.*)

GRACE. Well, Mr Ussher, I hope you are satisfied now. We are ruined; and my husband is becoming stranger in his behaviour every day. But for you, he might have been cured by this, and the estate in a very different condition.

USSHER. I have nothing, Mrs Tyrrell, to reproach myself with. I did all for the best.

GRACE. Yes, of course. That is the only satisfaction one ever receives for injuries done through gratuitous interference.

USSHER. Nothing has since happened to convict me of having acted wrongly. I have done you no injury.

GRACE. No injury? Well!

USSHER. You cannot lay to my account this quarrel with the tenants which is the cause of your present difficulties. Goodness knows I have done my best to mend it.

GRACE. (*impatiently*). Oh, that is only a temporary difficulty. But the estate will be ruined for ever by the great debt from which we should have saved it, if you had not interfered. (*Pause.*) Yes – I see now how it all will be. The child and I will be driven out, ruined, to battle with the world.

USSHER. Oh, don't think of such a thing, Mrs Tyrrell. It can never come to that.

GRACE (*sadly*). Ah, yes. You destroyed my last chance of saving our home. I might have kept it lovingly for Kit until he grew to be a man; but now I see it must go from us. I shall have to bid everything farewell – the familiar rooms – the garden where I found an occupation for my life – even those common useless things about the house I have been accustomed to look at for years. Oh, you don't know what it is – this parting from those everyday things of one's life.

USSHER. Yes, yes – indeed I do – and from my heart I feel for you.

GRACE. And yet you could have acted as you have.

USSHER. I acted only in good faith. Heaven knows that is the truth.

GRACE. The injury remains still the same.

USSHER (*with strong emotion*). If it is I who have injured you, Mrs Tyrrell, you must allow me to make amends.

GRACE. Alas, what amends are possible?

USSHER. Who can tell? I promise you, at least, you shall never, *never* bid farewell to your home.

GRACE. (*in a trembling voice*). If only what you say might come true. (LADY SHRULE, LORD SHRULE, *and* CARDEN TYRRELL *enter by door at right*.)

LORD SHRULE. Carden, I believe your servant was actually going to say 'not at home' to us, if I had not caught sight of you in the hall. Ha, ha.

LORD SHRULE. What a shame, Mr Tyrrell, to try and prevent me from seeing Grace. How do you do, Grace dear? (*Giving her hand apathetically to* USSHER) How do you do?

LADY SHRULE. (*shakes hands with* GRACE *and* USSHER). We should have been so disappointed.

TYRRELL. I assure you, Lord Shrule, my attempt to escape is purely an imagination on your part.

LORD SHRULE. Oh, you sly fellow, you think I do not know. You are just like your father when people used to call – although he would never run away from me, I can tell you.

TYRRELL. No more did I. I was only surprised to see you; that was all. When I heard the bell I thought it was Miles come from Dublin. I am anxiously expecting him now at any moment.

LORD SHRULE. Ah, it will be a pleasure to see Miles again. We have all heard of his University triumphs. How proud your poor father would have been.

TYRRELL. Yes, and how delighted to share his satisfaction with you.

LORD SHRULE. Poor Marmaduke, we were such friends – at our very last interview he asked me to keep you and your brother always in mind after he was gone. So I have always felt somehow like a father towards you both, you know, and with a father's privilege occasionally have given advice.

GRACE. Yes, Lord Shrule, and how I wish your good advice occasionally had been followed.

LORD SHRULE. Ah, we cannot help that, Mrs Tyrrell. Nothing will ever teach the young save bitter experience.

GRACE. I am sure there has been enough bitter experience; but it seems to have taught nothing at all.

LORD SHRULE. Well, well, I hope it won't be so. Eh, Carden?

TYRRELL. I do not see how my experience can teach me to act differently from my present way of acting. (*Aside to* USSHER) Miles ought to have arrived by this. Oh, I am nearly dead with anxiety to know the news he will bring.

USSHER (*aside to* TYRRELL). I hope there will be good news.

LORD SHRULE. Never mind, Mrs Tyrrell. Carden will come by degrees to see his mistakes.

GRACE. I fear we are now in so bad a way that it does not much matter whether he sees them or not.

LADY SHRULE. No – really, Grace, you do not say so?

GRACE. Oh, Lilian, we are ruined.

LORD SHRULE. Come, come, I am sure it cannot be as bad as that.

TYRRELL. Goodness me, of course not, Lord Shrule. On the contrary, in the near future we shall make a fortune.

GRACE. I say we are ruined, utterly, irretrievably.

TYRRELL. No – no –

USSHER. What noise is that? (*Listens, then opens door at right.*) Why, Miles has arrived.

TYRRELL. Miles – oh!

USSHER. There, Carden, for goodness sake be calm. (*Enter* MILES TYRRELL *by door at right.*)

MILES. Carden. (*He grasps his brother by the hand, then greets all the rest.*)

TYRRELL. What news, Miles? Will he wait?

MILES. (*turning away dejectedly*). I did my best, Carden. There is no hope, I fear.

GRACE. No hope? What is this new misfortune? Who won't wait?

MILES. The chief mortgagee.

GRACE. Is he going to foreclose?

MILES. He says so.

LORD SHRULE. Ha – this is a most serious matter.

TYRRELL. But Miles, didn't you explain to him all about the heather field?

MILES. Yes.

TYRRELL. Didn't you assure him that it would soon bring in what would more than pay his interest?

MILES. Indeed I did, Carden.

TYRRELL. Well?

MILES. Well, that only seemed to make him impatient with me. But I used every argument I could think of, and pleaded with him for nearly an hour in his office, until at last he had to get rid of me almost brutally.

TYRRELL (*with a look of humiliation and despair*). Oh ruin! ruin!

USSHER. No, no, Carden – it is not yet that. We must see how we can help you through this difficulty.

TYRRELL (*quietly*). With all your goodwill, Barry, what can you do now?

USSHER. Who knows? Just keep quiet, and do not distress yourself. Leave it all to me.

TYRRELL (*almost staggering*). Yes – such a severe blow – this. It has quite upset me. I am sure you will all excuse me. You, Barry, will see what you can do, won't you? Yes – (*He goes to door at right.*)

USSHER. Yes, Carden, I hope all will come well.

LORD SHRULE. How much of the property does this mortgage cover?

GRACE. Oh, pretty nearly all, I should think.

TYRRELL (*suddenly turning*). All, do you say? No – not all. This vulture cannot touch the heather field! My hope – it is my only hope now, and it will save me in the end. Ha, ha! these wise ones! They did not think the barren mountain of those days worth naming in their deed. But now that mountain is a great green field worth more than all they can seize, (*with a strange intensity*) and it is mine – all mine! (*Exit by door at right.*)

LORD SHRULE (*throwing up his hands*). Oh dear, oh dear, what infatuation!

GRACE. Yes indeed, it has caused us all to be cast adrift in the world. Oh, what is to become of me – what is – to become of me? (*She sobs in her handkerchief.*)

LADY SHRULE. Grace, you must not lose heart.

GRACE. Ah, the final misfortune has come.

LADY SHRULE. We shall try and help you, dear – there.

USSHER. Yes, we must lose no time now to see what can be done for Carden.

LADY SHRULE. You should indeed bestir yourself, Mr Ussher, and save him; for we have you to thank that he was left in a position to ruin himself.

USSHER. And have not you too, Lady Shrule, to thank yourself for the same thing?

LADY SHRULE. I ? How so, pray?

USSHER. Why did you and Lord Shrule disappear so suddenly on that day the doctors were here ? Your advocacy would doubtless have made them heedless of my objections –

LADY SHRULE. Ha – why indeed? You know, Shrule, I wanted you to –

LORD SHRULE. Well, well, I could not bear to act in such a way to the son of my old friend. But I suppose in my weakness I did wrong.

USSHER. No, Lord Shrule, you did right. You never could be suspected by anyone of doing otherwise.

LORD SHRULE. I hope not, Ussher! Still, I am inclined to think it might have been wiser then to have taken some definite step.

LADY SHRULE. I should think so. Just see what has happened since.

GRACE. Nothing less than the ruin of a helpless woman and her child.

LADY SHRULE. You have, indeed, incurred a nice responsibility, Mr Ussher.

GRACE. (*to* USSHER). What – what right had you to do my child and me this wrong?

USSHER. I only prevented what I thought a grievous wrong from being done to my friend.

GRACE. It was no wrong – it was for his good – for all our good. In your heart you must know I was right.

USSHER. I have often said, Mrs Tyrrell, I know nothing of the sort.

LADY SHRULE. Still, you must admit that his actions since more than justify Mrs Tyrrell in the course she adopted.

LORD SHRULE. Alas, I fear that is the case.

USSHER. I admit he is very wilful and extravagant, but no more. I cannot discover any mental infirmity. His mind has a perfect grasp of ideas.

GRACE. Don't talk of ideas. I have heard enough about them since I was married to give me a horror of them for the rest of my life.

LADY SHRULE. They have certainly caused the wreck of this household.

LORD SHRULE. Oh, I hope not. We must not be too pessimistic. – Who can tell? – perhaps the heather field may turn out a success after all!

GRACE (*with contempt*). The heather field.

LORD SHRULE. If it were to, there can be no doubt but that all would be saved. I wonder how it is going on. Have you been there lately, Mrs Tyrrell?

GRACE. Of course not, Lord Shrule. The very thought of the place fills me with despair.

MILES. That is a pity, Grace – a great pity, when so much depends upon the success of the heather field.

GRACE. No good can ever come of that abominable work.

MILES. You must not speak such words; no luck can come from such words.

GRACE. I cannot help it.

MILES. Oh, I know you have much to endure, but I cannot remain here and listen to such denunciation of what my brother holds nearest to his heart.

GRACE. I have only said the truth.

MILES. You cannot be certain of this truth. It is not right to speak such words. (*Exit by door at right.*)

LADY SHRULE. My poor Grace.

GRACE. Oh, Lilian.

LADY SHRULE. These troubles are driving you to distraction. You had better leave this place for a while. Will you not come and stay with us?

LORD SHRULE. Oh yes, won't you stay with us, Mrs Tyrrell? You might be saved much annoyance and worry.

GRACE. You are both so kind – I should like to for a little while, certainly. This house has become unbearable of late with debts and difficulties on every side.

LADY SHRULE. Oh dear, how terrible. You had better leave at once, Grace. Perhaps you might have some of your things seized. Anyhow, bring with you those that you most value. We will take care of them.

GRACE. Thanks, Lilian.

LORD SHRULE. Well then, that is agreed, Mrs Tyrrell. I am so glad we may be of use to you.

LADY SHRULE. We shall expect you this evening, dear.

GRACE. Yes, I shall get ready at once.

LADY SHRULE. And it is time for us to return home. Good-bye, Mr Ussher.

USSHER. Good-bye, Lady Shrule.

LORD SHRULE. Good-bye. (*Exeunt* LADY SHRULE, GRACE TYRRELL, *and* LORD SHRULE *by door at right.*)

USSHER (*gloomily*). Heaven help her – help them all. What is to be done? – Stay – I might go security, I would do anything to help them. – But would it really be of use? Other difficulties must follow these, so that my whole fortune would not suffice. I will think the matter over. – I wonder how the heather field is going on. No one

264

seems to have been there lately. (KIT TYRRELL, *carrying a small white bundle enters through door at back.*)

KIT (*placing the bundle on sofa*). Barry, the pony is splendid. I had such galloping over the heather field.

USSHER. Well, did you bring back any flowers?

KIT. They have not yet come out. All I could find there were these little buds in my handkerchief. (*Unties the bundle*) Look.

USSHER (*with a start*). What – buds of heather? Has your father seen these, Kit?

KIT. Yes, I told him I found them growing all over the heather field.

USSHER. You did, boy – and what did he say?

KIT. Nothing for a while. But he looked – he looked – well, I have never seen him look like that before.

USSHER. Ha – and then –?

KIT. Oh, then he seemed to forget all about it. He became so kind, and oh, Barry, what do you think, he called me, his 'little brother Miles'. So I am really his brother, he says, after all – (MILES TYRRELL, *in haste and violent trepidation, enters through door at back.*)

MILES. Barry, for pity's sake – (*sees* KIT *and suddenly checks himself, then brings* USSHER *over to fireplace*). Barry, something dreadful has come over Carden. He does not know me.

USSHER (*in a trembling voice, as he gazes fixedly before him*). The vengeance of the heather field.

MILES. Oh! for pity's sake, come to him. Come to him –

USSHER. Where is he?

MILES. Wandering helpless about the garden. Oh, heavens, what shall we do?

USSHER (*with suppressed terror*). Let us find him. (*He turns to go.*) (CARDEN TYRRELL *appears outside doorway at back. He has a strange, collected look.*)

USSHER (*starting*). Carden!

TYRRELL (*coming in*). Well, – Barry? – Why, what has happened to you since yesterday? My goodness, you look at least ten years older. (*Glancing at* MILES) Who is that? He was annoying me about something just now in the fuchsia walk.

MILES. Oh, I cannot stand this torture. Carden, dear Carden, look at me –

TYRRELL (*retreats like a frightened animal towards* USSHER, *keeping always his eyes fixed on* MILES). Barry, what is the matter with him? Don't leave me alone with him, Barry. Get him to go away.

USSHER. You need not fear him, Carden. (*He signs to* MILES, *who retires with an inconsolable expression and stands by fireplace.*)

TYRRELL. (*after a moment, mysteriously*). Barry –

USSHER. Yes, Carden.

TYRRELL (*looking cautiously around*). You remember our conversation yesterday.

USSHER. (*puzzled*). Yesterday? I did not see you yesterday.

TYRRELL (*with impatience*). We did not walk together on the cliff yesterday, when you advised me not to marry Grace Desmond? What do you mean?

USSHER. (*suddenly recollecting*). Oh, I remember, I remember. (*Then in a trembling voice*) But Carden – Carden, that was ten years ago. Don't you know that you are now married to her?

TYRRELL (*with a surprised baffled look*). I am? –

USSHER (*very gently*). Yes, indeed.

TYRRELL. Oh ! (*His expression for a moment grows vaguely painful, then gradually passes into one of vacant calm. After a short pause*) Barry, you are quite right.

USSHER (*joyfully*). I knew you would understand me, Carden.

TYRRELL. Yes, I will take your advice. I will not ask her to be my wife.

USSHER (*with cruel disappointment*). Hopeless – I see it is hopeless now.

TYRRELL (*unheeding*). I do not care for her any more. I know now I never cared for her.

USSHER. Do you? Why?

TYRRELL (*distressfully*). Oh, I have had such a dreadful dream.

USSHER. A dream?

TYRRELL. I must tell it to you. – Let me see, what was it? No – I cannot remember – no, – it has gone completely from me before the beauty of the morning. (*Looks out at back and stretches his arms*) Oh, is not this Spring morning divine?

USSHER. But – Carden, can you not see that it is evening?

TYRRELL. Ah, I must have been a long time asleep – a long, long time. Yet it looks like the morning. Yes, it seems as if it would always be morning now for me.

USSHER (*with interest*). Indeed – is that so?

TYRRELL. Yes – its genius somehow is always about me.

USSHER. And what do gou call this genius of the morning?

TYRRELL (*with a strange ecstacy*). Joy! Joy!

USSHER (*after looking at him for a while in wonder*). Then, you are happy, Carden?

TYRRELL. Oh, yes – so happy. Why not?

USSHER (*with hesitation*). You have no troubles, have you?

TYRRELL. Troubles –? No, except sometimes in dreams – but oh, when

I awake to the joy of this great beauty –

USSHER. Yet – great beauty – is it not for ever far away?

TYRRELL. No – it is for ever by me. (*Then as if suddenly recollecting*)
Ah, now I can tell you my dreadful dream. (*Slowly*) I dreamed that
my lot was to wander through common luxurious life – seeing now
and then in glimpses, that beauty – but so far away! And when the
vision left me – ah, you do not know the anguish I felt in looking
again at my lot in life.

USSHER. And this was only a dream?

TYRRELL (*fervently*). Thank heaven – only a dream! (*He goes to the
sofa, where* KIT *all this time has been playing with the heather
buds.*)

USSHER (*meditatively sorrowful*). And are beauty and happiness mere
illusions after all? (*Goes towards* MILES) I am dazed in the presence
of this awful misfortune.

MILES. (*approaching* USSHER). Oh, the misery of seeing him like this.
He thinks he is living in the old days.

USSHER. It has come upon him again – that eerie ethereal youth I
remember so well.

MILES. And for which he would yearn with such fond regret. But Grace
and the child – Oh, what is to become of them? I fear their ruin is
now certain and complete.

USSHER (*as if suddenly awakened*). Not so. – It may be possible to save
them now that there is no danger of further expenditure. And I *will*
save them. I will be security for the payment of all their debts. I will
save the estate, if it costs me every penny I have in the world.

MILES. (*grasping* USSHER *by the hand*). Oh, Barry, this is good of you.
(*They go towards the fireplace in earnest discourse.*)

TYRRELL (*placing a heather wreath on* KIT'S *head*). There – you are
like a young field-faun now.

KIT. What sort of thing is that?

TYRRELL. Why, one of the field-fairies fresh and clean as those soft
heather-shoots around your hair.

KIT (*delighted*). What – the fairies that live in green hillocks, and dance
by the river bank, in the valley over there? Oh, tell me of them
again.

TYRRELL. Yes, beautiful child-fairies that play with the water nymphs
– those sirens, you know, who sing in the wistful depths of the
stream. (*With a sudden transport*) Oh, we must go to Lorlei as last
year, where the river is lit with their gold. (*Pointing out at back*) See,
even now the sky is darkening as in that storm scene of the old
legend I told you on the Rhine. See, the rain across a saffron sun

267

trembles like gold harp strings, through the purple Irish Spring! (MRS GRACE TYRRELL *enters by door at right, dressed for going out, with her face thinly veiled and looking altogether younger and more handsome.*)

GRACE (*to* TYRRELL). I am just starting to visit the Shrules for some days.

TYRRELL. (*turns surprised*). Miss Desmond – Oh (*with emotion and signs of struggle*) Oh, where is that beauty now – that music of the morning? (*Suddenly arrested*) Such strange solemn harmonies. (*Listens.*) The voices – yes, they are filling the house – those white-stoled children of the morning. (*His eyes after a moment wander slowly to the doorway at back*) Oh, the rainbow! (*To* KIT) Come quick, See the lovely rainbow! (*They go to watch it hand in hand.*) Oh, mystic highway of man's speechless longings! My heart goes forth upon the rainbow to that horizon of joy ! (*With a fearful exaltation*) The voices – I hear them now triumphant in a silver glory of song!

GRACE. (*looking bewildered from* MILES *to* USSHER). What – what is all this?

USSHER. Ah, your fears have come true, Mrs Tyrrell. You have not heard –

GRACE. No. – What has happened? For heavens' sake, speak.

USSHER. The wild heath has broken out again in the heather field.

THE END

MAEVE

A PSYCHOLOGICAL DRAMA IN TWO ACTS

BY

EDWARD MARTYN

DRAMATIS PERSONÆ

THE O'HEYNES, Colman O'Heynes, Prince of Burren
MAEVE O'HEYNES, ⎫
FINOLA O'HEYENES, ⎭ his daughters.
HUGH FITZ WALTER, a young Englishman
PEG INERNY, a vagrant

In the dream of Maeve appear Queen Maeve, A BOY PAGE, CHORUS OF BOY PAGES, *ancient Irish harpers, chieftains, warriors, people, etc.*

The action takes place during the present time about and at O'Heynes Castle among the Burren Mountains of County Clare in Ireland.

ACT I

A ruined abbey in a green valley among mountains covered with layers of grey rock. At back a little removed is a cairn overgrown with grass. Gray limestones belonging to the ruin are strewn about the ground. At the left in the surrounding pasture of pale green, great leafless ash trees stand among boulders spotted with white and orange lichen. It is a sunny evening in the month of March.

(MAEVE O'HEYNES – *a girl of about three and twenty with a fair complexion, gold hair, and a certain boyish beauty in the lines and movement of her slim figure, rests thoughtful and attentive on one of the fallen stones. She wears a red frieze dress with a black jacket and folding linen collar, and has on her head a sailor's cap of black wool.*)

(FINOLA O'HEYNES – *a dark rather submissive-looking girl somewhat younger, dressed simply in an ordinary gown, sits near on another stone.*)

FINOLA (*reading from an old book*).
    'Every hill which is at this Oenach
    Hath under it heroes and queens,
    And poets and distributors,
    and fair fierce women'.

MAEVE (*rises and gazes before her as if in a dream*). And fair fierce women!

FINOLA (*closing the book, goes to her*). Maeve – what are you thinking of so earnestly?

MAEVE (*recalled to herself*). Visions – visions. – That is all.

FINOLA. Has this old West Connacht poem brought you visions?

MAEVE. Ah, the bard Dorban, who wrote it, was a poet! (*She sighs and covers her face with her hands.*)

FINOLA (*turning away*). I am sorry I thought of reading it to you.

MAEVE. Why, sister?

FINOLA. Because it seems to have called you back to your old self.

MAEVE (*smiling sadly*). My old self. As if I could ever have left my old self.

FINOLA. Oh yes, you were peaceful and contented a little while ago.

MAEVE. It seems so long ago, Finola.

271

FINOLA. Something strange has come over you now.

MAEVE (*with restlessness*). No, it is nothing. It is only the look of the evening.

FINOLA. But this is such a peaceful evening with that saffron sunlight over the ruins. Why should it make you anything else but peaceful?

MAEVE. Oh, Finola, when I see the ruins like that, I know the visions are near me.

FINOLA. Then, after all, it was not because I read that poem?

MAEVE. Yes – that, and the evening.

FINOLA (*looking at her anxiously*). Why should the visions make you so sad, Maeve?

MAEVE (*wistfully*). Such beautiful dead people! They used to walk in the oldest of these ruins before it was a ruin; they watched Goban, the great architect, building that round tower (*pointing to the right*), building his master-work. I see them now, and I see others who lived long before them (*turns and looks to the back*), and are buried in that green cairn. Oh, I am dying because I am exiled from such beauty.

FINOLA (*with great gentleness*). Darling, you must not think of these things. You know to-morrow –

MAEVE (*with a sudden chillness*). To-morrow, – why do you speak of to-morrow while it is still to-day, and I can still think of my love?

FINOLA. *To*-morrow when you are married, Maeve, it will be your husband who will be entitled to that love.

MAEVE (*significantly*). He has not yet returned.

FINOLA. Hugh will certainly return before night.

MAEVE. But he has not yet returned, Finola.

FINOLA. Do you really think he will not return?

MAEVE (*with a baffled look*). Oh, I don't know: but somehow I cannot believe that I am to be married to-morrow. (*Looks around.*) To leave all this for an English home –

FINOLA (*with increased anxiety*). Maeve –

MAEVE. The very stones, as I wander among them, seem to forbid it. (*Exit among the ruins at back.*)

FINOLA (*walking about in agitation*). Oh, why does not Hugh return? (*Then suddenly stopping.*) Here is father again. Poor father.

(THE O'HEYNES *enters from the left, leaning heavily on a stick. He is an old man, with thin, white dishevelled hair almost falling to his shoulders, wears a tall hat and clothes of a somewhat bygone fashion; while about his whole appearance there is just a suggestion of the peasant.*)

O'HEYNES (*restlessly*). Finola, I wonder will Hugh come after all?

FINOLA. Of course he will, father, Why have you been asking me this question all day?

O'HEYNES. Because he has been promising to come for ever so long, and he has not come.

FINOLA. Well – you know the reason.

O'HEYNES (*peevishly*). Yes – yes – legal business – always the same excuse.

FINOLA. You surely must understand that he had to consult the lawyers about many matters before his marriage with Maeve.

O'HEYNES. When he left here for England he said it would only be for a little time, and here he has been away more than two months.

FINOLA. The delay was very unfortunate, but necessary, I suppose. You see every sort of legal business is so tedious.

O'HEYNES. I don't know – I don't know. I distrust his excuses. He said he would certainly return to-day, and there, he hasn't after all.

FINOLA. But to-day is not yet over. Oh, you needn't fear. He will return before to-morrow.

O'HEYNES. Ah, this is the way you are perpetually making excuses for him, Finola.

FINOLA (*a little confused*). Father, why do you say so?

O'HEYNES. I understand it all. Another girl would not be so forgiving as you are, Finola.

FINOLA. I have nothing to forgive.

O'HEYNES. That is well, child. But, believe me, I had far rather he had married you than Maeve.

FINOLA. Oh, no. He always liked Maeve from the first, and no one else. I never at any time doubted that, father.

O'HEYNES. Well, this is certainly a queer way of showing his affection for her.

FINOLA. I suppose it would be, if there were no reasons for it.

O'HEYNES (*indignantly*). To think he should have put off coming until his very wedding morning. He deserves to lose her after leaving her all this time. Oh, the persistent ill-luck that has pursued me all through life.

FINOLA. I'm sure I can't think how you consider it ill-luck to be on the eve of having all your wishes fulfilled.

O'HEYNES. Ah, that is just it, child. I have so often been on the eve of having my wishes fulfilled: and then somehow the unforeseen has come about; and all my hopes have gone from me. I am surely the most unfortunate of men.

FINOLA. Father, dear, you must not despond in this way.

O'HEYNES. To think of all the anxiety your sister has caused me, Finola, and the trouble she put me to before she would accept this rich young Englishman. She must have been mad. As if the coming into this place of such a suitor was an everyday event to her.

FINOLA (*pensively*). He never for a moment interested her somehow. It was very strange, his coming – wasn't it?

O'HEYNES. Was there ever such good fortune? I advertise the fishing of my river in the papers. He arrives here last summer, and takes it at once. To be sure it is splendid salmon fishing – but that it should have brought such a tenant as Hugh Fitz Walter – and that he should have fallen in love with Maeve – well –

FINOLA (*with a sigh*). Well, father, you ought to be content with such good fortune.

O'HEYNES (*despondingly*). Ah, I am afraid it is too good to come to anything. But just think that after all *he* should be the one to wreck this good fortune – Oh, I am distracted. (*He begins to work his hands and tear his hair.*)

FINOLA (*alarmed*). Father, don't fret in this way. It is bad for your health. And you know there is no reason for it.

O'HEYNES (*feebly*). Oh child, if you could only realise how I have waited and waited for this – for the time when fortune would enable our family to resume its fitting position in the county! Hugh has at last promised me this fortune. Is it surprising that I should be anxious, when I see the danger of his failing me?

FINOLA (*inadvertently*). He is not the one who will fail you, father.

O'HEYNES (*with a quick suspicion*). You think Maeve is more likely to – eh? Where is she?

FINOLA. Oh don't trouble about her. She is safe.

O'HEYNES. I noticed she was taking to her old habits lately. I had again to forbid her to wander through the country at night.

FINOLA (*as if laughing the matter off*). You must not mind these wanderings of hers. They are very harmless, father.

O'HEYNES (*anxiously*). Does she still talk of this strange one she is in love with?

FINOLA. Oh that is nothing. Don't trouble about it.

O'HEYNES. I am not so sure of what you say, Finola. I'll take my oath she is thinking about some good for nothing fellow after all.

FINOLA. No – no, nothing of the kind. You don't understand her.

O'HEYNES. Indeed I don't, child.

FINOLA. It is not often easy to do so. She seems to live by the brain as we live by the heart.

O'HEYNES. She seems to me quite regardless of realities.

FINOLA. Those feelings and impulses which are in our hearts and which govern our affections, with her are all in the head. This sounds strange: but it is the only way I can account for her nature.

O'HEYNES (*surprised*). In the head?

FINOLA. Yes – that is why she appears so cold, and, as you say, regardless of realities. I even think if this one she loves were to become a reality, he would cease to fascinate her.

O'HEYNES (*curiously*). Have you ever found out who he is?

FINOLA. No – not altogether.

O'HEYNES. I wonder what put such an extravagant idea in her head.

FINOLA. I think I know.

O'HEYNES. Well, what is it?

FINOLA. Would you believe it, father, I think it is those books that belonged to Uncle Bryan.

O'HEYNES. You mean those books up in the top room. They are mostly about ancient Greece, aren't they?

FINOLA. Yes. She is always poring over them and looking at their pictures – white statues and beautiful wall ornaments which she told me were in Greece. And then she showed me other books too, with pictures of pillars and arches – all ornamented like those in the abbey here. Then I have seen her take the writings of Uncle Bryan and study them with all these pictures before her.

O'HEYNES. Poor Bryan's writings, do you say? I didn't think there were any here. I thought the Society he belonged to, took them all. (*With plaintive regret.*) My poor brother Bryan; he was a great scholar. They used to talk of him in Dublin. They said if he had lived to complete his book, it would have made him famous.

FINOLA. What was he writing about when he died, father?

O'HEYNES. Let me see – I think his work was to be called 'The Influence of Greek Art on Celtic Ornament' or something of the sort.

FINOLA. That must have been it; for Maeve is always talking of that, and of the brotherhood of the Greek and Celtic races, and of a curious unreal beauty besides, which she says the Greeks invented. She thinks she has discovered something similar in the Celt.

O'HEYNES. Is that what you say she is in love with?

FINOLA (*with earnest conviction*). I verily believe so, father. (*Then after a moment's consideration*) Still it often seems to me she must have some individual in her mind besides.

O'HEYNES. I thought that was the case.

FINOLA. Oh – not what you think

O'HEYNES. What then, child?

FINOLA. I don't know; – she speaks of his beauty as if it had some sort of likeness to the Celtic ornament she is so much in love with.

O'HEYNES. Ah, she must have discovered this in the writings of Bryan.

– He had all sorts of odd theories about everything, poor fellow.

FINOLA. Yes, and she is as full of theories. She says that, because Celtic ornament is as rare and delicate as the Greek, so her pattern of Celtic youth must, in the same way, equal the perfection of Greek youth.

O'HEYNES (*astonished*). My goodness, is the whole of life like this to her?

FINOLA. Ah, now you understand what I meant when I told you that everything with her seemed to be only in the head.

O'HEYNES (*seriously*). Yes, Finola, and nothing in the heart. She has no warm feelings of the heart. She was always cold and distant from her earliest childhood.

FINOLA. No, I would not say so much. I think it is only her imagination that has absorbed all the warmth of her nature.

O'HEYNES. What you say is the same thing, my dear. Whatever may be the cause, depend upon it, she has no feeling.

FINOLA. Oh, don't say that, father.

O'HEYNES. Oh no, she hasn't, Finola; and I don't wonder that this young man's affection should at last weary of her apathy.

FINOLA. It is not any want of affection that has delayed him, father.

O'HEYNES. I cannot believe any more in his affection. (*Querulously*) Why is he not here? Why is he not here?

FINOLA. You will surely see him very soon. For goodness sake, do not fret so. Go in, and try and rest.

O'HEYNES. Rest – I cannot rest. How can I rest with this anxiety gnawing at me?

FINOLA. Oh, this miserable pride and position. They are ruining your health and peace.

O'HEYNES (*with a sudden reviving of energy*). Not they, my girl, indeed – why do you say so? Why should what are good for every other man be bad for old Colman O'Heynes?

FINOLA. Yes, yes, father dear, I know. But somehow we have been so happy and united in our seclusion here. We are going to be divided.

O'HEYNES. How divided?

FINOLA. Maeve will soon leave us.

O'HEYNES. Ah – yes, of course.

FINOLA. Let that be sufficient. Let us at least not try to go out into the world.

O'HEYNES. Why not, Finola?

FINOLA. The world is such a great lonely place.

O'HEYNES. But my lost position – the lost dignity of our family. I have that to reassert. When my rich son-in-law comes there will be end of our poverty.

FINOLA. You are the Prince of Burren. – Is not the royalty of our race acknowledged? What place can *we* find in a grotesque world of plutocrats and shop-keeper peers? This change in our life seems unnatural to me. And then that wicked old Peg Inerny is always talking.

O'HEYNES (*sharply*). Eh – what does she say?

FINOLA. Oh, nothing definite – nothing but insinuations and mystery, till I feel quite terrified.

O'HEYNES. She has been the curse of our house; and now the infernal witch has bewitched your sister.

FINOLA. I don't think that – I hope not. Maeve is only fascinated by her strange tales – the past, always the past.

O'HEYNES. Ay, it was the same way with your poor mother and this Peg Inerny who was a servant here long ago, and put it into her head to call your sister by the name of Maeve. Peg Inerny, I know, had some sinister object for this.

FINOLA. Oh, no, no.

O'HEYNES. Ah – wait a while.

FINOLA (*with a scared look*). Father, don't forebode evil. Try and be contented – try and check this restlessness that is urging you to change your life. Let us go in. (*As they move to the left*) Look at our old castle. How spectral those giant ash trees rise up around it from the pale March grass. How peaceful they all live in the sunset. Would it not be misery to leave that peace for a world where there is at least no peace.

(HUGH FITZ WALTER – *a good-looking young Englishman of about five and twenty, dressed in a tweed suit – enters at the right.*)

HUGH (*eagerly*). So I have arrived, you see, at last.

O'HEYNES (*turning*). Who is that? – what, Hugh?

HUGH. It is I.

O'HEYNES. And so it is. – Heaven be praised. I thought you were never coming, Hugh. (*He shakes him by the hand.*)

FINOLA (*also shaking him by the hand*). I am so glad you have come – at last.

HUGH. But I wrote to you my reason for not getting here sooner.

O'HEYNES. Yes, I know, of course. But why should you have put off coming like this till the very last?

HUGH. Haven't I explained to you again and again how my affairs delayed me?

O'HEYNES (*peevishly*). Yes – yes – explanations. You have caused me, Hugh, the greatest anxiety for all that.

HUGH. I assure you, O'Heynes, this delay was sorely against my will:

and I am sorry you have had any anxiety on my account. Why you have, indeed, I cannot understand.

O'HEYNES. My mind has been a prey to all sorts of doubts and forebodings.

HUGH (*alarmed*). Good gracious. What is this for? Isn't Maeve well? How is she?

O'HEYNES (*impatiently*). Oh, she is well – well enough.

HUGH. You are hiding something from me, O'Heynes.

O'HEYNES. No – not at all.

HUGH. I, too, was anxious. That is why I hurried here at once after my arrival in the village.

O'HEYNES (*suspiciously*). Eh – why were you anxious?

HUGH. I had not heard about her from Finola for some days.

O'HEYNES. There is nothing the matter with her except what has come by your protracted absence.

HUGH (*frightened*). What has come to her? You alarm me.

O'HEYNES. Only a return of her strange ways that used to trouble me before her engagement to you. That is all.

HUGH (*with visible relief*). Oh – that is all.

O'HEYNES (*involuntarily*). She frightens me sometimes.

HUGH. In what way? (O'HEYNES *hesitates and looks confused.*)

FINOLA. Oh, don't worry her about such things. Hush, here she comes. (MAEVE *enters from the back*).

HUGH. Oh, Maeve, what is it –? (MAEVE *starts when she perceives him. He goes eagerly to her, but is checked by the chillness of her manner, then taking her hand which she gives apathetically*). I hope you are not angry, Maeve. I came as soon as it was possible for me.

MAEVE (*with some recovered composure*). Oh – for that – I am not angry in the least – I am not angry at all.

HUGH. You looked as if something disturbed you.

FINOLA. Hugh, it is only her surprise at suddenly seeing you.

O'HEYNES. Yes, indeed, when you have disappointed her so often. But, thank heaven, you have arrived safe at last. Come, Finola, come, now I can rest. I feel I want rest after all this suspense. Come, let us go indoors. (*Exeunt* O'HEYNES *and* FINOLA *at left.*)

HUGH (*to* MAEVE). Well, I am back at last; and you – you are so silent and forgetful there among those old stones.

MAEVE (*as if recalled to herself*). No. I am in reality thinking of this very thing.

HUGH. Of my coming?

MAEVE. Yes.

HUGH. It has no interest for you one way or the other?

278

MAEVE. Oh yes. But I can not understand father's reason for being so troubled about it.

HUGH. Of course not. As if I wouldn't return on the first opportunity to you. Why do you seem annoyed that I should tell you this?

MAEVE (*restlessly*). Somehow there seem such cross purposes in this world of ours.

HUGH. Cross purposes – how so?

MAEVE. Oh I don't know – persons seem to give others what those others don't want from them, but want from someone else.

HUGH. That is indeed a world of cross purposes.

MAEVE (*sadly*). Don't you see that it is just so with us here?

HUGH (*dejectedly*). You mean that I give what is not wanted.

MAEVE. Yes, and that another would give you what you want from someone else.

HUGH. Who is that other?

MAEVE. The one whom you once appeared to like best.

HUGH. You are the one I always likes best in the world.

MAEVE. The world did not think so.

HUGH. Indeed? – You puzzle me. Explain what you are saying?

MAEVE (*with a certain embarrassment*). I thought you liked my sister better than me.

HUGH. Than you? On no – impossible. I know you don't believe what you are saying.

MAEVE. But you appeared to be so much more intimate with her than you have been with me.

HUGH. Ah, that is just it. I have the greatest affection for Finola. I admire her goodness and unselfishness. She has indeed the disposition of an angel.

MAEVE. And yet you could leave her for one so less worthy, as I am.

HUGH. You shall not say you are less worthy; I can see no fault in you.

MAEVE. Oh, why did you ever leave Finola?

HUGH. You forget we were never more than friends. She is one of my very dearest friends.

MAEVE. And you were never engaged to her?

HUGH. Never. It was only when I despaired of your consent that I thought for a while of Finola. But it was no use. Your image always rose up between us. I soon understood that for me you were the only one in the world. (*Pause.*)

MAEVE (*absently*). The only one in the world. What happiness it must be to find the one who is so much as that.

HUGH. It may also be misery – that is, in a certain sense.

MAEVE (*a little surprised*). Really? How can it be misery?

279

HUGH. When we know that nothing of what we feel is returned.

MAEVE (*abstractedly*). I should not have thought that much mattered.

HUGH. Do you say this because I persist in loving you through all your contempt of my love?

MAEVE. Oh no – I was not thinking of you at all.

HUGH. What was your reason then for saying it?

MAEVE (*with a pensive deliberation*). I should have imagined that if one really loved, one would shrink from a return of love.

HUGH (*surprised*). You wouldn't like your love returned?

MAEVE. Ah no, for I think if it were, the beauty of love would come to an end in the lover.

HUGH. How very strange. But why should I think so? Yours is the reasoning of one who has never known love.

MAEVE. So you think I have never known love?

HUGH. Certainly. (*Pause.*) Have you?

MAEVE. Well, I can tell you truly that I have.

HUGH (*in a serious tone*). Is that really so?

MAEVE. Yes.

HUGH (*with a sudden suspicion*). Do you love someone now?

MAEVE (*quietly*). Yes.

HUGH (*growing excited*). Who is he?

MAEVE (*wearily*). Oh, what is the use of telling you?

HUGH. Who is he, I say? For pity's sake speak.

MAEVE. You would never understand.

HUGH (*bitterly*). I should understand only too well.

MAEVE. Look around you, then.

HUGH (*puzzled, looking around him*). Well? I see no one.

MAEVE (*scornfully*). I knew you would not understand.

HUGH (*wondering*). I see nothing but these ruins – that mysterious round tower – the stony mountains – and your gray castle through the leafless boughs of great ash trees.

MAEVE (*with a visionary look in her eyes*). And you see nothing but these?

HUGH. Oh, what is this mystery? Will you tell me?

MAEVE (*smiling ecstatically*). Among all these that you see – listen to what Gráinne says in the old poem –
'There lives a one
On whom I would love to gaze long,
For whom I would give the whole world,
All, all, though it is a delusion'.

HUGH (*downcast*). You are mocking me.

MAEVE (*gently*). Oh, no. – How can you think so? Are not all things beautiful that remind us of our love?

HUGH (*after looking at her calmly for some time*). Yes, you are right. How strange you are. I do not understand you. Among us simple men you seem like one of your golden fairies. What is the name you call them?

MAEVE. Tûatha dê Dannann, those tall beautiful children of the Dagda Môr. It is said they were the old people of Erin and were afterwards worshipped as gods.

HUGH. But you do not believe they are really gods?

MAEVE. Oh, no – only a race whose great beauty still haunts our land. (*Sadly*) They were too beautiful to compare with me.

HUGH. They could not be more beautiful than you are. You don't know how beautiful you are to me. No – if you knew, you would not be so indifferent. Ah, I realise but too well how little you care for me. You would never have consented to be my wife but for your father: you are doing it all for your father – not for me.

MAEVE. Oh, why do you go back to all that? Have I not consented? And is not that the main thing?

HUGH (*resignedly*). Yes, – I suppose I must be satisfied. I must only trust to time for winning you completely.

MAEVE (*with mysterious significance*). Let us all trust to time.

HUGH (*brightening*). May I put my trust in time?

MAEVE. You must ask that question of Time himself.

HUGH. Oh, I am confident of his answer.

MAEVE. And I too, am confident in Time. (*Exeunt leisurely at the left.*)

(*As they are going,* PEG INERNY – *a little old woman in a ragged red frieze petticoat, a black frieze cloak raised up to partially cover her head, and with dark woollen stockings worn away at the bare soles of her feet – enters stealthily from among the ruins at back. Muttering indistinctly she follows the two for a while, then squats down on a stone, and gazes fixedly at the cairn.*)

(*After a pause* MAEVE *and* FINOLA *enter at the left.*)

FINOLA. Oh, Maeve, why do you come out here again?

MAEVE (*joyfully*). He is gone. Until to-morrow, at least I shall be free.

FINOLA. Poor Hugh.

MAEVE. He is gone; and I will make the most of my little liberty. I have to say good-bye to beauty. How this moonlit night – this Irish night comes like a fawn!

FINOLA (*perceives* PEG INERNY *and stands as if transfixed*).

MAEVE. What's the matter, Finola? (*Turns and looks.*) Oh, it is only Peg Inerny.

FINOLA. Come away, Maeve, for heavens' sake come. I have left father sleeping in the hall; and if he awakes he is sure to call me, and ask where you are.

MAEVE (*not heeding Finola*). Peg, Peg, I have not seen you for many days. What has brought you here to-night?

PEG (*rousing herself slowly and looking steadily at* MAEVE). I come to take a last farewell of my Princess on the night before her wedding day.

MAEVE (*with a rigid melancholy*). Yes, I shall never return here, Peg.

PEG. Do you think you will ever leave, Princess?

FINOLA. Oh, what is that she says? I am terrified.

MAEVE (*carelessly*). You are always alarmed at one thing or another, Finola.

FINOLA (*uneasily*). No – no – but didn't you hear her?

PEG (*to* FINOLA). Princess, do not fear a poor old woman.

FINOLA. Why will you always call us princesses?

PEG. Isn't your father a prince? The Prince of Burren?

MAEVE (*impatiently*). A prince indeed. It is a mockery now to call him that.

PEG. The O'Heynes is none the less a prince whatever he may have done to put shame on his race.

MAEVE (*helplessly*). Oh, what a misfortune it was.

FINOLA (*expostulating*). Maeve – darling.

PEG (*slyly*). They told me my Princess Maeve was content to marry her young Englishman.

MAEVE (*with suppressed scorn*). Ha – no one ever troubled before to consider whether she was or not.

PEG. He is so rich – so rich with his grand English house and possessions.

MAEVE. Yes indeed – and that is how the whole tragedy has come about.

PEG. I was sure you cared not, Princess, for this world's riches.

MAEVE (*sadly*). Heaven knows I never had any greed of them.

FINOLA. Oh Maeve, I thought you had done with these complaints once and for all.

MAEVE (*pained and irresolute*). So I, too, thought – once perhaps. But to-day in the abbey – it was so beautiful. Something seemed to come back to me.

PEG. It was haunting you, Princess? The day-ghost, eh?

MAEVE (*with a wan look*). The day-ghost. Oh the wistful pleading of a day-ghost!

FINOLA (*frightened*). Why do you say that, Maeve?

MAEVE. Ah – if you saw him – but you never have, Finola.

FINOLA. Saw him – good heavens, where?

MAEVE (*pointing to the round tower*). In the master-work of Goban – in the mountains too.

PEG. Your love is dreaming among the rocks of these mountains, Princess.

MAEVE (*with a sort of ecstasy*). Oh, how I have grown to love these stony mountains.

PEG. They are the pleasure haunts of many a beautiful ghost.

MAEVE. The many beautiful buried in that cairn.

PEG. Oh what a world there is underneath that cairn.

MAEVE (*pensively*). Yes, the great beautiful Queen Maeve who reigned over Connacht hundreds of years ago – she is buried in that cairn you say?

PEG. Haven't I often told you so, Princess?

FINOLA. But I have always understood that Queen Maeve was buried at Rathcroghan in County Roscommon.

PEG. No, Princess, she is here.

FINOLA (*inquiringly*). Can you know that?

PEG. Can I know? I can know many things. (*With a low laugh.*) Indeed I ought to know where Queen Maeve is.

MAEVE. Why you especially, Peg?

PEG. Haven't I dwelt in her palace, child?

FINOLA (*timidly approaching* MAEVE). That is a strange thing to say.

PEG (*continuing with a sort of inward satisfaction*). Yes, I have dwelt in her palace. Ha – ha – does anyone think that I could bear my miserable outcast life in the world if I could not live the other life also? Oh, my sweet ladies, you don't know the grandeur of that other life.

MAEVE (*eagerly*). Tell me, do tell me of that other life.

FINOLA. Maeve – take care – don't ask such a thing.

MAEVE (*impatiently*). Oh Finola, you mustn't prevent me in this way. (*To* PEG INERNY) Tell me.

PEG. A life among the people with beautiful looks.

MAEVE (*suddenly delighted*). With beautiful looks!

PEG. Yes, Princess – Oh, just so graceful and clean as you are yourself. I often think you must be one of them.

MAEVE. Tell me more about those people.

PEG. They are now ruled over by the great Queen Maeve.

MAEVE (*puzzled*). But – she is dead, isn't she? Didn't you say she was buried in the cairn?

PEG (*with an enigmatical grimace*). Yes, yes, Princess – but not dead – Oh, I never said that she was dead.

MAEVE. What new and wonderful tale are you now telling me?

PEG. Haven't I told you before that Queen Maeve has ever been watchful of you?

MAEVE (*surprised*). No – you have not. What does this mean?

PEG. Just fancy, Princess, it was she who had you called after herself.

FINOLA (*excitedly*). Maeve, don't believe her. How is this possible?

PEG. Ah, Princess Finola, didn't you ever know that I was once a servant in the Castle?

FINOLA (*restraining herself*). Yes, I believe you were. It was a very long time ago, was it not?

PEG. When your beautiful sister here was born.

FINOLA. Well then, supposing you were, what has that to do with Queen Maeve naming my sister?

PEG (*slyly*). Oh – only 'twas I made them think of calling her Maeve.

FINOLA. But you said Queen Maeve did so?

PEG (*with veiled significance*). Haven't I told you of the other life I lead, sweet Princess Finola?

FINOLA (*starts, then looking awed and mystified at* PEG INERNY, *says in a trembling voice*) Maeve, she is a wicked woman. It is not right to hold any intercourse with her.

MAEVE (*who has been listening with a troubled expression*). Ah me, I am the most miserable one in the world.

FINOLA (*terrified*). Dearest, for pity's sake don't – don't give way to such a feeling.

MAEVE (*despairingly*). My father – oh, my father.

PEG. I know it was for his sake alone that you promised to marry this Hugh Fitz Walter.

MAEVE. Yes, father will become rich and great – but my heart will break.

FINOLA (*anxiously*). No – no, Maeve, you must remember how good and kind Hugh is. He will surely never cause you unhappiness.

MAEVE. How could he be anything but unhappiness to me, when I can only think of my beloved?

PEG (*insidiously*). That one who haunts the mountains and the beautiful old buildings, Princess –

MAEVE. My beloved whom I am leaving for ever!

FINOLA (*throwing her arms around her sister*). Hush – you must not think of him any more, Maeve.

PEG. Ah – you cling to her like ivy, my Lady Finola. You were the one made for clinging. You were the wife that would have been best for the Englishman.

MAEVE. Oh, if he could but understand that this is so.

PEG. They never can, Princess. Dwellers in the valley are always looking at the heights above them.

MAEVE (*sadly*). I am no longer on those heights. I have fallen from them miserably, and have become (*looking at* FINOLA) like the ivy in the valley.

PEG. Not yet – you are still on the heights. No, you are still like the tall smooth larch on the top of the mountain.

MAEVE (*dejectedly*). Ah, no, not any longer.

PEG. Come then, to the mountains, Princess – there you will believe it.

FINOLA (*restraining her*). Maeve, Maeve, do not go. It will kill father if he hears you have wandered away to-night.

PEG. See how bright it is. The night is lit for your visit. (MAEVE *appears to hesitate*.) Beware of the ivy clinging around the larch, Princess Maeve. It will kill the fairy growth of the larch.

MAEVE (*restlessly*). Let me go, Finola, let me go.

FINOLA. I will not, Maeve.

MAEVE. Let me go to the mountains for this last time; I promise to return soon.

FINOLA. Oh, sister, do not go there to-night.

MAEVE. How white the moon rays dance upon the mountains.

PEG. It is the mountains, Princess, that are white with the dancing feet of the fairies.

MAEVE (*desperately*). I must go there to-night.

FINOLA. You shall not, Maeve.

MAEVE (*gazing fondly on the mountains*). O beauty of my day-dreams come forth from the mountains.

PEG. Princess, what is it that you see?

MAEVE (*with transport*). My love, like an exhalation from the earth to the stars!

PEG (*moving towards the back*). Come, Princess, come.

MAEVE. I am coming.

FINOLA (*with sudden determination*). Then I shall go too. I could not bear the suspense of your absence. (*Distant voice of* THE O'HEYNES *is heard several times calling* 'FINOLA'.) Good heavens, there is father calling. (*Runs to the left and listens in great agitation while the calling is repeated*). Yes, father, yes, father. (*Exeunt* MAEVE *and* PEG *quickly at the back.*) If he finds she has gone he will be so distressed. I must not tell him. Oh, Maeve, why, why have you gone? Yes, father – coming – coming. (*Exit at left.*)

285

ACT II

The exterior of O'Heynes Castle. At the left a large square tower with its two roof gables facing right and left, and Irish battlements which carry two high chimneys, one at front and one at back of roof. On ground level at front is the pointed Gothic entrance-door, over which a square-headed window lights a room above, while on the side facing the right above a hall window, is another square-headed window belonging to the same upper room. Around great leafless ash trees grow upon the pale green grass. Some way off at the right is the cairn with the abbey ruins beyond; and stony mountain ranges, as in the first act, form a background to the whole scene.
It is a frosty night with a very bright moon.
(FINOLA O'HEYNES, *closely muffled, comes out through the door of the castle.*)

FINOLA. Maeve. Are you there, Maeve? (*Pause.*) Maeve. (*Goes to the right and peers about.*) I don't see any sign of her. Oh dear, oh dear, I wonder does she intend to come back. (*With an anxious and undecided look*) I don't know which way to search for her. Stop – I will try this path leading to the mountain. (*Exit at back behind the Castle.*)

(MAEVE, *looking very pale and listless, enters from the right.*)

MAEVE (*gazing forlorn around the scene*). Oh, moon and mountain and ruin, give a voice to my infinite sadness! (*Pause.*) (FINOLA *re-enters from behind the Castle.*)

FINOLA. O sister, you are here!

MAEVE (*slowly*). Yes.

FINOLA. Thank heaven, you have returned. (*She advances towards her.*)

MAEVE. I said I would return, Finola.

FINOLA. Oh, I was so frightened. Aren't you perished without a cloak on, this bitter night?

MAEVE (*wearily*). Is it so cold?

FINOLA (*surprised.*) Cold? You must feel this biting frost air?

MAEVE. No – not particularly.

FINOLA (*feeling the hands and face of* MAEVE). Why, Maeve, you are like ice.

286

MAEVE (*as if remembering*). Like ice. How beautiful to be like the ice!

FINOLA. Oh, come in, come in from the cold.

MAEVE. No – let me wait here, in the moonlight.

FINOLA. Darling, you will get dreadfully ill – and on your wedding morning too.

MAEVE (*with a shudder*). What – it is not yet the day?

FINOLA. Midnight has just passed – yes, this is your wedding day.

MAEVE (*mournfully*). Oh, so soon – so soon.

FINOLA. Far better had it been sooner, my poor sister.

MAEVE. Oh, don't say that, Finola.

FINOLA. Yes, yes, this long delay since your engagement has brought the old trouble upon you again.

MAEVE (*with a scornful smile*). Do you think I was ever really reconciled to my fate?

FINOLA. And yet – and yet – you seemed happy for a while.

MAEVE. No – never really. I was only talked into a false sort of happiness, Finola.

FINOLA (*expostulating*). Oh, how can you say that?

MAEVE. Yes, I deceived myself there among you. You all seemed so happy, and were so kind and indulgent to me, that I wished to believe this marriage was for the best.

FINOLA. And you never really believed it?

MAEVE. Never – I was soon certain that I never did.

FINOLA. When was that?

MAEVE. When he went to England to arrange with his lawyers, and this family happiness that encircled me gradually disappeared –

FINOLA. Do you think so? I am sure father and I have never changed.

MAEVE. Perhaps not, but you understand, I was left more to myself and had time to think over what I had done. (*Despairingly.*) Ah then I saw that I never could be reconciled to my fate.

FINOLA. Darling, you should not have encouraged such a thought. It will leave you, when you are married and away from here.

MAEVE. Oh, the sacrifice – I make it for father's sake.

FINOLA. Be sure your sacrifice for father's sake will have its reward.

MAEVE. It is a cruel sacrifice. And yet it must be –

FINOLA. Poor Hugh. At all events he is unchanged.

MAEVE. I too am unchanged, Finola. Don't you see it after what I have told you?

FINOLA. I suppose so. But have you always disliked him? You do not hate him?

MAEVE. Oh, but if you were to see him, Finola, in the light he appears to me –

287

FINOLA. How does he appear to you, dear?

MAEVE (*with sudden vehemence*). A bandit – a plunderer!

FINOLA. Maeve, what are you saying?

MAEVE. Yes, I say a bandit, like his English predecessors who ruined every beautiful thing we ever had.

FINOLA (*frightened*). Sister, how can you accuse him of that?

MAEVE (*bitterly*). Yes, he has come finally to ruin every beautiful thing.

FINOLA. He, who is so generous? Why, instead of destroying, is he not restoring the dignity of our ancient Celtic house?

MAEVE (*scornfully*). Yes, I know what such restoration means. It is bought at too great a price, I can tell you. It is like that great restoration of a family's pride by Strongbow, who first brought our humiliation upon us.

FINOLA. No – I cannot see the likeness, Maeve.

MAEVE. Don't you remember the conditions of the English noble whom the Irish king Diarmid called to his aid?

FINOLA. Was it not, if Strongbow regained for Diarmid his kingdom he was to marry the king's daughter Eva?

MAEVE. Yes, and then become heir to Diarmid. – He succeeded in regaining the kingdom and the conditions were fulfilled, weren't they?

FINOLA. They were.

MAEVE. And thus with the power that was given him he subdued and ruined the ancient splendour of Erin. The old, old story! Poor Eva, you were sacrificed – a sweet symbol of your country in her subjection.

FINOLA. That may be, but still I can't understand in what way Hugh is to injure our country.

MAEVE. By killing the last flame of her life.

FINOLA. The last flame of our country's life? How is that?

MAEVE. Yes, the last light of her life.

FINOLA. What is this last light?

MAEVE (*with a child's smile and as if forgetful of all sorrows*). The fairy lamp of Celtic Beauty!

FINOLA (*after a moment, in a very gentle voice*). Dearest, it is impossible he ever could do this thing.

MAEVE. Is he not destroying my chosen way of life – that life which alone may keep the flame alight? Am I not the last?

FINOLA. The last? Why should you think that you are the last?

MAEVE. Listen and I will tell you, Finola. You have heard Peg Inerny speak of her other life, and of having dwelt in the palace of Queen Maeve?

FINOLA (*nervously*). Yes, what of her?

MAEVE. This very night after I had left her upon the mountain I thought I saw her beckoning to me in the abbey. I followed her while she went past the round tower to the cairn which now was glowing against a sky that had turned crimson. With a gesture the old woman seemed to open the cairn, and then stood transformed in a curious region of fresh green suffused with saffron light, so that I saw her tall, and beautiful, and marvellously pale of face, and crowned with a golden diadem not so golden as her hair. And I heard her say these words in ancient Gaelic:- 'Last Princess of Erin, thou art a lonely dweller among strange peoples; but I the great Queen Maeve have watched thee from thy birth, for thou wert to be the vestal of our country's last beauty. Behold whom thy love hath called to life. Mark him well, for already his hour of dissolution hath come' And I looked and saw him who was beauty standing by the round tower. With a feeling of nothingness, I fell upon my knees and bent down to the earth. When I looked again he was not there. Then a company of ancient Celts bore a covered form upon their shoulders; while a choir of rose-crowned boys sang dirges with violet voices of frail, lace-like beauty. And they buried their dead one by the round tower, and over his grave they raised a great ogham stone. And again I heard the voice of the Queen:- 'They have buried thy dead beauty, Princess. Thou hast killed him by deserting thy chosen way of life; for there are no more who live for beauty'. Then in my desolation I seemed to lose consciousness of all save these last words of the queen: 'Yet, princess, I will come and comfort thee again to-night'. And with a start I discovered that I was sitting alone in the moonlight by the round tower. And I looked, and I could not find the great ogham stone that they had raised over my beloved.

FINOLA. And so you were only dreaming after all?

MAEVE. Yes, it must have only been a dream – for my beloved is not dead.

FINOLA. Nor will Queen Maeve come to you again to-night.

MAEVE. Do not be so sure of that, Finola.

FINOLA (*in a frightened voice*). Oh heavens! there she is.

MAEVE (*starting*). Who?

FINOLA. Peg Inerny.

(PEG *enters from the right.*)

PEG. My noble ladies.

FINOLA (*angrily*). What do you want?

PEG. Oh, I never thought you could be so sharp, Lady Finola.

FINOLA (*with the desperation of terror*). Go – you are here for no good

289

purpose.

MAEVE (*deprecatingly*). Finola.

PEG (*to* FINOLA). Won't you give me the liberty of a wild beast to walk about at night, my dear?

FINOLA (*shrieking*). Go, I say, or I will let loose the dogs of the castle upon you.

MAEVE. Finola, for goodness sake, what are you saying? What wrong has she ever done to any of us?

FINOLA. Oh yes, don't I know her evil intentions towards you?

MAEVE. I feel sure she has never done me harm.

PEG (*to* MAEVE). Sweet Princess, you'll rejoice for the gentleness you have shown me.

FINOLA (*to* PEG). I will call my father up if you don't leave at once. Come, sister, come into the castle.

PEG. Good-night, sweet Maeve – sleep – sleep – and dream. (*Exit at right.*)

MAEVE (*yearningly*). And dream – Oh that I could dream again to-night, that dream!

FINOLA. Don't think of it any more, dearest. Come in to rest.

MAEVE. No – let me stay a while longer here.

FINOLA. But you will be frozen, Maeve. I wonder you ever awoke again after falling asleep in the abbey.

MAEVE. Let me stay, Finola, I do not feel the cold.

FINOLA. It is because you are already so cold.

MAEVE. My love is so divinely cold.

FINOLA. Ah, that is a strange sort of love.

MAEVE (*wistfully*). He is the only one I have ever loved. Let me stay. I hear him coming.

FINOLA (*frightened*). You hear him – ?

MAEVE (*pointing towards the abbey*). Yes, there – far away – coming on the wings of the March wind. Don't you hear?

FINOLA. I hear the bitter wind, Maeve, through our old ash trees.

MAEVE (*smiling in reverie*). The fairy March wind which races at twilight over our fields, turning them to that strange pale beauty, like the beauty of a fairy's face. – Oh, it is fit that my beloved should ride on such a steed.

FINOLA. Dearest, you must go to rest. He will never come. He is dead.

MAEVE. He is not dead. He will come. I know he will. But the way is long. A long – long way.

FINOLA. A long way, indeed, without beginning and without end.

MAEVE. It began from the land of everlasting youth.

FINOLA. You have often told me of that land, Tir-nan-ogue, is it not?

MAEVE. The Celtic dream-land of ideal beauty. There he lives in never-fading freshness of youth. (*With a steadfast visionary look.*) I am haunted by a boyish face close hooded with short gold hair – and every movement of his slender faultless body goes straight to my heart like a fairy melody. Oh, he has a long way to journey:- for that land of beauty was never so far away as it is to-night.

FINOLA (*sadly*). It never was nearer, my poor sister. Come, I will see you to your rest.

MAEVE. I must rest alone, Finola. You must not follow me to my room.

FINOLA . Why not, dear?

MAEVE. Oh, do not. Leave me to myself.

FINOLA (*with a sigh*). Very well, if you wish it.

MAEVE (*going*). Good-night.

FINOLA . Good-night, dear.

MAEVE (*quickly turning and throwing her arms around* FINOLA). Good-night –good-bye – Oh my darling, good-bye.

FINOLA (*consolingly*). My poor Maeve, it is not yet the time for parting.

MAEVE. Who knows where I must go, when my beloved shall come. (*Exit hurriedly by door leading into the Castle.*)

FINOLA (*wonderingly*). What does she mean by those words? (*With a reassured air*) Oh, she is tired, poor sister. That is what it is. And I suppose her mind is confused with her imaginary difficulties. But all will come well in good time. (*Exit by door leading into the Castle.*) (*Pause.*)

(MAEVE *appears at the window of the castle, above the hall-window facing the right, and slowly opens the casement.*)

MAEVE (*leaning out*). Oh, the beautiful frosty night! I cannot keep it from me. The greatest beauty like the old Greek sculpture is always cold! My Prince of the hoar dew! My golden love, let me see you once more in that aureole of crimson sky! (*With an infinite longing*) Oh that the beauty I saw in my dream could return to me now. (*With sudden terror*) But to-morrow, how shall I face the misery of to-morrow? Oh pity me, pity me – (*Calmer*) And yet I have always known that my beloved would deliver me from bondage. (*With a gradually weaker voice as she sinks upon a chair*) But I am weary of waiting – weary –weary – it is hard to resist the longing for sleep. (*She sighs as she reclines back out of sight in an angle of the window.*) (*Pause.*)

(*There is a soft music of harps, while the aurora borealis arises and glows in the sky. Soon a ghostly procession is seen to emerge like vapour from the neighbourhood of the cairn. Presently as it advances it grows more distinct and then is discovered to consist of* QUEEN

291

MAEVE, *tall, pale faced and fair haired, in a golden crown and gold embroidered robes; of* BOY PAGES *in garlanded tunics and wearing wreaths of roses upon their heads; of ancient Irish harpers with their harps; of chieftains and warriors in conical caps; of people, etc.)*

(As they approach near to the castle, MAEVE *enters from the door at its front, and stands looking on in wonder. They halt; and the harpers cease playing on their harps.)*

CHORUS OF BOY PAGES (*Singing in broad solemn unison*).

> Every hill which is at this Oenach
> Hath under it heroes and Queens,
> And poets and distributors,
> And fair fierce women.

(The harpers recommence their music.)

MAEVE (*with a thrill of happiness*). Ah, that song of Dorban I know so well. And this is Queen Maeve again. (*The harpers cease their music.*)

CHORUS OF BOY PAGES.

> Hast seen our warriors? In their hands are white shields
> Ornamented with white silver signs –
> They wield blue flaming swords
> And carry red horns with metal mountings.

MAEVE (*listening*). Now they are chanting the lay of Fiachna son of Reta.

A BOY PAGE (*singing alone*).

> Obedient to the settled order of the battle,
> Preceding their prince of gracious mien
> They march across blue lances
> Those troops of white warriors with knotted hair.

CHORUS OF BOY PAGES.

> They march across blue lances
> Those troops of white warriors with knotted hair. (*The harpers recommence their music.*)

QUEEN MAEVE. Princess I come, as I have promised.

MAEVE (*approaching and falling on her knees*). My Queen – Oh save me, my queen.

QUEEN MAEVE. O last of my daughters in the land, what help can I give you?

MAEVE. My beloved – where is he?

QUEEN MAEVE. He is coming over the mountains. He is coming to you over the mountains.

MAEVE (*rising*). Yes, I knew he was coming on the fairy March wind.

QUEEN MAEVE. Your love is so great that you divine his coming? And yet you can suffer bondage?

MAEVE. How shall I escape the stranger's bondage?

QUEEN MAEVE. I will take you to the land of joy.

MAEVE. To Tir-nan-ogue? – O Queen, do you rule in Tir-nan-ogue?

QUEEN MAEVE. The empire of the Gael is in Tir-nan-ogue. There during life he is at peace in the building of beauty from the past.

MAEVE. And so the land you reign in is the home of living men.

QUEEN MAEVE. Each man who comes to his ideal has come to Tir-nan-ogue.

MAEVE. And thus we see you so young and so beautiful after all those two thousand years!

QUEEN MAEVE. Your fame also shall remain beautiful and young.

MAEVE. Of what kind is the happiness that makes Tir-nan-ogue happy?

QUEEN MAEVE. Happiness in the present as sweet as the remembrance of happiness.

MAEVE. Then shall my happiness be great indeed.

QUEEN MAEVE. You remember much happiness?

MAEVE. I remember beauty.

QUEEN MAEVE. Those who love beauty shall see beauty.

MAEVE. The immortal beauty of form!

QUEEN MAEVE. Form that will awaken genius!

MAEVE. Form is my beauty and my love! (*The harpers cease their music.*)

CHORUS OF BOY PAGES.
> Their strength, great as it is, can not be less,
> They are sons of queens and kings,
> On the heads of all a comely
> Growth of hair yellow like gold.

A BOY PAGE.
> Their bodies are graceful and majestic,
> Their eyes with a look of power have the eye-ball blue.
> Their teeth are brilliant like glass,
> Their lips are red and thin.

CHORUS OF BOY PAGES.
> Their bodies are graceful and majestic,
> These sons of queens and kings. (*The harpers recommence their music.*)

MAEVE. So Fiachna is made to sing when the poet tells how the hero came from the land of the gods. I love that poem!

QUEEN MAEVE. I have all the poems – the greatest those that are lost. Come into my land; and they that made them shall sing them, and their music shall turn all things to beauty.

MAEVE. Queen, I have seen that land afar.

QUEEN MAEVE. You also have seen Tir-nan-ogue?

MAEVE. In my dreams, in my day-dreams.

QUEEN MAEVE. Daughter, it is passing sweet when our day-dreams come true.

MAEVE. Oh let me see the beloved of my day-dreams.

QUEEN MAEVE. Your Prince of the hoar dew, when he comes, will give you rest.

MAEVE. Rest without pain or fear of bondage?

QUEEN MAEVE. Rest in beauty – a beauty which is transcendently cold.

MAEVE. Oh let me see that beauty. I have sought it in vain on earth.

QUEEN MAEVE. He is coming, he is coming over the mountains. You shall speak to him when he is come.

MAEVE (*with a sudden disconsolate look*). I will never speak to him.

QUEEN MAEVE. Why, wayward child?

MAEVE. Queen, I cannot, The sight of such beauty will make me speechless.

QUEEN MAEVE. Then shall you find peace in his beauty.

MAEVE. But oh, my queen, let me see him.

QUEEN MAEVE. You shall see him in the Northern lights of Tir-nan-ogue.

MAEVE. And his beauty shall be my joy in an ideal land.

QUEEN MAEVE. Beauty in the midst of all beautiful things.

MAEVE. Oh take me to that land.

QUEEN MAEVE. I am waiting for you, poor weary child.

MAEVE. The land where my day-dreams will come true!

QUEEN MAEVE. See, the Northern lights are passing before the dawn. We must not tarry.

MAEVE. I am ready, my beautiful queen.

QUEEN MAEVE. Then come with the Northern lights, beautiful ice maiden!

MAEVE. I shall see my beauty – my love – ! (*Half swooning she falls on the neck of* QUEEN MAEVE.) (*The harpers cease their music.*)

CHORUS OF BOY PAGES.

> Noble and melodious music thou dost hear;
> Thou goest from kingdom to kingdom
> Drinking from goblets of massy gold,
> Thou wilt discourse with thy beloved.

A BOY PAGE.

> We have carried from the plain Mag Mell
> Thirty caldrons, thirty horns for drinking
> We have carried from it the lamentation sung by Mear,

Daughter of Euchaid the Dumb. (*The harpers recommence their music.*)

CHORUS OF BOY PAGES.

What a marvel in Tir-nan-ogue
That mead should fall with each shower,
Drinking from goblets of massy gold,
Thou wilt discourse with thy beloved.

(*During this song all, including* MAEVE, *have gradually moved off towards the cairn and faded away with the aurora borealis, so that, when the music ceases, no trace of them remains. A faint grey light of dawn now prevails; and then the whole scene, at the approach of sunrise, is discovered to be completely white with a thick coating of hoar frost.*

After a while HUGH FITZ WALTER, *muffled and carrying a large bunch of flowers, enters from the left.*)

HUGH. I can wait no longer. I must come to her castle with the first light. How fine it looks decked out with the hoar frost! Oh, I hope she is safe and well; let these be my morning offering before she awakes. (*He lays the flowers by the doorway of the castle.*)

(THE O'HEYNES, *also muffled, enters from the left.*)

O'HEYNES (*looking in the direction of Hugh*). Ah! you too, are out early this morning.

HUGH. Yes. Somehow I felt I had to come.

O'HEYNES. What a blessing you are here at last, Hugh. (*He grasps him by the hand.*)

HUGH. I wish I could have returned sooner.

O'HEYNES. I wish you could have. Well, let that be.

HUGH. But why are you also about at this hour of the morning? I did not expect to see any one stirring.

O'HEYNES (*peevishly*). I could not sleep these hours past with thinking and thinking. Then something made me get up, and see what would happen.

HUGH (*anxiously*). What would happen? Heavens! what do you expect to happen?

O'HEYNES. Oh nothing, nothing, I suppose. Only my mind will not let me rest.

HUGH. Do you know I too was very uneasy about things last night.

O'HEYNES (*suspiciously*). You, why? What reason could you have had?

HUGH (*with rather a forced laugh*). Oh, none of course. How could I?

O'HEYNES. Of course not – of course not. But come in to the fire, Hugh, and warm yourself. There has been a great frost last night.

HUGH. Yes, the whole country is white, as if it were covered with snow.

O'HEYNES. A March frost soon melts before the sun. See, it is already rising. The day is going to be a glorious one.

HUGH. There is an old saying – 'Happy is the bride the sun shines on'.

(*As they go towards the door of the castle,* FINOLA *enters from it.*)

FINOLA. Oh, what lovely flowers!

HUGH. I brought them for Maeve. She is not yet awake?

FINOLA. No. I gave orders she was not to be disturbed. It was very late last night when she went to rest; and she seemed so tired.

HUGH. Then I would not have her disturbed for worlds. Will you bring her these flowers, Finola, when she awakes?

(PEG INERNY *enters from the right.*)

PEG. When she awakes –? Ah, – my Princess Maeve – do you think she will care for such flowers now?

HUGH (*in a subdued voice*). Why not? Why do you say she would not?

PEG. Oh, it's a cold morning, a cruel cold morning.

FINOLA. Go away from this place. – Let me never see you again.

PEG. I have never before been refused the shelter of O'Heynes Castle.

HUGH. O'Heynes Castle is never the better for your presence. I understand you are always importuning Miss O'Heynes.

O'HEYNES. Come, we must not be hard to the old woman on such a day as this. Go round to the kitchen, Peg, and get something to eat.

PEG. Yes, some food. I want some food and warmth, Prince – I have been out all night, and I am famished.

O'HEYNES. Well, then, get all you wish. The Castle hall is open to everyone in honour of my daughter's wedding to-day.

HUGH. Yes, we must try to make everyone happy to-day – even this wicked old woman.

PEG (*with a sinister look*). I suppose you also, my brave Englishman, think you ought to be happy.

HUGH. Why – of course. Don't you know I am to be married to-day?

PEG (*almost contemptuously*). You married to the Princess Maeve?

HUGH (*bridling up*). Yes.

PEG (*mockingly*). Well, well, how queer that you should think so!

FINOLA (*with a scared expression*). There is misfortune in those words.

O'HEYNES. Peg Inerny, you are awakening my forebodings again.

PEG (*humbly*). Oh, Prince, I can't say otherwise.

HUGH (*indignantly*). What old woman's talk is this?

PEG (*with a quiet prophetic triumph*). You think I am only an old woman; but I tell you that Erin can never be subdued.

HUGH. I should like to know what that has to do with the matter?

PEG (*smiling insidiously*). Perhaps the Englishman may think that he already holds her? Ah, she will slip like a fairy from his grasp. (*She

296

laughs low and sardonically.)

FINOLA (*excitedly to* PEG). Leave the place at once, you wicked woman. Oh, drive her away, Hugh, before she says any more.

HUGH (*advances to* Peg, *who draws herself up defiantly. He then steps back, saying, with a forced laugh*) What do I care for her. I shall soon be married and far away!

PEG. Take care, my fine Englishman, if your Irish Princess hasn't already slipped from you like a fairy.

O'HEYNES (*nervously*). What do you mean, Peg Inerny?

PEG. Oh, my Prince, just before dawn upon the mountains – I saw her.

HUGH (*with a look of terror*). You saw her?

PEG (*with a smile of ecstasy*). Yes, I saw my Princess Maeve!

HUGH (*turning perplexed to* O'HEYNES *and to* FINOLA). But – but didn't you say she was there in the castle?

O'HEYNES (*with a helpless look*). I thought so. I am sure I thought so. Didn't you say she was here, Finola?

FINOLA (*in a hollow voice*). Yes, father. (*As if petrified she now slowly retreats towards the castle door, keeping her eyes always fixed on* PEG.)

HUGH. Oh that Maeve should be wandering over the mountains on such a night as this.

O'HEYNES (*confusedly*). I knew some misfortune was coming. What has happened?

PEG (*with increasing ecstasy*). If you had only seen her, as I saw her upon the mountain – she was so beautiful – so happy. You would have died at the sight of such beauty, my Englishman.

HUGH (*with a look of bitterness and despair*). As if I required to be persuaded of her beauty!

PEG (*quietly*). And you will never see it again. (*Exit* FINOLA *by door leading into the castle.*)

HUGH (*suddenly subdued*). Never again – why never again?

PEG. It has gone to where he is.

HUGH (*wildly*). He – he – who is he? Speak at once. Don't you see you torture me?

PEG. The beauty that she loves.

HUGH (*growing quieter*). Ah, I understand – only that.

PEG (*calmly triumphant and ecstatic*). Like the glory of the Northern lights was his face upon the mountains. And when she saw him, her own face shone like a star.

HUGH (*as if transfixed*). Oh what does all this mean? (*Recovering himself.*) Ha – Ha – it is nothing. Of course you are only raving. That's what it is. Anyone can see that.

O'HEYNES (*with an agonised look*). She has given utterance to my worst forebodings. Tell what you saw next, Peg Inerny.

PEG. The dawn came then; and Princess Maeve went out from my sight with the stars! (*Short pause.*) (*Cries of 'help' are heard within the Castle. Then* FINOLA, *with a scared face, appears at the window over the entrance door, and throws the casement open violently.*)

FINOLA (*wailing*). Oh heavens, oh, my heavens – oh – (*looks across the room towards the window facing the abbey at right, and after a moment's awful silence says in a voice of terror*) – Maeve – she is sitting there at the open window – dead.

THE END

THE TALE OF A TOWN

PLAY IN FIVE ACTS
BY
EDWARD MARTYN

DRAMATIS PERSONÆ

JOSEPH TENCH, the Mayor.

JASPER DEAN, DANIEL LAWRENCE, THOMAS MURPHY,
VALENTINE FOLEY, RALF KIRWAN, JAMES CASSIDY,
MICHAEL LEECH, Aldermen of the Corporation
JOHN CLORAN, the Town Clerk.
GEORGE HARDMAN, an English Lord Mayor.
MISS MILLICENT FELL, an English girl, his niece,
engaged to marry Alderman Dean.
MISS CAROLINE DEAN, MISS ARABELLA DEAN
maiden aunts of Alderman Dean.
MRS BELLE CASSIDY, *wife and first cousin of Alderman Cassidy,*
sister of Alderman Leech, and cousin of the Deans.
MRS SARAH LEECH, *wife and first cousin of Alderman Leech, sister*
of Alderman Cassidy, and also cousin of the Deans.
MRS COSTIGAN, *an elderly woman, caretaker of the Town Hall.*
A PARLOUR MAID, *at Alderman Dean's house.*
A WAITER, *at the Hotel.*
Several Town Councillors, People, etc.

The action takes place during the present time at a
coast town of West Ireland.

ACT I

(The Meeting Hall of the Corporation.)
(MRS COSTIGAN sets down a large bucket in front, and then leisurely begins to sweep the floor).
(JOHN CLORAN enters carrying some papers.)

CLORAN *(with importance)*. What are you doing here, Mrs Costigan? Don't you know the Corporation are now due to meet?

MRS COSTIGAN. I'm tidying the room a bit for them, Mr Cloran.

CLORAN. You ought to have had that sweeping done long ago.

MRS COSTIGAN. Have the Corporation never been behind with their work?

CLORAN. Of course not – what do you mean? Are not they always discussing resolutions?

MRS COSTIGAN. What resolutions, Mr Cloran?

CLORAN. I'm too busy now, ma'am, to explain them.

MRS COSTIGAN. I think you'd find it hard enough to explain them, indeed.

CLORAN. That'll do, Mrs Costigan. It isn't the business of the town clerk to argue with the charwoman of the Corporation.

MRS COSTIGAN. Oh, you're a proud man to be town clerk; but I can tell you this Corporation you think so fine, isn't respected much in the town.

CLORAN. You are, no doubt, a sound authority as to the feeling of our town, ma'am.

MRS COSTIGAN. I'm in the way of hearing many complaints, Mr Cloran; and believe me if you don't begin to do the people some good, none of you will long remain where you are.

CLORAN. Oh, indeed, I suppose your associates, the proletariat, are discontented because there is not more unanimity among the members of our Corporation. Well, what do you expect? You don't suppose that where there are so many men of equal intelligence, ability, and push, ma'am – you don't suppose, I say, that they will sink their individual opinions to follow the opinion of one of their number. The idea is out of the question.

MRS COSTIGAN. If they valued the good of the town, you'd think they'd all have the one opinion.

301

CLORAN. You're quite mistaken, my good woman. All their opinions for the good of our town are of equal value. That's what it is; and so one cannot prevail over the other. What we want is a superior opinion to be offered. What we want is a leader. There's the desideratum. A man whose superiority will unite us to act in the best interests of our town – and believe me, we will find him, if we have not found him already. I think we have.

MRS COSTIGAN. You mean young Mr Jasper Dean?

CLORAN. The very man – you know he has been elected Alderman for a ward. To-day he is to take his seat here for the first time, as a member of our Corporation.

MRS COSTIGAN. Oh, I have heard the boys talking about him. They say he is a great scholar.

CLORAN. Of course – no end of a superior young man, English education, and what not – besides he has one thing especially in his favour.

MRS COSTIGAN. What's that, Mr Cloran?

CLORAN. He is in a better position, socially, than any others of the Corporation.

MRS COSTIGAN. A real gentleman, I suppose –

CLORAN. Just so – very well to do in the liquor trade – that's to be highly honoured in Ireland, ma'am. But there – I hear the members coming.

MRS COSTIGAN. Oh, I suppose it would never do for them to see me at all. (*Exit carrying her sweeping brush and bucket.*)

CLORAN. She's always trying to push herself forward the ignorant old woman. I'm sure she'd like to sit with the Corporation. (*Enter* ALDERMEN JAMES CASSIDY *and* MICHAEL LEECH.)

CLORAN. Good morning, gentlemen –

CASSIDY. Good morning, Cloran –

LEECH. Isn't the Mayor here yet?

CLORAN. No, Alderman Leech – he is very late to-day..

CASSIDY. Any news, Cloran – ?

CLORAN. Not a word, Alderman Cassidy –

CASSIDY. No sign of their granting our demands for compensation – ?

CLORAN. There is just a communication I received. I shall lay it before the Corporation to-day. It leave matters pretty nearly where they were, sir.

LEECH. This English town is behaving outrageously towards us.

CASSIDY. And apparently no steps will be taken by our Corporation. (*Alderman* RALF KIRWAN *enters.*)

KIRWAN. You are quite right. We must expect nothing from our

302

Corporation . Can you imagine a headless body with all its limbs pounding and hacking at each other. That's our Corporation, sir.

CASSIDY. You forget, Kirwan, that you are one of those limbs.

LEECH. Very true, James, very true –

KIRWAN. Yes, Cassidy – and you are the head which once thought to control them, but which they pulled off with such ease.

LEECH. That is altogether a false metaphor, Kirwan. A decapitated head can no longer be a member of a Corporation; and James is still one of our Corporation.

KIRWAN. Oh, this is a very strange body you know. Its decapitated head still keep bobbing about just because it is so light and hollow, for it hopes some day by dint of bobbing to bound up again upon the shoulders of this Corporation.

CASSIDY. I am sure by the position I hold in this town that I am entitled more than anyone to lead.

LEECH. Quite so, James – it is most impertinent of you, Kirwan.

CLORAN. Gentlemen, gentlemen – ah gentlemen, I can aver there is none of you but is entitled to lead.

KIRWAN. No, no. Cloran – we want a leader. By the way, is not young Mr Dean, our new alderman, very enthusiastic on this question of our civic rights?

CASSIDY. I am sure we all enthusiastically desire that Anglebury should pay what is due to us.

KIRWAN. Yes, yes – I know all about that. But tell me, Cloran, hasn't he been rousing quite an agitation among the electors of the wards?

CLORAN. He has, Alderman Kirwan. He is a fine young man; and the people believe him.

KIRWAN. I shouldn't wonder if he were just the man to unite this distracted Corporation.

CASSIDY. Why do you say so?

KIRWAN. Well, he appears to have the faculty of inspiring confidence. Then, you see, he has been away a good deal, and has not become mixed up in the miserable factions of this town. Besides he must have some brains, for by all accounts he distinguished himself at Oxford University.

CASSIDY. Oh, not particularly –

LEECH. Oh, not at all, I assure you –

KIRWAN. Then why does every one say he did?

LEECH. He became engaged to an English girl over there.

KIRWAN. Oh, come – that can scarcely be a reason for his reputation of University distinction.

CASSIDY. No, indeed – except that through the influence of this Miss

303

Millicent Fell he seems to have grown most fastidious in his tastes. Anyway she has had a civilizing influence with him.

KIRWAN. A droll way, certainly, of becoming civilised –

CASSIDY. Why do you say that? I hear she is a person of much refinement.

KIRWAN. Strange that their refinement should never have made them civilize themselves! Woman is the last wild animal that man will civilize.

LEECH (*puzzled*). Dear me – then I suppose Jasper's fastidiousness must be false when it arises only from her influence.

CASSIDY. Yes – I shouldn't wonder if that is why Jasper's fastidiousness makes him appear only a prig after all. He is perpetually condemning the want of honesty and principle in this town.

KIRWAN (*ironically*). No doubt a very sufficient reason for thinking him a prig –

CASSIDY. There are other reasons as well.

KIRWAN. Are there? He is young you know, and, I am sure, will improve. Everyone believes he has stuff in him.

CASSIDY. I tell you he is quite an ordinary young man.

LEECH. Of course – James, and I ought to know him. We are his relations, you know.

KIRWAN. Yes – it is easy to see you are his relations. (ALDERMAN VALENTINE FOLEY *enters*.)

FOLEY. Good morning, good morning – I hope you are all very well. I hope you are beginning to feel disposed to act in concert at last.

KIRWAN. Certainly – if only some one would come with an uncontentious proposal.

FOLEY. In honour and conscience I feel bound to take some action at the meeting to-day.

CASSIDY. Whether you obtain general support or not, Alderman Foley, will largely depend upon the nature of your action.

FOLEY. You have read my article in the 'Weekly Denouncer'?

KIRWAN. It was full of fury, as usual, against the enemies of our town.

KIRWAN. The sense of our wrongs fills me with uncontrollable indignation. It is nothing but the sense of our wrongs that keeps me before the public at all.

CLORAN. Indeed, Alderman Foley, the people do say that you have a mission among them.

FOLEY. I am naturally austere. I could never appreciate what people call the comforts and good things of this world.

KIRWAN. Bosh –

FOLEY. What 'bosh' – ? I tell you I am austere, and have a mission to

304

guard the public interests. You're not going to stultify yourself by advocating carelessness of public interests.

KIRWAN. Certainly not – I am very indignant at what I see.

LEECH. It is impossible not to feel indignant at the manner in which our sea-port has been ruined for the advantage of that English sea-port.

FOLEY. But still you and Cassidy here have voted against every measure for re-establishing our line of American steamers which that very English sea-port filched from us.

CASSIDY. We certainly dreaded injuring the English line of steamers to America.

LEECH. There are so many interests involved, you know.

KIRWAN. Of course, when certain members of our Corporation hold shares in the English line –

FOLEY. Then loyalty to our town is not to be expected.

CASSIDY. Loyalty – what do you mean?

LEECH. I thought loyalty was a term that only could be used in connection with something English.

KIRWAN. Curious that no one in this country can understand its meaning, except in such a sense –

FOLEY. Upon my honour and conscience, it is a word that is hateful to me from its perpetual association with that callous and perfidious town of Anglebury. I cannot understand our citizens supporting any of her institutions.

CASSIDY. That is not the point. What is really serious and blameable is that the town of Anglebury has not fulfilled her bargain.

LEECH. The bargain she agreed to when she took the packet station from us –that is what makes our townsmen of all parties indignant.

CASSIDY. Especially, too, when the Anglebury Corporation itself appointed a Commission to enquire into the justice of our claims, and when it has been seeking ever since to evade the recommendations of that Commission – I cannot understand this at all.

KIRWAN. I can, though. Has not the English Commission reported against the English themselves?

FOLEY. Well, now that the Commission has defined our rights, and said that we are entitled to the money due by that bargain, why, in all honour and conscience, don't we legally enforce payment?

KIRWAN. Because the man has not yet come, who will persuade our Corporation to do that, or anything else useful. (*Enter* THE MAYOR *and* ALDERMAN THOMAS MURPHY.)

MAYOR. Well, of course, Alderman Murphy, you may bring forward your motion; but I fancy it will meet with a great deal of opposition.

MURPHY. I will carry it in spite of the opposition.

KIRWAN. That's what every mover of contentious matter thinks.

MURPHY. Oh, it's a pity, isn't it, Alderman Kirwan, that you never move any resolution yourself. It's a pity you can't make a speech, isn't it?

KIRWAN. There's quite enough of talk. I only care for action.

MURPHY. No – you only care for criticising people. That is the passion of middle-aged persons.

KIRWAN. Not at all – shall I tell you what is the passion of middle age?

MURPHY. Well – what is it?

KIRWAN. Glancing down every column of the newspaper to see if your name occurs any where in it –

MURPHY. Oh, I suppose you mean that I –

KIRWAN. Yes – that is the essential passion of middle age. (*Enter* ALDERMEN DANIEL LAWRENCE *and* JASPER DEAN, *followed by other Aldermen and several Town Councillors. Then the public crowd into the place allotted to them.*)

LAWRENCE. My dear Jasper Dean, I haven't seen you for a long time. How well you're looking! I never saw you looking so well in my life. I am delighted you have become a member of our Corporation. We want men of your position and education.

DEAN. Indeed, between you and me, Alderman Lawrence, public life in our town sadly lacks that higher tone which comes from proper education.

LAWRENCE. It is for you to import that higher tone into it, my dear fellow. (THE MAYOR *and Corporation all now take their places.*)

MAYOR. Mr Cloran, will you read the minutes of the last meeting?

CLORAN. Yes, your Worship – (*Reads from a large book.*) At the last regular meeting, present, the Worshipful the Mayor, Alderman –

MURPHY. That'll do. Let us get on to the business of to-day.

LAWRENCE. Really, Alderman Murphy –

MAYOR. Order, order –

FOLEY. What is the good in taking up our time by reading all these minutes?

KIRWAN. They might have been read in less time than this dispute will take.

ALL. That'll do. Enough –

CLORAN. Then, I am not to read them, your Worship?

MURPHY. Of course, not –

MAYOR (*looking around*). Well, I suppose not –

CLORAN. Names of aldermen present and minutes taken as read – (*Laughter, during which he hands the book to* THE MAYOR.)

MAYOR. Is it your wish, gentlemen, that I sign these minutes which Alderman Murphy won't have read?

306

LAWRENCE. It is most illegal.

MURPHY. Oh, illegal be –

KIRWAN. Sign them, sign them, and let us get to work.

MAYOR. Well – I suppose I must. (*Signs the minutes in the book.*) Mr Cloran, have you written as you were ordered, to the authorities in Anglebury?

CLORAN. Yes, your Worship – in accordance with your resolution at last meeting I wrote, and have received this answer from the town clerk.

MAYOR. Well – read it then. Silence, gentlemen –

CLORAN. (*reading the letter*). – 'Sir – In reply to your communication in which you demand on the part of your Corporation a definite answer from our Corporation to your repeated claims, I am directed by our Corporation, in the first place, to remind you that it is very unusual for us to state definitely beforehand the course of action which we may eventually deem prudent to pursue. Our Corporation wish you to understand that our well-known integrity as English gentlemen (*laughter*) and generosity in our dealings with other bodies have ever hitherto rendered such a demand as yours super-fluous, and that we might have been led to expect from the union of hearts, which has recently arisen between our two towns, a complete disappearance of all doubt as to the possibility of our acting in any other than a just and generous spirit towards you. Finally, I am expressing the very general feeling of our Corporation when I now demand of you such trust in this matter of dispute as past experience should warrant you in bestowing upon us, and remain, etc., etc'.

MURPHY. We will certainly give that pack of rogues such trust as experi-ence warrants us in giving them, which means just no trust at all.

KIRWAN. Our position is not advanced one jot by that letter.

FOLEY. They will never pay this money unless they are made to.

LAWRENCE. The English are an honourable, upright people. I am sure they would pay anything that was really due.

MAYOR. Oh, I am afraid experience does not warrant any such expectation.

LAWRENCE. They never disappoint one's just expectations.

MURPHY. Well, I hope they won't disappoint yours. That's all.

LAWRENCE. What do you mean, sir?

MURPHY. Don't you expect the appointment of solicitor to the English Corporation who are wronging us? Haven't you been sniffing after it for ever so long?

LAWRENCE. How dare you, sir? Mr Mayor, I protest. I protest in the name of my honourable profession. (*Uproar, and cries of 'place hunter' –.*)

MAYOR. Order, order – (*Continued uproar –*) Order, order – let us now proceed to discuss what action we shall take in reference to the letter you have just heard read.

MURPHY. Mr Mayor, before we go into that matter, I have a resolution to propose. I beg to propose the following. (*Reads from a slip of paper.*) 'Resolved – That our Corporation shall immediately cease to employ for the printing of its notices and advertisements, that journal owned by the Member of Parliament for this town, inasmuch as he has outraged the majesty of our people by voting for a Government inspection of their public expenditure and accounts'. Mr Mayor, I think this a most important matter –

LAWRENCE. Mr Mayor, I protest, I protest.

FOLEY. What for, I want to know?

LAWRENCE. This is a most improper resolution.

MURPHY. Alderman Lawrence, what do you mean, sir?

LAWRENCE. I thought it was settled that nothing of a political nature was to be discussed at our meetings.

KIRWAN. A wise rule where no two persons can agree on politics –

LAWRENCE. Of course – besides this resolution contains a most serious breach of parliamentary privilege, and renders us liable to severe penalties.

FOLEY. Oh, come, what a great attorney you are with your discovery of mares' nests, and your bogus threats of the law. I think this is a good resolution, and ought to be passed.

LAWRENCE. No doubt you think so, when its passing means that you must get all the printing and advertisements for the 'Weekly Denouncer'.

FOLEY. I repudiate your insult to my civic integrity with indignation and disdain.

MAYOR. This is only another of his place-hunting tactics. (*Laughter and cries of 'order' –*)

MURPHY. Order, order –

LAWRENCE. Tactics or no tactics, I know what I will do, if this disgraceful resolution is passed.

MURPHY. (*with suppressed fury as he puts his face close up to that of* LAWRENCE). What will you do, Daniel Lawrence, you brute? What will you do, Daniel Lawrence, you brute? (*Uproar.*)

MAYOR. Order, order, gentlemen – (*Gesticulates and raps the table with his knuckles.*) Order, order, please, gentlemen –

KIRWAN (*laughing*). Mr Mayor, you are making more noise yourself than all the others put together.

MAYOR. Oh, gentlemen, I beg of you – let us get at once to our business.

At this rate we shall never finish. There are many of us who want to catch the four o'clock tram-car to the sea-shore.

MURPHY. But what about my resolution – ?

MAYOR. Does anyone second Alderman Murphy's resolution?

FOLEY (*a little embarrassed – after a short pause*). – Mr Mayor, I had intended to second it, but after the pitiful aspersions cast on my civic integrity in connection with this resolution, I would not stultify myself by giving it the smallest support, so I have no option but to remain neutral under the circumstances.

MAYOR. Oh well then, as no one else appears to support it, I suppose it falls to the ground. Now let us consider the letter.

LAWRENCE. Before we proceed – ahem –

MAYOR. What is it, Alderman Lawrence?

LAWRENCE. I wish to propose a resolution.

MAYOR. Oh, man alive, we shall be here all night.

LAWRENCE. It will not take a minute, Mr Mayor.

MAYOR. Well, well – go on, Alderman Lawrence.

LAWRENCE. (*reading*). – 'Resolved – That at the forthcoming Unionist celebration in our town, we lend the Meeting Hall of the Corporation to the Unionists for the holding of their assemblies and conferences'.

MURPHY. What is that I hear? What is that brazen, shameless resolution?

MAYOR. Order, order – (*Uproar.*)

KIRWAN. This is an odd resolution from one who objected to the last resolution for being political.

LAWRENCE. Alderman Kirwan, you are as great a rebel as –

MAYOR. Order, order –

KIRWAN. I am in favour of suppressing all political party demonstrations. Party politics prevent us from uniting for the interests of our town.

MAYOR. I am afraid your resolution, Alderman Lawrence, is as inadmissible as the other one.

LAWRENCE. This is disgraceful. Why shouldn't I be allowed to propose so worthy and respectable a resolution?

KIRWAN. You have proposed it. Now find a seconder.

CASSIDY. I wish to make an explanation, Mr Mayor. Under ordinary circumstances I would have seconded this resolution, but at present –

MURPHY. Oh, sit down. (*Confusion.*)

MAYOR. Order, order – gentlemen, I beg of you – I trust this incident is over. Alderman Lawrence's resolution, for want of a seconder, falls to the ground. Let us now proceed to business. Gentlemen, you have heard this letter from the town clerk of the English

Corporation. What are your opinions of it?

LAWRENCE. Mr Mayor, I submit that this is an affair in which we ought to proceed with the greatest caution. (*Murmurs and applause.*) We cannot foretell what may be the consequences, if we rush into any rash action. Our substance and our safety, I may say, depend upon our English neighbours. Are not our savings invested in the very line of steamers with which some mischievous persons among us propose to interfere?

CASSIDY. Very true – no one of any standing would wish to interfere with the English line of steamers.

LEECH. Yes, it would be a disreputable thing to do, and be fatal to our interests.

LAWRENCE. Of course, it would – but to put the question of our interests altogether aside, think of the regard and loyalty we are bound to show towards Anglebury.

LEECH. To be sure – I forgot that. It is a far more important consideration than our mere interests.

FOLEY. I repudiate it altogether. What have we to be loyal for, I should like to know?

LAWRENCE. This is perfectly disgraceful coming from one of our Corporation. What have we to be loyal for? As if the reason were not patent to everyone!

KIRWAN. Of course – because some of us have investments in the English line of steamers.

FOLEY. Mr Mayor, long ago I considered that I had gauged to the bottom of this controversy. By my article in the last number of the 'Weekly Denouncer' I demonstrated the reckless municipal folly of which every member of our Corporation was guilty except myself. (*Sensation.*) My opinions on this question before us to-day, are well known; and if every member only could fall in with them, it would be easy to save our town. I am not going to stultify myself by pretending to be infallible. At the same time it is hard to think that those who don't agree with me are not mad –

MURPHY. What an odd thing that you should be the only sane man in this town!

FOLEY. But don't you agree with me?

MURPHY. Mr Mayor, one moment –

FOLEY. I am in possession of the meeting.

MURPHY (*shouting*). Mr Mayor, I have some observations to make. (*There are cries among the Corporation and people for* MURPHY *and* FOLEY. *Those for* MURPHY *preponderate; and* FOLEY *sits down.*)

310

MAYOR (*thumping the table*). Silence, silence –

MURPHY. Mr Mayor, this matter before the Corporation would be easily settled if only we could agree to one thing. We must fight for the restoration of the American line of steamers to our town –

LAWRENCE. You want to ruin us by dissevering our connection with our English neighbours. Separatist principles mean ruin.

MURPHY. Our town is ruined by Unionist principles.

MAYOR. Gentlemen, I cannot allow this wrangling.

CLORAN. Ah, gentlemen, don't –

CASSIDY. Mr Mayor, I have long been convinced that we shall never obtain our rights until some one of family and position is made leader –

LEECH. That's true, James – very true, James – (*Murmurs.*)

CASSIDY. There is only one person in this town of sufficient position to lead. I ought to be the head of the family –

MURPHY. Who the dickens cares for you or your family? (*Uproar.*)

MAYOR. Gentlemen, gentlemen, order – for goodness sake order –

DEAN. Mr Mayor, may I saw a few words?

MAYOR. Certainly, Alderman Dean – silence, gentlemen, please –

DEAN. Mr Mayor, if one so new at municipal business as I am, might presume to advise gentlemen so experienced, I would suggest that each of us should keep more strictly to the questions before us.

KIRWAN. Hear, hear –

DEAN. We have really nothing to do now with any question except whether we shall decide or not decide to enforce payment of what is due to us. All the other matters may be discussed again at their proper time. We must first run down the thief, and when we have recovered our property, each man may fight for whatever he wishes afterwards. (*Cheers.*) I am glad that, so far, all seem to be of my opinion.

LAWRENCE. Not all, by any means, Alderman Dean –

MURPHY. Yes, all, except a few place-hunters.

KIRWAN. Is our town to miss every advantage for the sake of a few officials? (*Cheers.*)

DEAN. Mr Mayor, we are the owners of property in this town. We have nothing to do with officials. What interest can it be to us whether this or that official is or is not making money by our connection with Anglebury? There is nothing particularly interesting in the fact of other people making money. We ought therefore not to consider such people at all.

LAWRENCE. Alderman Dean, I'm afraid you're not a sound politician. I thought you were a different man. sir.

311

DEAN. My only thoughts are for the general good of our town. (*Cheers.*)
I hope our different representatives of popular feeling will be patient
while I explain what I know to be the real interest of our citizens,
and what our citizens will afterwards acknowledge as their best
interest.

LAWRENCE. Well, what is this grand discovery?

DEAN. It is that each of us should sink his particular plan of action in
a combined effort for the general good of our town. (*Cheers.*)

LAWRENCE. We are far too independent for that.

DEAN. It is because we are becoming so independent, that we see the
necessity of being united. (*Cheers.*)

MURPHY. Very true, very true –

DEAN. Our aim must be that higher usefulness which is so necessary for
spirited public action. We must for once cease to think of ourselves
as individuals, and think of ourselves only as so many members
belonging to the body of our town. (*Hear, hear.*) It is very encouraging to know that you agree with me. Well, then, admitting what
I say is right, how ought you to meet the present crisis? How do we
stand in our public capacity? We are the Corporation of a Town
unrivalled for its natural advantages, and possessing the supreme
fortune of being the nearest port in Europe to America. (*Hear, hear.*)
Mr Mayor, until some years ago we enjoyed the results of that good
fortune. There was direct communication between our town and the
United States. Our town was the most important packet station in
the three Kingdoms. The American mails arriving here could be
delivered in London much sooner than it was possible to deliver
them when landed at any other port. Mr Mayor, we were deprived
of our American packet station. We were deprived of it by that
English town which now enjoys the advantage in our stead.
(*Groans.*) What ever are our differences of opinion, we must all
agree to that. (*Hear, hear.*)

LAWRENCE. Mr Mayor, I do not agree to it. I agree to nothing.
(*Murmurs.*)

DEAN. I need not dwell now upon the treachery of those among our
Corporation who at that time took bribes from the English for their
votes which deprived us of our packet station. They would never
have dared to vote thus against the wishes and sentiments of our
fellow-citizens, if it had not been for this indemnity which
Anglebury then agreed to pay us, and which it was alleged would
bring us such wealth as we never before enjoyed, even when in
possession of our packet station. For it was agreed that we were to
receive a percentage on all harbour rates in Anglebury, where the

shipping was known to be enormous. Not one penny of that percentage or indemnity has ever since been paid. That is the state of affairs which we have met to consider to-day. (*Hear, hear.*) Many of us, Mr Mayor, differ widely in our municipal opinions. For reasons which I need not enter into, several of my colleagues and I myself are now opposed to the agitation for restoring to our town her packet station. But there is one point upon which we all of us – even the most extreme of each section – agree as one man, and it is, that our rightful percentage should be paid to us.

LAWRENCE. Indeed sir, what is really due ought to be paid. We are all agreed to that. But what is it that is really due? (*Oh, oh.*)

DEAN. To hear Alderman Lawrence admit even so much, is satisfactory. Every citizen who has the interest of our town at heart must feel the justice of our claim, now that he has read the report of the Commission of Arbitration which Anglebury herself appointed to enquire into the merits of our dispute. What has the report of these financial experts said, Mr Mayor? It has said that for several years past we have been practically swindled out of a large sum of money.

LAWRENCE. Strong language, strong language, Mr Mayor –

MURPHY. Not one bit too strong – go on, Alderman Dean. We are all with you. (*Hear, hear, and cheers.*)

DEAN. Well, Mr Mayor, we have made several appeals to our rich debtor for payment. In what spirit has she received these appeals? We have all heard her town clerk's last letter to-day. Is it a candid letter? Is it the answer of a town that wishes to act justly? (*No, no.*) Are we to be thus put off and played with by the stranger, while our town is daily impoverished by the stranger's defalcations? (*Tremendous cheers.*) No, sir, our free and independent Corporation, I am sure, will never consent to such treatment of our town. After all what have we but our town? Do we not stand or fall together? If she is ruined, will not we – yes, every class among us – be ruined also? (*Hear, hear.*) We must therefore cast to the winds that deference to England which makes us weak. We must be strong and self-sacrificing and ready to sink all our feelings of class and other differences in a firm resolve to unite for obtaining our just rights. We have only to agree upon taking legal proceedings, and the Law will very soon compel our debtor to disgorge –

MURPHY. I'll unite with anyone to do that.

FOLEY. So will I, upon my honour and conscience.

DEAN. Then let me appeal to all members of our Corporation to join hands. While we are disputing about one private interest or another, our town is fast sinking into hopeless decay. Nothing but united

313

action to obtain this rich subsidy can save her fortunes.

SEVERAL VOICES. We are all with you. We are all ready to unite.

DEAN. I am overjoyed to hear it. For I look upon our obtaining this subsidy to be so necessary that although, as you know, I am opposed to the restoration of the packet station now to our town, and have always with my family been a loyal supporter of our connection with Anglebury port, still, if the authorities in that port persist in denying us justice, and in casting us back upon civic ruin, then I for one do solemnly declare, that I am prepared to shake off all my loyalty towards so perfidious a people, and to fight till death for the existence of our beloved town. (*Tremendous and prolonged cheering and enthusiasm.*) Mr Mayor, I beg to move that immediate legal proceedings be taken for the recovery of this debt of so many years' accumulation.

MURPHY. I beg to second that resolution. (*Cheers.*)

LAWRENCE. Mr Mayor, it is with very considerable pain that I have listened to the able speech of my respected and cultured young friend, Alderman Dean. I feel it is a disadvantage to all the respectable people of our town and a disadvantage to his own family that such rare abilities as his, should not be used in a cause more fit for reputable approbation. I feel that such abilities are eminently calculated to forward those most sacred principles of loyalty to Anglebury. Indeed my ears could hardly make me believe that he advocated action so discourteous towards a Corporation whose friendship is of paramount importance to us. (*Murmurs.*) I sincerely trust that our Corporation will do nothing to alienate the sympathy of our valued English friends. (*Uproar.*)

SEVERAL VOICES. Put the resolution. Put the resolution.

LAWRENCE. Will I not be listened to?

MURPHY. We have heard too much from you long ago.

LAWRENCE. Mr Mayor, I protest. (*Uproar, during which he is forced to sit down.*)

CASSIDY (*to* LEECH). It is very extraordinary how Jasper has brought the Corporation with him.

LEECH (*to* CASSIDY). Most extraordinary – because he really hasn't much in him, you know.

CASSIDY (*to* LEECH). I think his arguments quite wrong. However, I suppose we cannot go against such an unanimous burst of civic opinion.

LEECH (*to* CASSIDY). Oh, no – besides he is one of the family; and it wouldn't look well if we took an active part in opposing him.

MAYOR. Let all who are in favour of the resolution say 'aye'.

SEVERAL VOICES. Aye, aye –

MAYOR. The contrary say 'no'.

LAWRENCE. No – (*Laughter.*)

MAYOR. The 'ayes' have it. (*Taking out his watch.*) We shall catch the four o'clock tram-car after all. (*Laughter and wild excitement – several gather with congratulations around* JASPER DEAN, *while all move out of the room.*)

CURTAIN

ACT II

(Drawing-room in JASPER DEAN'S *house.)*
(THE MISSES CAROLINE *and* ARABELLA DEAN *are seated by an afternoon tea-table.)*

ARABELLA. Is it not time that Millicent arrived, Caroline?

CAROLINE. She should be here now very soon.

ARABELLA. And Jasper not here – won't she think it odd if he is not at home to receive her when she comes?

CAROLINE. Millicent Fell is a sensible girl, Arabella, and knows that the administration of our town is more important to an alderman than even the welcoming of his intended bride. Jasper, no doubt, has much to transact at the Corporation on this his first day of civic life.

ARABELLA. I hope he will mind his health and keep always on the winning side.

CAROLINE. Arabella, you are in the habit of talking irrelevantly. The one important thing is that Jasper should take a leading position in the government of our town.

ARABELLA. I am sure I should like our dear nephew to do what suited him best. Ever since he lost his parents and came under our care, my one thought has always been for the happiness of our brother's child.

CAROLINE. Of course – I know that. However you don't seem to realise what his wealth and education entitle him to. Arabella, he should become the leader in our municipal deliberations.

ARABELLA. I hope they won't cause him trouble.

CAROLINE. Cause him trouble? – no, the Corporation will be quite different when he has infused into it that higher tone he speaks of.

ARABELLA. What sort of a thing is 'higher tone,' Caroline?

CAROLINE. Oh, you know what it is, of course, Arabella. Jasper is always talking about it, since he went to Oxford. It is the higher tone, you know. Something superior and English you know – wait – I hear people coming. (*Enter* MRS BELLE CASSIDY *and* MRS SARAH LEECH.)

MRS CASSIDY. Caroline, we thought we should find Jasper at home. We want to hear about his first experience at the Corporation.

MRS LEECH. Indeed that wasn't what brought you here at all, Belle.

MRS CASSIDY. I don't understand you, Sarah.

ARABELLA. We expect Jasper at any time.

CAROLINE. But what is Sarah hinting at?

MRS CASSIDY. Goodness only knows. She is always making a history out of nothing.

MRS LEECH. You know you have come on a visit of inspection, Belle.

MRS CASSIDY. Inspection of what – ?

MRS LEECH. Why, the bride-elect, of course – is she here, Caroline? Where are you hiding her? (*She screams with laughter.*)

CAROLINE. Millicent has not yet arrived. The boat was late; so she missed the early train from Dublin this morning.

ARABELLA. But she has telegraphed that she is coming by a later one. She will be here this afternoon.

MRS CASSIDY. Oh, then, it is likely we may see her.

MRS LEECH. I wonder what she is like.

ARABELLA. We have never seen her. But Jasper raves about her.

CAROLINE. You know, of course, that he became engaged to her when he was in England. She is the niece of Mr George Hardman, the Mayor of Anglebury, which, they say, owes us this subsidy.

MRS LEECH. How very queer – perhaps the wedding may lead to a settlement of the question?

CAROLINE. A good marriage usually settles everything, Sarah.

MRS CASSIDY. What sense you always have, Caroline!

MRS LEECH. You both must be dying of curiosity to see her.

CAROLINE. We are most anxious to become acquainted with her; and it is for that very purpose that Jasper has asked her over to stay with us.

MRS CASSIDY. Of course, Caroline – what could be more natural than that he should be anxious for your approval of his choice?

CAROLINE. He need not fear that we shall not appreciate her; for she is an heiress with a fine fortune. Besides, by the most trustworthy accounts, she is a very superior English girl.

ARABELLA. And an ardent and earnest politician too – so Jasper says.

MRS LEECH. Oh my gracious – that means a radical, doesn't it?

CAROLINE. Sarah, the English radicals are now quite respectable.

MRS LEECH. Well, I suppose you understand all about it.

MRS CASSIDY. Yes – Caroline always understands and has such care for the credit of our family, likewise.

MRS LEECH. That's a hit at me. Do you hear her, Caroline? What have I done?

CAROLINE. Don't ask me, Sarah. Ask your conscience.

MRS LEECH. One would think I was a stranger who had come into the

317

family, and not a first cousin to my husband and sister to Belle's husband, and, I may say, some sort of cousin more or less near to all the rest of the family. And then again think of Belle being sister to my husband and first cousin to me, and our husbands first cousins to each other – think of all that, and isn't it queer that she should find such fault with me.

ARABELLA. I suppose it is the privilege of near relationship, my dear.

MRS CASSIDY. No – but I am greatly distressed at Sarah's general want of dignity. It seems extraordinary in a person who, after all, is so much one of the family.

CAROLINE. I should have thought that one would feel more impressed by the fact of belonging to such a family.

MRS CASSIDY. It is not everyone has your sense, Caroline.

MRS LEECH. Ah, I am afraid she has too much.

CAROLINE. One cannot have too much.

MRS LEECH. You will do something very foolish soon, Caroline,

ARABELLA. Ha, ha, that is what I have always thought.

CAROLINE. That is what the foolish always say to persons of sense.

MRS LEECH. Is it a sensible thing, Caroline, at your age to think of getting married?

CAROLINE. Who ever said I thought of such a thing? How dare you, Sarah Leech?

ARABELLA. Goodness, gracious, we're going to have a family quarrel.

MRS CASSIDY. Sarah, you have no right to make such insinuations about Caroline.

MRS LEECH. Ah – I didn't know there was any harm. She has so much money, you know; and all the family have been talking of her and Alderman Foley –

MRS CASSIDY. Hold your tongue, Sarah Leech. Don't mind her, Caroline. I never mentioned your name with that of Alderman Foley. Never – I wouldn't do such a thing, Caroline.

CAROLINE. You are always most inaccurate in your assertions, Sarah Leech. You have even less sense than Arabella, with all your mischievous cunning.

MRS CASSIDY. It is not everyone has your sense, Caroline. Jasper was indeed fortunate to have found a guardian in you.

ARABELLA. I am sure the luck was all on our side. The dear boy has been such a source of happiness to us.

CAROLINE. Yes, Arabella, in spite of all you have done to spoil him –

MRS LEECH. Never mind, Caroline. *You* made up for all Arabella's spoiling by your lecturing of him.

318

CAROLINE. I don't understand such impertinent remarks, Sarah. It was my duty to direct his education, and form his mind to a sense of his family responsibilities.

MRS CASSIDY. Of course, Caroline – and now you must feel much satisfaction with the result of all.

CAROLINE. I hope I have rendered him fit to take the lead in our municipal life, Belle.

MRS LEECH. If he really is what you want to make him, Caroline, I'm afraid he'll never take the lead anywhere. (*A loud knocking at the street door and a violent ringing of the bell are heard.*)

MRS LEECH. That must be she. (THE MAID *enters.*)

THE MAID. Miss Fell. (MISS MILLICENT FELL *enters. Exit* THE MAID.)

CAROLINE (*to* MILLICENT). We are delighted to see you, my dear.

MILLICENT. Thank you. You are very kind. How do you do? (*To* ARABELLA.) How do you do?

ARABELLA. These are our cousins, Mrs Belle Cassidy and Mrs Sarah Leech.

MILLICENT. How do you do? How do you do?

MRS LEECH. (*aside to* MRS CASSIDY). Look at her. Isn't she very queer? Did you ever see such clothes?

MRS CASSIDY. She has an emphatic manner, Sarah.

MRS LEECH. Yes, she said, 'How do you do?' as if the fate of the world depended upon it.

ARABELLA. Jasper says you are very fond of Ireland, Miss Millicent.

MILLICENT. Oh yes, I love dear Ireland, and the dear Irish.

CAROLINE. How very fortunate for Jasper my dear.

ARABELLA. Jasper is the head of our family.

MRS CASSIDY. Well, he certainly is by primo-geniture, although there is another more qualified in many ways to lead.

ARABELLA. Belle, you and your husband were always jealous of Jasper.

CAROLINE. That will do now. He happens to be the head. And his education gives him a further right to take the lead.

MRS LEECH. But what thing is he to take the lead in, Caroline?

CAROLINE. He is to take the lead, Sarah; and if you had any sense of the family dignity, you wouldn't always ask such questions. (*Enter* ALDERMEN JAMES CASSIDY *and* MICHAEL LEECH.)

CASSIDY (*perceiving* MILLICENT). Oh, Michael, what a remarkable fine woman –

LEECH. You're right, James. She is. What taste you have!

CAROLINE. James, this is Miss Millicent Fell.

MILLICENT (*to* CASSIDY *and* LEECH). How do you do? How do you do?

CASSIDY. You must find our town, Miss Fell, rather poor looking after your handsome opulent English cities.

MILLICENT. Oh, I think it is charming. I think everything you do is so charming.

LEECH. We do our best though conscious of our inferiority.

CASSIDY. We are doing our best to introduce your grand English customs into our town.

MRS CASSIDY (*approvingly*). Have you come from the Corporation, James?

CASSIDY. Yes, yes – the proceedings are finished.

ARABELLA. I wonder Jasper isn't here.

CASSIDY (*laughing*). Oh, Jasper – he has been carrying all before him.

CAROLINE. Why – what has he done? How has he comported himself?

CASSIDY. He has succeeded in uniting for once the whole Corporation.

LEECH. Yes – it seems a wonderful thing; but he has done it. I am sure no one ever would have thought he could.

CAROLINE. Ha – I thought so. You see my training has already borne fruit.

MILLICENT. I always knew he only wanted an opportunity to prove himself great.

ARABELLA. He was always great.

CAROLINE. No, Arabella, he was great only after the education I gave him.

CASSIDY. What a sensible woman Caroline always is.

LEECH. Yes – sound common sense, James – sound common sense –

MILLICENT. Oh I hate reservations in admiration. Why should we not say what we feel is so?

MRS LEECH. Because we may afterwards be disappointed perhaps.

CASSIDY. You have, doubtless, had many opportunities, Miss Fell, of judging the abilities of Jasper.

MILLICENT. Yes – we have been acquainted in England for some time.

CAROLINE. Jasper has made some advantageous acquaintances at Oxford, you know.

MILLICENT. My cousin, George Hardman, junior, was a friend of his there. He brought him during one vacation to stay at his father's, the mayor's house. That is how I first met Jasper.

CAROLINE. You always live at Anglebury with your uncle, the mayor. Don't you, my dear?

MILLICENT. Oh, yes – he is like a father to me.

MRS LEECH. Better than many fathers, I should think, when he has found so good a husband for you.

MILLICENT. Found a husband for me – I don't understand you.

MRS LEECH. Oh, then, you found him for yourself. She is an independent young lady. Isn't she, Caroline?

CAROLINE. Sarah, you forget you are one of the family.

CASSIDY. Sarah, you are perpetually saying the most embarrassing things. (*A noise of voices is heard outside.*)

ARABELLA. Here is Jasper coming. (*Enter* ALDERMEN JASPER DEAN *and* RALF KIRWAN.)

DEAN (*at the door to* KIRWAN). That's just it. Don't you see? We'll have them in such terror now that they must give in to us. (*Perceiving* MILLICENT *and advancing.*) Millicent, how glad I am to see you! When did you arrive? How are you?

MILLICENT. I am very well, Jasper. So you have made a most successful first appearance at the Corporation.

DEAN. Indeed I have. This is my friend, Alderman Kirwan. Let me introduce you, Millicent.

KIRWAN (*bowing*). He has exceeded our wildest expectations, Miss Fell.

DEAN. Would you believe it the whole Corporation has risen, like one man, to my speech? Now I lead the town.

MILLICENT. I do not wonder. This was bound to happen some day.

DEAN (*amorously*). Millicent, I have longed that some day you might feel proud of me.

MILLICENT (*with great tenderness*). Oh, Jasper, I am so proud of you.

CAROLINE. And now, my dear Jasper, you must tell us exactly how it all happened.

ARABELLA. Yes, we are dying to hear from your own mouth the narrative of your triumph.

MILLICENT. Do tell us Jasper, how it all happened. What was the question that led to your success?

DEAN. Oh, the simplest question in the world –

KIRWAN. In fact so simple that it is surprising no one else ever made a success of it before –

MILLICENT. Ah, Alderman Kirwan, you require genius to show the way.

MRS CASSIDY. Well, let us hear what the question was.

MRS LEECH. Yes, indeed – I wonder none of you ever thought of asking that before.

KIRWAN. To be sure – that is the way with you ladies. You always leave the most important matter for the postscript.

MRS LEECH. Oh, you mustn't include me, Alderman Kirwan. I thought of it. But as they generally snub me, I was afraid to ask.

DEAN. I thought you all knew that to-day the Corporation were to consider our claims against Anglebury.

MILLICENT. Oh, I have often heard my uncle speak about this. He says there is nothing in your claims.

DEAN. He says that; does he?

MILLICENT. Yes – why Jasper.

DEAN. Because to-day our Corporation had to consider a letter on our claims from the town clerk of Anglebury.

MILLICENT. I suppose this letter explained the whole matter.

DEAN. Well, the curious thing about it was that it explained nothing at all.

MRS CASSIDY. How very odd – !

DEAN. In fact none of us could make out what it meant.

KIRWAN. Except, vaguely, that we had nothing to expect in satisfaction of our claims –

LEECH. Yes – I think the Corporation seemed somehow convinced of that.

KIRWAN. Convinced or not they were hopelessly at variance about what course to pursue, until our friend here united and directed their energies by a most effective speech.

CASSIDY. That is very true.

LEECH. No one can deny that, James.

ARABELLA. How noble of you, Jasper – !

CAROLINE. What did you say, Jasper, that it should succeed so wonderfully in uniting the Corporation?

DEAN. Oh, I simply explained that we had a legal right to the payment of our claims which the report of the Commission had strengthened and defined; and then I vehemently urged that the law should be set in motion to enforce this payment.

KIRWAN. It seems very simple; doesn't it?

CASSIDY. Yes, indeed – and the wonder is that no-one ever before could do what he has done.

CAROLINE. None of the rest have his education. See the magnificent education that I gave him.

KIRWAN. Pshaw – education had nothing to do with it. The more of this quack modern education, the worse discernment, the worse literature, the worse taste –

MRS LEECH. What does he mean? None of us can understand him.

CASSIDY (*evasively*). Oh, Kirwan, questions of literature and taste have never been subjects of serious attention to the *elite* of our town.

KIRWAN. Then what is all the education for?

CAROLINE. Education should lead to practical results – not to things of such mere sentiment as you mention. They are unworthy of a person of sense.

KIRWAN. What do you mean by practical results?

CAROLINE. Oh, you know what they are. The obtaining of

appointments, for instance –

MRS LEECH. Yes, indeed – but for appointments I should like to know what would be the use of any education.

DEAN. Sarah, you have often a crude way of expressing what is dimly in the minds of the family.

MRS CASSIDY. Sarah is unfortunately a great trial to us all.

MRS LEECH. Ah – there I am snubbed again, and I said nothing more than Caroline said, after all.

CAROLINE. You are greatly mistaken, Sarah. I would not limit the usefulness of education merely to obtaining appointments. I think a most legitimate outcome of its usefulness consists in its fitting a man to take the lead amongst his fellows.

MRS CASSIDY. (*tentatively*). James, don't you think that others, perhaps, might have hesitated before they sought leadership by the *means* which Jasper used?

LEECH. Well indeed, I must confess the same idea crossed my mind too.

MILLICENT. I was waiting to see if anyone had doubts about these means.

CAROLINE. (*to* MILLICENT). What, my dear – aren't you satisfied?

MILLICENT. Well you know it *was* a strong measure.

CASSIDY. So I thought at the time.

CAROLINE. Did you? Well if you did, why didn't you prevent Jasper? What is the use of your pretending to lead, if you could not do even that much for the family?

MRS LEECH. I knew Jasper's action would soon be criticised by the family.

KIRWAN. Well, I can tell you all that he has done a splendid work.

DEAN. Yes, it is splendid for the first time to feel one's power. It is splendid to put one's soul into men, and make them act to forward one's most cherished ideas. Isn't it so, Millicent? But why are you looking so solemn?

MILLICENT (*with a faint smile*). Oh, Jasper – of course, I desire everything that is for your good.

DEAN. And don't you think my success to-day for my good?

MILLICENT. Well, I don't know. It is all so sudden.

DEAN. Oh come, let us have no hesitations. I am in such spirits this evening.

KIRWAN. I hope nothing will happen to damp your spirits.

DEAN. I shall not allow anything to do so, I can tell you.

CAROLINE. Don't you think, Jasper, you had better consider before you do anything rash.

DEAN. Don't be afraid, Aunt Caroline. I shall do nothing rash. Come,

Kirwan, to the study. I want to show you the rough draft I have made of a letter which our solicitor can send to Anglebury. (*Exeunt* JASPER DEAN *and* RALF KIRWAN.)

CAROLINE. James, I wonder you did not tell us at once what this question was.

CASSIDY. You mean the question upon which Jasper took the lead.

CAROLINE. Of course –

CASSIDY. Oh, I forgot at the moment. It didn't seem necessary somehow.

LEECH. We thought, Caroline, that you knew there was to be a discussion about our claims against Anglebury.

CASSIDY. Besides, I believed the only thing you would be interested to know was that Jasper took the lead.

MRS CASSIDY. Yes indeed, Caroline, you always have been saying that he must take the lead.

CAROLINE. To be sure I have. At the same time it is essential that the means by which he is to take the lead, should be considered.

MRS LEECH. Ah, that is something new. Fancy, something new from Caroline –

MRS CASSIDY. To be sure we have never heard Caroline say this before, although she has often said that Jasper should lead.

CAROLINE. But of course the importance of the means being strictly respectable was always understood.

MRS LEECH. Isn't it queer that so important a matter should only have been understood? Fancy, I have caught Caroline. (*She laughs immoderately.*)

CAROLINE (*furious*). Sarah, I wonder you are not ashamed to make such an exhibition of yourself.

MRS CASSIDY. Come away, Sarah. You have no idea of behaving with dignity.

LEECH. Yes – on the whole we had better go.

CASSIDY. Good-bye Caroline. Of course a woman like you could not fail to have considered always the importance of the means.

LEECH. Of course Caroline's judgment is never at fault. (*Exeunt amidst general leave takings* ALDERMAN JAMES CASSIDY, MRS CASSIDY, ALDERMAN MICHAEL LEECH, *and* MRS LEECH.)

MILLICENT. I do not feel comfortable about Jasper.

CAROLINE. You mean about this action he has taken to-day.

MILLICENT. Yes – I wonder will it lead to a breach with his English friends.

ARABELLA. Why should it? Why should people quarrel with him because he does what he thinks right?

CAROLINE (*not heeding her*). I wonder will they resent it.

MILLICENT. It would be dreadful if they did. It would ruin his prospects.

CAROLINE. Do you really think so, my dear?

MILLICENT. We should be completely ostracised in England, and should be obliged to live over here altogether.

ARABELLA. You ought not to think that a misfortune, my dear. You who love dear Ireland and the dear Irish –

MILLICENT. O yes, a misfortune, of course –

CAROLINE. It would be dreadful for his family, if Jasper were in any way to incur the disapprobation of any respectable friends.

ARABELLA. The family, the family again – that's all you think of. What is the family compared to Jasper himself?

CAROLINE. I'm afraid, Arabella, your excitement is getting beyond your control. (*Exit* ARABELLA *in a temper.*)

MILLICENT. I wish I could be certain what is best to do.

CAROLINE. Does your uncle, the mayor, know of this resolution of our Corporation?

MILLICENT. Not yet, I should think –

CAROLINE. Perhaps, my dear, you might write to him. Just say that Jasper has no intention of acting in a hostile manner against Anglebury.

MILLICENT. Would it be safe to say that? Perhaps I had better telegraph the bare facts to him at once.

CAROLINE. Perhaps that would be best. There are forms of telegram there on the writing-table.

MILLICENT. (*as she writes.*) I should not be surprised if this telegram brought him over here at once.

CAROLINE. I'm sure I hope it may. His presence and advice would be of great advantage to us in this emergency.

CURTAIN

ACT III

(The same scene as in the last act.)
(Enter ALDERMEN JASPER DEAN *and* VALENTINE FOLEY.*)*

FOLEY. Well – I will just come in for a moment. I cannot stay long now.

DEAN. Why – where have you to go?

FOLEY. I was hurrying to the office of the 'Weekly Denouncer' when you stopped me.

DEAN. Oh, wait a while. I want to speak to you about this public meeting.

FOLEY. I suppose you know it is settled to take place the day after to-morrow. You have heard of our solicitor's letter: haven't you?

DEAN. I should think so. He lost no time in writing to the English corporation. That was good business, Foley.

FOLEY. Yes – the letter was a fine plain-spoken one.

DEAN. We are really united at last.

FOLEY. We are, and have the law on our side as well: so we will force those stubborn English down on their knees.

DEAN. My goodness, what an awakening this will be to them!

FOLEY. They have always counted on our disunion for doing whatever they wished to our town.

DEAN. Very true – it was time that this fatal disunion should cease. Have you written your article yet?

FOLEY. I have, and upon my honour and conscience, I think I have exposed the whole situation in a convincing light.

DEAN. I am glad to hear it. You are a power, Foley.

FOLEY. Power – what is my power to yours? What an enviable position, Dean, you have got yourself into!

DEAN. I don't know. It will require a great effort to keep up to the level of the work.

FOLEY. If only I had your luck in hitting upon this vein, I wouldn't much mind what effort the work entailed.

DEAN. Oh, my dear fellow, the strain may become almost unbearable.

FOLEY. You don't mean to say you are already beginning to tire of the work.

DEAN. No- no, Foley, of course not – I only mean that I hope I shall be able to keep all of you united, and as enthusiastic for the cause as I am myself. That is all.

FOLEY. Never fear us. Upon my honour and conscience, we shall stand by you to a man. At this monster meeting of our citizens when you are to be in the chair –

DEAN. Who said I was to be in the chair?

FOLEY. Why, who else could be in the chair? We wish this meeting to be unanimous as an expression of our citizens' approval. Nothing short of that will give the Corporation full confidence in its action. What better man could we have in the chair than he who united the Corporation?

DEAN. Oh – if you put it that way, of course I shall take the chair. (MILLICENT FELL *enters.*)

MILLICENT. Fancy the news I have for you, Jasper –

DEAN. What can it be, Millicent?

MILLICENT. My uncle is coming here to-day.

DEAN. Mayor Hardman from England – ?

MILLICENT. Yes, he sent a telegram saying he will arrive by the mail this morning.

DEAN. I shall be very glad to see him.

FOLEY. He must have learned very quickly the news here.

MILLICENT (*to* DEAN). This gentleman – what does he say?

FOLEY. Oh – nothing – nothing, I assure you Miss –

DEAN. Millicent, let me introduce my friend Alderman Valentine Foley to you. He is the proprietor and editor of the 'Weekly Denouncer', and is our ablest man on the Press.

MILLICENT. To be an able man on the Press is to personify everything that is beautiful in modern civilisation, Alderman Foley.

FOLEY (*modestly*). Well – the Press does give somehow distinction to even the most ordinary man.

MILLICENT. It should be an efficient means for intellectualising your town.

FOLEY (*suddenly inspired*). Miss Fell, what an intellectual influence you might be to us!

DEAN. Like the most earnest of her townspeople she is in deep sympathy with our town.

MILLICENT. I really do love your town you know.

FOLEY. Miss Fell, I have heard of your riches. I now see you are rich in sympathy also.

MILLICENT. Sympathy is of greater value than money.

FOLEY. Yes – I always have thought that. Upon my honour and conscience I really despise money.

DEAN. Such a sentiment is sure to make an impression on so generous a nature as that of Miss Fell.

FOLEY (*ardently*). My fondest dream would be to make a favourable impression on Miss Fell.

MILLICENT. Gracious, what do you mean?

FOLEY. I would not stultify myself by pretending to deny how proud I should feel to stand in the good graces of such a lady. Good-bye Miss Fell. I hope I may be honoured by meeting you soon again. I must go to my office, Dean, and have the programme for the meeting printed at once. Good-bye for the present. (*Exit.*)

MILLICENT. That's a very forward fellow. He gives me the idea of an adventurer. Oh, Jasper, you are so superior to those people around you. My uncle has such a high opinion of you.

DEAN. I hope I shall never disappoint either of you. But tell me, Millicent, why is your uncle coming here so suddenly?

MILLICENT. Shall I tell you? Well – I will be straightforward. Yes – we English are a straightforward people. Well, I telegraphed to him yesterday evening.

DEAN. *You* telegraphed to him?

MILLICENT. Yes, Jasper – don't be angry.

DEAN. I am not angry. Only surprised – but why did you do this?

MILLICENT. I was guided by my woman's instinct, Jasper.

DEAN. Explain. I do not understand.

MILLICENT. Something told me that you were going to act injuriously to yourself.

DEAN. To myself – ?

MILLICENT. Yes – are you not taking part in a movement against our town? Is not that injurious to you?

DEAN. I don't see it.

MILLICENT. Well, anyhow I thought it best that you should have the benefit of my uncle's advice. He is such an able man, and you know how high an opinion he has of you.

DEAN. As I said before I shall be very glad to see him. It will be interesting to hear what he has to say. I am sure his sense of justice will force him to acknowledge our claims.

MILLICENT. I am sure he would be the last person to do anything unjust.

DEAN. When he comes, you will soon see that I am not acting injuriously to myself.

MILLICENT. I hope so.

DEAN. You will see this difficulty arranged, Millicent. You need not fear that I will do anything to make me less worthy of you.

MILLICENT. No, no, Jasper, I am not thinking for a moment of such a

328

thing.

DEAN. As it is I am not worthy of you, nor ever could be: but I shall always try not to become less so.

MILLICENT. Jasper, you have a noble nature. It is because I admire your character and talents that I am now so anxious. I would not for worlds you did the slightest thing to tarnish them.

DEAN. There is really no necessity for all this fear, Millicent.

MILLICENT. In this movement you are surrounded by so many adventurers.

DEAN. Indeed I beg your pardon. I am surrounded by the most considerable men in the town. But, Millicent, let us not talk about these subject. You are my chief interest in life. Let me hear about you and your interests.

MILLICENT. My greatest interest is your welfare, Jasper. (MISS CAROLINE DEAN *enters*.)

CAROLINE. Oh – I am interrupting an agreeable conversation. I shall retire.

DEAN. Not at all, Aunt Caroline, not at all – it is time for me to go to my committee meeting now. I shall not be long away, Millicent. (*Exit*.)

CAROLINE. I hope you have been reasoning with him, my dear.

MILLICENT. I tried to; but he seemed not to mind me.

CAROLINE. I am sorry to say his manners are not of the best.

MILLICENT. Oh, I think they are very well.

CAROLINE. Is it his manners? No, my dear, I regret that with all his education, he has never acquired the art of making himself agreeable to the ladies.

MILLICENT. So much the better, Miss Dean – I am sure I don't know what you would have him do.

CAROLINE. It is hard, of course, to lay down special rules. But generally speaking he is too serious – too candid. He is not sufficiently gay and complimentary.

MILLICENT. So much the better – one cannot do better than be perfectly natural.

CAROLINE. If one merely follows nature one becomes a perfect savage. No –one must cultivate the graces. I could never teach him to enter a room properly, my dear. He never would learn to bow and smile pleasantly at the door when coming in. He never was ready with repartee, and light persiflage. It is such brilliancy that dazzles the eyes of the ladies.

MILLICENT. I don't want him to do such things at all. They are quite unnecessary.

CAROLINE. It's well you think so my dear; for I suppose you would now find it hard to change him. He has become more and more undisciplined of late.

MILLICENT. Indeed I am afraid he is being urged on by a band of adventurers.

CAROLINE. Where it will end goodness knows! Just imagine the misfortune if he were to sully his family's reputation for respectability.

MILLICENT. I really don't know what to think. It will be a great relief when my uncle arrives.

CAROLINE. From what I hear of his ability and sense, I should certainly like to consult him.

MILLICENT. He ought to be here now at any moment.

CAROLINE (*goes to the window*). Yes the train has arrived. I see them wheeling the mails to the post-office. (*A bell is heard to ring.*) Ah – the hall-door bell – this must be he. (THE MAID *enters.*)

THE MAID. Mr Hardman, ma'am. (GEORGE HARDMAN *enters. Exit* THE MAID.)

HARDMAN. My dear Millicent –

MILLICENT. I am so glad you have come. This is Miss Caroline Dean.

HARDMAN. Miss Dean, you are, if I mistake not, our friend Jasper's gifted and devoted Aunt Caroline, who has done so much to make him what he is.

CAROLINE. Oh Mr Hardman this is too great praise from such a noted judge of character as you are.

HARDMAN. I say no more than what common report says.

CAROLINE. And common report says you have wonderful discrimination for public affairs.

HARDMAN. I have had great experience, my good lady – great experience. That is all.

MILLICENT. Uncle, dear, we have need of all your experience in this affair of Jasper.

HARDMAN. You are right, my dear. I feel it is a serious business. I just left my things at the hotel and hurried across to consult at once.

CAROLINE. We are anxious to have your advice. What is thought of the matter?

HARDMAN. Well – your telegram, Millicent, caused a great shock to us.

MILLICENT. And to think that Jasper should have been the cause of bringing about this decision of the Corporation –

CAROLINE. What is your opinion of this decision, Mr Hardman?

HARDMAN. I think it will bring ruin and discredit upon your good town.

CAROLINE. I am glad to hear you say so, Mr Hardman.

MILLICENT. Glad, Miss Dean – ?

CAROLINE. Yes, because your uncle's opinion was mine from the first.

HARDMAN. Oh there can be no doubt about what I say. Don't you see how your town must suffer, if her business connection with Anglebury is in any way injured?

CAROLINE. I quite agree with you. For where does she obtain fashion, wealth, or importance except from Anglebury?

HARDMAN. How could the business of this good town subsist by itself?

CAROLINE. It is surely much more honourable for our commercial life to be connected with yours, than for it to seek a precarious and petty independence.

HARDMAN. What admirable common sense:– How seldom a woman is found with such grasp of a situation!

CAROLINE. Ah, Mr Hardman, my life has been passed in managing affairs of all kinds.

HARDMAN. It is easy to see in the brilliant Jasper Dean the influence of a modern Cornelia.

CAROLINE. If Jasper were only to hear you speak, I feel certain that he would be led by you.

HARDMAN. I must see Jasper. I must see the others. I must reason with them. Like every Radical I have a great belief in argument.

MILLICENT. Oh how delightful it will be to have an argument! I do love argument for its own sake!

CAROLINE. I am sure, my dear, you have a great deal to say to your uncle: so I will leave you for the present. Mr Hardman will, of course, stay for lunch.

HARDMAN. You are very kind.

CAROLINE. Till then you will excuse me. (*Exit.*) –

HARDMAN. A very worthy old lady –

MILLICENT. She seems much afraid that Jasper will injure himself.

HARDMAN. And she is right, my dear. You did well to inform me at once of his mischievous conduct.

MILLICENT. You frighten me. Do you think it is so very serious?

HARDMAN. Do *you* think he may be brought to reason?

MILLICENT. I am sure I don't know. He seems very determined.

HARDMAN. I suppose you are aware, Millicent, that if he persists, he will be banished from all social and political life in Anglebury.

MILLICENT. Yes uncle, I feel that what you say is true.

HARDMAN. Are you prepared to share his banishment, Millicent?

MILLICENT. I love Jasper. You know I have promised to marry him.

HARDMAN. I know, my dear. That is all very well. But are you prepared to relinquish the whole of your active political life, and social influence in Anglebury, and to bury yourself for the rest of your days in Ireland? Are you prepared to do this? For this is what it means.

MILLICENT. It would certainly be a dreadful wrench in my life.

HARDMAN. I should think it would indeed. Why your career which has begun so well, would come to a premature and ignominious end. What use to you is your Girton education and those ideas about the higher mission of woman, if you are going to sever all your political ties and sink into obscurity?

MILLICENT. Oh, uncle, why prophesy such a miserable fate for me?

HARDMAN. I am only stating sober fact, Millicent. It therefore behoves you to get Jasper off this work of his, as soon as possible.

MILLICENT. But if he won't – ?

HARDMAN. I have confidence in you, my child. I know you will act prudently. Let us hope there will be no necessity for us to consider the possibility of his refusal. He is devoted to you; and you could persuade him to do what none other could.

MILLICENT. I am afraid I shall never be able to persuade him in this matter. He is so much convinced that he has justice on his side.

HARDMAN. But you must prove to him that he hasn't.

MILLICENT. That is not easy, when he is so clever, and well informed on the whole question.

HARDMAN. I don't care how clever and well informed he may be, if he has not right on his side.

MILLICENT. Do you really believe uncle that he is not in the right?

HARDMAN. Why, of course I do, my dear. Is it not the present wish of our municipality and citizens to do justice to this town?

MILLICENT. Yes, justice to our Irish neighbours is now the cry with us in England.

HARDMAN. Yes – justice, of course, in all things where our town has nothing to lose or suffer –

MILLICENT. Oh in that case I perfectly see how Jasper can not have justice on his side.

HARDMAN. You understand, Millicent that if it were a question of one party or class in this town being benefited by us at the expense of another party or class, then, of course we should not hesitate to do justice. But to expect us to be at any loss ourselves in the matter – well, that is outside of practical sense, you know.

MILLICENT. Yes – we are full of sympathy with our Irish neighbours. We really and truly love Ireland. But we must above all things remember that we are English, and as English we must in no circumstances whatever injure the least of our interests. Is not that our position, uncle?

332

HARDMAN. That is truly our position, child. We are a conscientious people with a manly sense of justice and fair play.

MILLICENT. And still I cannot understand why other nations will persist in vilifying us.

HARDMAN. It is perfectly simple, my dear. Don't you see that the fate of all philanthropists – whether nations, corporations, or individuals – is to be misunderstood at first.

MILLICENT. But it seems to me that we are always misunderstood here.

HARDMAN. (*throwing up his hands*). What a country –! what a country –! the more we English try to understand Ireland, the more sacrifices we make for her, the more ungrateful and difficult she becomes. But we must be patient, and go on doing such good solid work to benefit this town as we have steadily done in the past.

MILLICENT. Yes – I clearly see how unjustifiable is this agitation which Jasper has stirred up.

HARDMAN. Of course – besides, Millicent, supposing the claims of this town were really just, do you think for a moment our ratepayers would consent to the extra rate which the payment of those claims would impose on them? Why, if our Aldermen were to suggest such a thing, they would never again be elected to the Corporation.

MILLICENT. As if you could expect men to relinquish their municipal position for any principle however just –

HARDMAN. Don't you understand, then, how the whole movement is quite outside the domain of practical politics? It would be fatal for you, my dear, to identify yourself in any way with it.

MILLICENT. Oh to think that Jasper whom I love, should involve me in such misfortune – !

HARDMAN. You must not allow him to, Millicent. You can change him, you *must* –

MILLICENT. But how, uncle – ?

HARDMAN. If he knows that you are not prepared to share the life he is fashioning for himself –

MILLICENT. Oh that life would be dreadful.

HARDMAN. Very well then – he will do anything rather than lose you. You must arrange this matter at once. Can you see him soon?

MILLICENT. I think so. He ought to be here soon again. (THE MAID *enters followed by* ALDERMAN FOLEY. *Exit* THE MAID.)

HARDMAN. I want to put some of my papers and things in order at the hotel, and will return after a while to lunch.

MILLICENT. Alderman Foley, this is my uncle, Mr Hardman.

HARDMAN (*shaking hands with* FOLEY). I am proud to meet you, sir. How do you do?

333

FOLEY. You are welcome to our town, Mr Hardman. We shall make your path easy to tread over here. I will see to that.

HARDMAN. You will –

MILLICENT. Alderman Foley owns and edits the 'Weekly Denouncer'.

HARDMAN. Oh, of course – I know –

FOLEY. You were going to your hotel. Well, don't let me detain you. I know you have business.

HARDMAN. Oh nothing that cannot wait – I am delighted to have an opportunity of conversing with you, Alderman Foley.

FOLEY. There – my dear sir – another time – you had better go to your hotel now. It is all right, I assure you. I shall see you very soon again.

HARDMAN. Agreed then, Alderman Foley. I hope we shall meet soon again. Millicent, try to have that matter settled before I return. (*Exit.*)

FOLEY. I hear Jasper Dean is not at home. Do you know when he is likely to return?

MILLICENT. He said he would be here when his committee meeting was over.

FOLEY. Ah – committees and office work – how delightful is the atmosphere of this place after such sordid drudgery!

MILLICENT. Do you think so, Alderman Foley? I consider committees always interesting.

FOLEY. Well, I find women are never so charming as when we men come from some dry, ugly, occupation, such as economics, politics, or law. That is why lawyers and the like are so fascinated by female society.

MILLICENT. I must say I always preferred men of the recognised professions.

FOLEY. Yes – they are certainly preferable to the others – to poets and men of letters for instance who are occupied with such sublunary visions, that female society, instead of being a delightful relief, would seem to them – well something quite the opposite.

MILLICENT. Poets and men of letters aren't, somehow, of much practical use to women. I know I always disliked them. Their work, for one thing, doesn't lead to salaried appointments.

FOLEY. But journalists are not men of letters, I am proud to say.

MILLICENT. No – journalism is one of the recognised professions.

FOLEY. Then I am proud to be a journalist. I am proud to belong to a profession that gives me a right to your approbation.

MILLICENT. You are too complimentary, Alderman Foley.

FOLEY. Impossible to one so adorable as you are –

MILLICENT. I do not understand you.

334

FOLEY (*kneeling*). I mean, I adore you. Will you accept my heart and hand?

MILLICENT. Alderman Foley, are you mad?

FOLEY. Yes madly in love with you –

MILLICENT. But aren't you aware that I am engaged to marry Alderman Dean?

FOLEY. Oh – that is only detail. You can change your mind.

MILLICENT. Sir, you offend me. I shall not stay in the room an instant longer.

FOLEY. Do you mean to say you absolutely refuse me?

MILLICENT. Of course I do. If you don't go away, I shall scream. (ALDERMAN JASPER DEAN *enters. She rushes to him.* FOLEY *rises quickly and strikes an attitude.*)

DEAN. What is all this about?

MILLICENT. Oh Jasper he has dared to propose to me.

DEAN. What audacity –

FOLEY. What do you mean by audacity?

DEAN. How dare you behave in this outrageous manner?

FOLEY. I will not stultify myself by arguing with you in your present state of excitement –

DEAN. You disgraceful bohemian, if you don't clear out of this at once, I'll –

FOLEY. What, will you have the brutality to use physical violence?

DEAN. (*rushing at him*). I'll break every bone –

FOLEY (*flying*). Oh don't, don't – (*He flies out.* DEAN *rushes after him as far as the door. There is then heard a noise outside as of a person falling down stairs, then a bang of the street-door.*)

MILLICENT. (*excitedly*). There, you see the kind of people your policy has brought you among. I am insulted by one of your party.

DEAN. My dear Millicent, I am so sorry you have been subjected to such annoyance.

MILLICENT. This comes of going against your class. The impudent fellow – how dare he? – and he was so complacent to my uncle just now.

DEAN. Then Mr Hardman has come?

MILLICENT. Yes – and now I see the reason why this fellow wanted him out of the room, and kept assuring him of his good will.

DEAN. What is that? Has he gone over to your uncle?

MILLICENT. He was pretending to, I suppose.

DEAN. Then your uncle is against us?

MILLICENT. What else can he be, when he knows you will ruin yourself and this town? Here you are surrounded by adventurers. I was sure

335

Foley was an adventurer. I told you so.

DEAN. Indeed I am astonished at his behaviour. My opinion of him is quite changed. I am sure none of my other colleagues –

MILLICENT. They are all the same. They are not of your class.

DEAN. They are the leading men of our town.

MILLICENT. Never mind Jasper. This is a movement against the best class of your town's people whose interests are bound up with Anglebury. It was always believed that you would take the lead here in a manner approved of by your English friends.

DEAN. No man approved of by Anglebury could ever take the lead in this town.

MILLICENT. That is a great mistake, Jasper. If the people are properly managed by local men of position, they can easily be made instrumental for forwarding the convenience and interests of Anglebury. But you have taken it upon yourself to go against the traditions of your family. If you continue, we shall be ostracised by all our English friends.

DEAN. I don't know why you should be so certain of that.

MILLICENT. My uncle says so. He says I shall be banished from all circles of political activity.

DEAN. If your friends are so worthless as to turn against you because I act justly –

MILLICENT. Justly – you cannot think, Jasper, that you are acting justly?

DEAN. Why not Millicent – ?

MILLICENT. My uncle says you have not justice on your side; and I myself feel – I know you haven't.

DEAN. That is only your opinion, my dear Millicent.

MILLICENT. We English cannot do injustice.

DEAN. I wish you had never done any here.

MILLICENT. But Jasper don't you know that justice to Ireland is now the cry that is vitalising our party in England?

DEAN. I know – a word to vitalise a party – a name that is shouted and then forgotten when it has served its turn –

MILLICENT. Jasper I will not argue with you. I have confidence in my uncle.

DEAN. It would be better for you if you had confidence in me.

MILLICENT. I cannot Jasper.

DEAN (with a sigh). Yes – I suppose that is the way. The man of fame who influences thousands, cannot often command the confidence of his nearest and dearest. It was so with Marcus Aurelius. On the other hand the quite obscure man is often an oracle in his home.

MILLICENT. Jasper dear I always thought you were very clever. I now

336

think you are only misled by some evil influence. Oh Jasper if you really loved me, you would not seek to destroy the interests of my life.

DEAN. I want you to find all your interests here, Millicent.

MILLICENT. I could not bury myself in Ireland.

DEAN. Why not, Millicent – ? Could we not work together? And heaven knows there is much work to do. Our interests would be the same. I don't know how I could imagine greater happiness for us both.

MILLICENT. No Jasper, it would not be happiness. You see it so, because you are talking of what only interests yourself.

DEAN. But I thought you loved this country. Do you not?

MILLICENT. Oh yes – of course – but you must understand that you cannot take me from my surroundings, from my pursuit of educational ideals, from the aim of life in England which fascinated our generation of girl students. You cannot do all this without destroying my happiness.

DEAN. And do you believe that I could find my happiness in the course *you* would have me follow, of placing England before Ireland?

MILLICENT. That is not it, Jasper. I want you to see that the best interest of Ireland is never to oppose in any way England. It is a fatal policy. Oh, Jasper, I entreat of you to abandon it.

DEAN. Millicent, you do not know what you are asking. Even if I agreed with you, and were inclined to abandon my policy, I could not – without incurring suspicion and contempt.

MILLICENT. What does it all matter with these people here – people I am sure like this Foley for the most part? Is not anything better than to be ostracised by our friends in England? Dear Jasper, let us leave this place. Let us go to England. Let us amid the riches and prosperity of England forget altogether this poor mean place.

DEAN. I love this poor mean place better than your England that has made it poor and mean. But it will not remain so. We are at last united, and we shall enforce payment of those riches we know are our due.

MILLICENT. Jasper, you do not love me. You would not talk like that if you loved me.

DEAN. I love you, Millicent. You do not believe what you say.

MILLICENT. True love refuses nothing.

DEAN. Nothing – except a betrayal of honour –

MILLICENT. No, not that – I would only awaken your conscience before it is too late. That conscience will surely yet force you to abandon this false idea of honour.

DEAN. I can not tell what may happen in the future; but now my conscience is at rest.

MILLICENT. You will see that there is no justice on your side. You will yet see that false honour was but a destroyer of true love.

DEAN. My love is the same. It is yours that is failing, or you could not put me to this cruel test.

MILLICENT (*after a short pause*). Jasper, if that is so, we had better go our different ways.

DEAN. What do you say? You are not serious, Millicent. You must not mind my words. I did not mean –

MILLICENT. I had better no longer be an obstacle to your ambition, Jasper.

DEAN. Millicent – dear Millicent, you are not serious. You would never leave me.

MILLICENT. Will you abandon your policy for my sake, Jasper?

DEAN (*with a struggle*). I – I cannot. (GEORGE HARDMAN *enters*).

DEAN (*starting*). Oh, Mr Hardman –

MILLICENT. Uncle, I must no longer remain a guest in this house.

HARDMAN (*looking from one to the other*). Is that so, my dear? Come then, you had better stay with me at my hotel until to-morrow when we shall return to England. (MILLICENT *and* HARDMAN *bow to* JASPER, *and exeunt.*)

DEAN (*bewildered*). What is this? I cannot believe – what have I done? I have lost her. Oh, I have lost her.

CURTAIN

ACT IV

(A sitting-room in the principal hotel of the Town.)
(GEORGE HARDMAN anxious and restless walks to and fro.)
(THE WAITER enters.)

THE WAITER. Alderman Daniel Lawrence wants to see you, sir.

HARDMAN. He has come at last. (*To* THE WAITER.) Show him up. (*Exit* THE WAITER. ALDERMAN DANIEL LAWRENCE *enters.*)

LAWRENCE. My dear Mayor, I'm so glad to see you. How well you are looking. I never saw you looking better in my life.

HARDMAN. Thank you, Alderman Lawrence, thank you. I am very glad to see you. I hope you are well.

LAWRENCE. As well as can be expected in these anxious times, Mayor –

HARDMAN. Anxious times indeed they are. I wish especially to consult you about the unjustifiable agitation that is going on in this town. You are an able man, Alderman Lawrence – a man of the world and of affairs. You know your town well. How do you think this agitation will end?

LAWRENCE. I think it will succeed.

HARDMAN. You do?

LAWRENCE. That is my opinion.

HARDMAN. You are a staunch friend of ours. What is your advice?

LAWRENCE. I advise payment before the law is set in motion: otherwise you will have enormous costs to pay as well.

HARDMAN. Oh, this is impossible.

LAWRENCE. Why – ?

HARDMAN. No member of our Corporation could propose such a thing without being municipally discredited for life.

LAWRENCE. Well, I don't see what else you can do.

HARDMAN. Really, Alderman Lawrence, one would think that you were holding a brief for the other side. Why, you say things that completely upset my policy.

LAWRENCE. Quite so – your preconceived policy, my dear Mayor – there is nothing English politicians dislike so much as being told what they do not want to hear. At the same time I feel I would only

339

be misleading you, if I told you otherwise. All our townspeople are so united, that I see no escape for you.

HARDMAN. Well, they say of us Englishmen that we never know when we are beaten; and I for one don't mean to allow our townspeople to be mulcted of extra taxation without making a fight for it. You know this town well, Alderman Lawrence. Cannot you think of some device?

LAWRENCE. I declare you give me a most difficult task.

HARDMAN. Just consider now. You are a man of great acumen. I always maintain that Anglebury has not appreciated your merits as it should have.

LAWRENCE. Well indeed I would not have mentioned the subject: but now that you have touched upon it, I will say to you as a friend, that Anglebury has done nothing to encourage me, considering the extremely unpopular part I play here from time to time in her interest.

HARDMAN. You know the post of solicitor to our Corporation is just vacant. The emoluments are very handsome.

LAWRENCE. I know, my dear Mayor. I know.

HARDMAN. The appointment will surely be given to the lawyer who does the best service to Anglebury.

LAWRENCE. Quite so – I have often thought what a pleasant thing it would be to have that appointment.

HARDMAN. Besides – remember there is a very handsome retiring pension.

LAWRENCE. Yes – I have always considered a pension as the fine flower of an appointment.

HARDMAN. And still with such a prize before you, can you not find a means of winning it!

LAWRENCE. My dear Mayor, how you torture me!

HARDMAN. Come – come, Alderman Lawrence, there is no time to be lost.

LAWRENCE. Well really I am put to the pin of my collar. Well –have you seen the Corporation yet?

HARDMAN. Only a few of them, and then not in a business way –

LAWRENCE. Perhaps it might come to something, if you were to meet them in a body?

HARDMAN. Or perhaps one by one – just casually, you know. Who are the most likely to be influenced? What kind – for instance – is Foley, the editor?

LAWRENCE. A great mountebank with a popular reputation for asceticism –why do you ask?

HARDMAN. Oh nothing – only he protested great friendliness.

LAWRENCE. I don't think you would do any good by trying to tamper with the Corporation singly. You see popular excitement has risen to such a pitch that not one of them, even if he were inclined, would dare to take your advice. The only one I would suggest to be got at singly would be Jasper Dean. If he could be induced to abandon the movement, then, I am sure, there would be such a scramble among the rest for leadership that everything else would be forgotten.

HARDMAN. I am afraid it's no use with Jasper Dean.

LAWRENCE. You think so.

HARDMAN. I am afraid so.

LAWRENCE. Well in that case all I can suggest is that you meet the Corporation in a body, and try the efficacy of argument. You may not think much of this; but I really don't see any thing else to be done.

HARDMAN. Where can I meet them?

LAWRENCE. Why here – can you not invite them to meet you?

HARDMAN. Certainly – I should be very pleased.

LAWRENCE. You might put your views to them quietly and with tact.

HARDMAN. Yes – I am sure I could influence them, if they have any reason left.

LAWRENCE. I think it is worth trying. The Corporation is sitting at present. Suppose I were to go now and ask all the members to meet you here when their business is finished.

HARDMAN. Or do you think it would be better if I were to go and meet them? What do you think?

LAWRENCE. Oh, no, that would be too public and formal. The meeting ought to be friendly merely – convivial, you understand. You know all our Corporation: don't you, my dear Mayor?

HARDMAN. Well, I know some of them, Alderman Lawrence.

LAWRENCE. Do you know Cassidy – a pretentious fellow who is dying to be recognised as the head of the family?

HARDMAN. What family?

LAWRENCE. Well you may ask. But you mustn't on any account appear ignorant of the importance its members attach to it. I mean Jasper Dean's family – a lot of very worthy people a hundred years behind their time, and with no sense of the movement of the world or the realities of things.

HARDMAN. No – I don't think I ever met Cassidy.

LAWRENCE. Do you know Kirwan – a bitter fellow? Take care of him.

HARDMAN. Why – ?

LAWRENCE. I really believe he is honest. He's no use.

341

HARDMAN. Oh – yes I've met him.

LAWRENCE. And a scurrilous person called Murphy, who thinks everyone a fool but himself –

HARDMAN. Yes, yes, I've met him too. But he is very able; isn't he?

LAWRENCE. Unfortunately he is. Well, my dear Mayor, now that you know the foibles of these men, it might be useful to your purpose if you said something to each, that would flatter his vanity.

HARDMAN. I see – I see. Now you are beginning to suggest something. Does anything else occur to you?

LAWRENCE. I fear you do not help me much in my suggestions. Well – let me see – if this conference should fail –

HARDMAN. Don't prophesy failure, Alderman Lawrence.

LAWRENCE. I do not wish to, I assure you. Still we ought to be prepared to meet every contingency: and I was thinking that if you do not succeed in persuading them to abandon the holding of this meeting, it might perhaps be possible to create a noisy opposition.

HARDMAN. You mean at the meeting?

LAWRENCE. Yes – it is a very dangerous proceeding, as there is such a huge majority against us. Still there are in this town reckless, determined fellows who for money would make a desperate attempt to break up the meeting.

HARDMAN. Do you think you could manage this?

LAWRENCE. I am sure I could, if you supply the means.

HARDMAN. Of course I will. What satisfaction it is to deal with a practical man like you, Alderman Lawrence, after the worry these mischievous theorists give me here.

LAWRENCE. Ah, my dear Mayor, I as a professional man cannot but become practical when I discern a prospect of leaving this meagre place for a sphere of emolument in so rich a garden as England. (THE WAITER enters.)

THE WAITER. The Misses Dean, sir. (Exit.) (Enter MISS CAROLINE and MISS ARABELLA DEAN.)

CAROLINE. Mr Hardman, how is your dear niece? How do you do, Alderman Lawrence?

LAWRENCE. How do you do, Miss Dean? How well you're looking. I never saw you looking better in my life.

ARABELLA. We haven't yet got over our surprise at the departure of Miss Fell.

HARDMAN. I shouldn't have thought there was anything to be surprised at under the circumstances.

CAROLINE. Is she very distressed, poor thing?

ARABELLA. Poor Jasper is dreadfully distressed.

342

HARDMAN. I never thought he would have brought this trouble upon her. However she struggles against her grief.

CAROLINE. I am very angry with Jasper.

HARDMAN. He might have been more generous to his affianced bride.

LAWRENCE. Yes, and to such a charming young woman into the bargain –

CAROLINE. I always respected your sound common sense, Alderman Lawrence. Can you not help us in this difficulty?

LAWRENCE. That is exactly what I am now trying to do, Miss Dean. I am going to bring the Corporation here for a conference with Mr Hardman.

CAROLINE. That is the only useful move I have heard of in this agitation.

LAWRENCE. I have great hopes of its success. (*Exit.*)

CAROLINE. I can assure you, Mr Hardman, that this trouble you are suffering, is none of my doing.

HARDMAN. I know that perfectly well, Miss Dean.

CAROLINE. Goodness knows I have always tried to instil sound political principles into my nephew. It is not my fault if he has listened to other advice.

HARDMAN. We must not yet despair of saving him from his bad advisers. (MILLICENT FELL *enters.*)

CAROLINE. My dear, how I feel for you!

ARABELLA. It must be very disappointing when something prevents one from settling one's self.

HARDMAN. I tell her that perhaps she would do better if she were to marry some steady man in England.

MILLICENT. Indeed it seems that Jasper doesn't care about raising my social and political station.

CAROLINE. As if the principal object in marriage was not to improve one's social position –

ARABELLA. Yes, Caroline, I hope you will do nothing yourself to belie what you say.

CAROLINE. Arabella, I wonder you can make so inappropriate a remark. It is as bad as your sympathy with Jasper.

HARDMAN. It is certainly odd that he should become an object of sympathy under the circumstances.

ARABELLA. Well, all I know is that he is dying to be reconciled to Miss Fell.

HARDMAN. Is he? Then what steps will he take towards a reconciliation? (THE WAITER *enters.*)

THE WAITER. Alderman Dean.

MILLICENT. Oh, I will not – I cannot see him. (*Exit.*)

THE WAITER. Am I to show him up, sir?

HARDMAN. Yes – stop a minute. I expect several gentlemen to see me here soon. When they come, bring some refreshments. (*Whispers to* THE WAITER.) You understand. (*To* CAROLINE *and* ARABELLA.) And you will have tea also: won't you ladies? Yes, bring tea also, waiter. (*Exit* THE WAITER.) Now we shall see if Jasper means reconciliation. (ALDERMAN JASPER DEAN *enters.*)

DEAN. So you have invited the Corporation here to see you, Mr Hardman. I was overjoyed when I heard Lawrence give your message. I couldn't even wait until our business was finished, to come here.

HARDMAN. Are the Corporation coming, also, Jasper.

DEAN. Of course they are. They will finish directly. You have raised hopes in all of us.

HARDMAN. I have not yet lost hope, Jasper.

CAROLINE. You must know, Jasper, the sorrow your conduct has brought on Miss Fell.

DEAN. Oh how is she? I am truly sorry. I haven't had a moment's rest since she left us.

HARDMAN. She is a proud girl and feels the humiliation.

DEAN. What do you mean by humiliation? It was none of my doing. That's certain.

HARDMAN. Whose doing was it then, if not yours, Jasper?

CAROLINE. Alas! whose indeed – ?

DEAN. No one has a right to reproach me for doing my duty.

HARDMAN. We all have a right to feel grieved at your mistaking your duty.

DEAN. How can you sincerely believe I have mistaken my duty?

CAROLINE. Is it the duty of a man with your family and position to join anti-English agitators?

DEAN. Why not, if they are in the right – ?

ARABELLA. To be sure, Jasper – the winning side is always in the right.

HARDMAN. You cannot really believe they are in the right? Before having committed yourself, you might have consulted the other side. You would then doubtless have realised that there was not such unqualified justice in your movement as you imagined.

DEAN. I know all the arguments of your side, Mr Hardman, and consider none of them sufficient.

CAROLINE. But taken together wouldn't they be more than sufficient? I now say nothing of the disgrace to your family, and the loss of this charming girl who is so devoted to you, and to your best interests in life.

344

DEAN. Ah, she is the only argument that might influence me, if it were possible I could change.

HARDMAN. If she were the only argument, I would not press you, Jasper. You would not be justified in abandoning your colleagues merely for the sake of private affection, however deep.

CAROLINE. What an elevated impartial mind – ! Jasper, you should be led by Mr Hardman.

HARDMAN. I don't wish to influence anyone in the least. I am merely anxious that you, Jasper, should listen to me, and then I know your sense of right and justice will lead you to take a correct view of the case. (THE WAITER *enters carrying a large tray on which are tea things, liquor, glasses, etc.*)

THE WAITER. The gentlemen of the Corporation are below, sir.

HARDMAN. Very good – show them up. (THE WAITER *lays the tray on a table and exit.*)

CAROLINE. Dear me, here come Belle Cassidy, and Sarah Leech too. I wonder what they want by coming?

ARABELLA. Don't you know that Belle must always watch James when he goes to an entertainment, for fear he might take too much intoxicating liquor.

CAROLINE. Oh – and of course Sarah knows that Belle always abuses her behind her back. So she is afraid to leave her.

DEAN (irritated). That is the way with the family! (*Enter* MRS CASSIDY MRS LEECH, MAYOR JOSEPH TENCH, ALDERMEN DANIEL LAWRENCE, JAMES CASSIDY, MICHAEL LEECH, RALF KIRWAN, THOMAS MURPHY, VALENTINE FOLEY, *and various other Aldermen and Town Councillors, then the Town Clerk,* JOHN CLORAN, *and* MRS COSTIGAN, *who peeps in at the door.*)

LAWRENCE. My dear Mr Hardman, I suppose it is superfluous for me to introduce our respected Mayor and Corporation.

HARDMAN. Indeed we are no strangers. Gentlemen, you are welcome. How is my courteous friend, Alderman Murphy? Ah, if we only had your wise head and strong will in *our* Corporation – ! And here is our ascetic of the new journalism, Alderman Foley? How do you do sir? Ah – Alderman Kirwan, you dislike us English. We don't deserve it. How do you do? (*Shakes hands with other members of the Corporation.*) How do you do? How do you do, Alderman Cassidy? How do you do, Alderman Leech? You both belong to the family: don't you? Ah, what a family – !

LAWRENCE. A family with so many wise heads that each is capable of taking the lead –

CLORAN. That's right, sir. True for you sir –

HARDMAN. Gentlemen, won't you have some refreshments? Here is your excellent wine of the country. Ha – ha – (*they help themselves now to liquor.* MRS CASSIDY *prevents* CASSIDY *from doing so.*) Ladies – the tea is waiting for you.

FOLEY. I will, if you please, take the beverage of the ladies.

CAROLINE. Sarah, I think you had better preside over the tea.

MRS CASSIDY. Yes, Sarah is never so satisfactory as when she is given lots to do.

MRS LEECH (*pouring out the tea*). Ah, it's well they see some good in me.

FOLEY. Woman never looks so charming as when presiding at the social tea-table.

MRS LEECH Alderman Foley, what do you mean? I declare you are getting quite complimentary. Are there any more for tea? (*Pours in the milk*). There, sugar yourselves, and I'll milk you all round.

CAROLINE. Sarah, you are talking too much.

MRS CASSIDY. It never does to excite Sarah.

LAWRENCE. What a satisfaction it is for us all to meet together in this rational enjoyment of a social prosperity. I assure you ladies and gentlemen, the world was made for prosperity. And what a splendid world it is! How truly exhilarating to expand one's chest and breathe in the air of prosperity!

MURPHY. Yes, and what a fine big tone it gives to the lungs!

KIRWAN. And how impressively a commonplace thought comes from the sound-board of a fine pair of lungs!

FOLEY. In fact after brains the best things to have are fine sounding lungs.

MURPHY. A great deal better than brains, as far as public pay goes –

MRS COSTIGAN. (*coming in*). The people don't want to give any pay. The people never like to pay anything. They think their representatives are not acting –

CLORAN. Costigan, what are you going here? Retire, woman.

MRS COSTIGAN. *MRS* COSTIGAN, if you please – Cloran. (*She retires outside the door.*)

HARDMAN. Who is this person trying to create a disturbance?

CLORAN. No one of consequence, sir – she only came into the hotel, thinking this was a public meeting.

HARDMAN. Well, gentlemen, I am sorry that by your remarks to my worthy friend, Alderman Lawrence, you appear to be wanting in that unanimity which renders public life durable and influential.

KIRWAN. On the contrary, Mr Hardman, we are all unanimous, with the sole exception of Alderman Lawrence.

HARDMAN (*facetiously*). Why can you not agree with him and thus be wholly unanimous?

FOLEY. (*who has all along been making himself remarkable by his attentions to* CAROLINE). Come, this is not the place for arguing. Remember, gentlemen, we are in the presence of ladies.

MRS LEECH. What does he mean?

CAROLINE. It is the height of bad taste to argue with Mr Hardman and Alderman Lawrence. (*Murmurs.*)

FOLEY. It is disgraceful to make this noise at any remarks of a lady. I will not allow it. I beg to take this lady under my protection.

MURPHY. What – are you losing your head, Foley?

KIRWAN. Not in the least – he has his wits very much about him.

FOLEY. Madam – Miss Dean, allow me to escort you from among these unruly fellows. (*Cheers.*)

HARDMAN. Gentlemen, I beg of you –

CLORAN. Ah, gentlemen, don't be excited.

FOLEY. I shall have something to say about this in the next number of the 'Weekly Denouncer'. (*Laughter. Exeunt* FOLEY *and* MISS CAROLINE DEAN, *who leans on his arm. The other men again help themselves to liquor, and* MRS CASSIDY *again prevents* CASSIDY.)

MRS LEECH. Isn't Caroline very queer?

MRS CASSIDY. What does she mean by making a fool of herself in this way with Alderman Foley?

ARABELLA. Caroline has always had such sense.

HARDMAN. Dear me, this misunderstanding is most unfortunate. However, gentlemen, I dare say you know that literary people are always somewhat flighty, and not to be depended upon. Let us hope that this incident may have no further disturbing effect upon our unanimity, and social enjoyment.

DEAN. It is a most strange incident, and puzzles me.

KIRWAN. I hope it may not lead to disunion.

HARDMAN. Oh; think of it as a union that may lead to a union with Anglebury.

TENCH. Such a union rests altogether with your Corporation, Mr Hardman. You have only to accept the report of your Commission of Arbitration.

HARDMAN. Oh, the Commission – it was not fairly constituted?

DEAN. It was constituted by yourself, Mr Hardman.

HARDMAN. Well – at all events it was not unanimous in its decision.

DEAN. No, but a large majority agreed –

HARDMAN. I do not think majorities always infallible. One of the dissentients from this majority is a most able man with a great

347

knowledge of the question.

KIRWAN. I thought it was an article in your political creed, Mr Hardman, that the majority must always be right.

HARDMAN. So it is , my dear sir. But this is not exactly a case in point.

KIRWAN. Of course – when England is attacked by a fever of justice, Ireland is never a case in point.

HARDMAN. Well gentlemen, if you are going to deride every word I say –

DEAN. Oh we ought to hear courteously whatever Mr Hardman has to say, gentlemen.

MURPHY. Come, come, that's very well. But what I want to know is why were we brought here at all? I was quite against coming.

TENCH. We came because we would wish to settle amicably with Mr Hardman.

DEAN. And I am sure we are quite ready to hear any argument from him. We would give it our best consideration. But up to this he has brought forward no real argument. What can we do?

HARDMAN. You can listen to what I have to say now.

DEAN. I am most anxious to. You can only expect to convert us by a valid argument.

MURPHY. One would think, Alderman Dean, that you were anxious to be converted.

DEAN. You misunderstand me, Alderman Murphy.

MURPHY. Well, what does all this mean?

DEAN. You surely must admit that if Mr Hardman brought forward a valid argument, we should be bound in conscience either to refute it satisfactorily, or to act according to it.

LAWRENCE. Upon my word that is very fair, and quite what I should expect from Jasper Dean.

HARDMAN. It is the right spirit in which to meet me; and I am confident of your favourable judgment, gentlemen, when you hear what I now have to say. This is what I have to say, gentlemen. I think you are under a misconception as to the true point of dispute between us. I mean you all seem to have forgotten the large sums of money that Anglebury has repeatedly subscribed to your charities. Have we not also sent money to you for public works in times of distress? I should think that what we have given in those ways ought more than compensate for what may be owing to you.

MURPHY. Not at all – not at all – you owe us a hundred times more than you ever gave us in charity.

HARDMAN. That is a matter for calculation, sir, and not for mere assertion.

348

DEAN. I seem to have overlooked somehow this argument. I wonder is there any real force in it.

KIRWAN. You are no expert, Dean. It is enough that a body of financial experts has decided the case.

DEAN. I suppose so. If it were otherwise, and I were doubtful of our right to this money, I should never have rest.

MURPHY. Look here, Alderman Dean, if this movement is ever broken up by any man, that man will be you.

DEAN (*indignantly*). What right have you to say this, Alderman Murphy? (*Sensation.*)

CASSIDY (*to* LEECH). It's disgraceful that one of the family should be attacked by a creature like Murphy?

LEECH. I don't think he would venture to attack you like that, James. Jasper I knew wasn't the man to lead.

HARDMAN. Every man must be morally responsible for his actions. I always admired Jasper Dean, because in addition to his great talents, I believed him to be thoroughly conscientious.

KIRWAN. Well – well – if one isn't conscientious one's self, the next best thing is to praise another's conscientiousness.

HARDMAN. Not conscientious – what do you mean sir? We English are a conscientious people. Our public men are among the few public men in the world, who have a conscience.

KIRWAN. No doubt they have; but it takes so much to awaken their conscience.

MURPHY. Nothing short indeed than putting the Englishman with his face to the wall, and kicking him till he roars –

MRS CASSIDY. I declare I never heard such language as this in all my life.

CLORAN. Ah gentlemen don't – and think of the ladies, gentlemen.

HARDMAN (*blandly*). Oh do not hinder discussion. This is nothing beyond the limit of legitimate argument.

MURPHY. I don't mean to give anyone offence. I merely wish to state that we have our knife now in the throat of Anglebury, and that we intend to turn it round and round and draw a fine pailful of the blood she has sucked out of our town. (*Commotion.*)

MRS CASSIDY. I declare Jasper, you should repudiate this. I am shocked.

MRS LEECH. Belle is always shocked when there is a chance of prosperity to the town.

ARABELLA. Jasper, take care and keep on the winning side. Belle only talks like that because she thinks it fashionable.

DEAN. There is nothing to be gained by using strong language. I am perfectly certain that, if my conscience is not convinced in the

349

justice of this movement, violence of language will not make it so.

MURPHY. Conscience be – it isn't your conscience, man. It's the lady upstairs –

DEAN (*furious*). Sir, how dare you?

KIRWAN. Gentlemen, gentlemen, I beg of you –

CLORAN. Ladies, ladies – think of the ladies, gentlemen.

KIRWAN. Where is the use of this quarrelling? Where is the use of strong language to Mr Hardman?

HARDMAN. Oh, pray do not mind me. I am not in the least offended.

KIRWAN. I know. There it is. The English do not mind anything provided they gain their point. That is the secret of their success. We insult them. We make street demonstrations against them. We think we are enraging and annihilating them. But it doesn't harm them. They don't mind. There is only one thing they mind, and would at all hazards prevent. But we are prepared to do anything except that one all important thing whereby we could wring from England all we want.

HARDMAN. And pray what is that all important thing?

KIRWAN. To unite.

MURPHY. Why man, aren't we all united? Come, let us talk no more, but act. (MRS COSTIGAN *re-enters*.).

CLORAN. Oh my, there's Costigan again. Stand outside, Costigan.

LAWRENCE. Why would you turn her out? Let her stay – this venerable type of the people!

HARDMAN. Of course – I always like to have the people with me.

MRS COSTIGAN. Hooray for Lawrence and Hardman who won't shut out the people –

SEVERAL VOICES. The people for ever – the people for ever –

CASSIDY. I am for giving the people practical advantages.

LEECH. That's right, James. Sound common sense, James –

CASSIDY (*to* MRS COSTIGAN). Come, ma'am, let me give you some refreshment. (*He leads her to the liquor to which he helps her. He is then about to help himself, but is prevented by* MRS CASSIDY.)

LAWRENCE. Gentlemen, gentlemen, I should like to make a settlement between you and Mr Hardman. Do not be so exacting in your demands. Remember that politics, especially in this town, are subject to strange and sudden shiftings. Take my advice and come to terms when you can.

MURPHY. There will be no shifting as long as we are united.

LAWRENCE How long will you be so? Do you think you are really united?

MURPHY. The citizens' meeting to-morrow will answer you that.

TENCH. It will be the largest and most unanimous ever known in our town.

KIRWAN. And my friend Alderman Dean will be in the chair.

DEAN (*starts and looks scared*). What's that? What –

MRS CASSIDY. I think – perhaps – a more experienced member of the family might be found –

ARABELLA. Hold your tongue, Belle Cassidy. Don't try to push your old husband before my Jasper.

CLORAN. Ladies, ladies – ah don't ladies –

MRS LEECH. Gracious, what has come over Arabella? She'll be turning dynamiter next.

MRS COSTIGAN (*having meanwhile repeatedly helped herself to the liquor*). Who's talking of dynamiters?

CLORAN. Oh my – Costigan too –

MRS COSTIGAN. Hic – I never approved of dynamite. I think the whole thing is immoral. Hic – still at the same time I think no Irishwoman should be discouraged –

CLORAN. For shame, woman – out you go. Come along –

MRS COSTIGAN. Hooray! I'm the voice of the people. Hooray – what – you Corporation – are you turning out the people? I'm a respectable woman – (*She is hustled out by* CLORAN, *who also exits.*)

MRS CASSIDY. I'm sure after this it's time we ladies took our departure. Come James.

MURPHY. I know I'm going off. I haven't any more time to waste here. (*Exit.*)

LAWRENCE. My dear colleagues of the Corporation, where are you going to? Where are you going to at all?

HARDMAN. Oh, gentlemen – listen to me. Your demands are outside the pale of practical politics.

KIRWAN. That's the first English answer to every Irish demand.

TENCH. I am afraid, Mr Hardman, we cannot stay any longer.

DEAN. Gentlemen do not go.

KIRWAN. Not go, Dean – what is the meaning of this?

DEAN. Don't you think we might settle with Mr Hardman?

TENCH. I don't think it is possible now to settle with Mr Hardman.

LEECH. James, you will have to take the lead after all.

CASSIDY. I am prepared to take the lead. Gentlemen, permit me to lead you out of the room. (*Exit.*)

LEECH. That's right James. (*Exit after him.*)

MRS CASSIDY. James has taken the lead.

KIRWAN. I suppose somebody must walk first out of the room.

HARDMAN (*as the Corporation are bowing and departing*). Well, gentlemen, I hope we part good friends, in spite of all differences of opinion. Good-bye, gentlemen, good-bye, ladies, good-bye.

KIRWAN. Oh – we shall be such friends, Mr Hardman, as the sheep can be with the shearer. (*Exeunt all except* GEORGE HARDMAN, DANIEL LAWRENCE *and* JASPER DEAN, *who lingers near the doorway.*)

HARDMAN (*exchanges glances with* LAWRENCE. *Then after a moment says*) Jasper, you will stay and dine with us: won't you? (MILLICENT FELL *appears at the door.*)

MILLICENT. Uncle, have they gone? (*Sees* DEAN.) Oh – (*She is about to retire.*)

DEAN (*vehemently*). Millicent, Millicent, don't go. Listen to me.

MILLICENT. What is it, Jasper?

DEAN. I must speak to you. Come. (*Exeunt* JASPER DEAN *and* MILLICENT FELL.)

LAWRENCE. My dear Mayor, what a charming girl your niece is! An English girl is certainly the most perfect type of womanhood in the world.

HARDMAN. Quite true Alderman Lawrence – but tell me, how do you think things are going?

LAWRENCE. I think Miss Fell a splendid young English woman. (*They sit down together in deep consultation.*)

ACT V

(Drawing-room in JASPER DEAN'S *house.)*
*(*THE MAID *enters and ushers in* MRS BELLE CASSIDY *and* MRS SARAH LEECH.)*

THE MAID. I will tell Miss Dean you are here, ladies. *(Exit.)*

MRS LEECH. Now confess, Belle, you are just as curious as I am to know what Caroline is contemplating.

MRS CASSIDY *(loftily)*. I am coming to visit a relation. Is there anything extraordinary in that?

MRS LEECH. Ah – you know best, Belle.

MRS CASSIDY. Sarah, you are too inclined to build up stories upon no foundation.

MRS LEECH. Well, if you think her extraordinary manner towards Alderman Foley yesterday no foundation –

MRS CASSIDY. Stop, Sarah. Caroline is a woman of far too great common sense for any foolish tenderness.

MRS LEECH. Oh indeed I know there is no tenderness in her. She only wants to get married. That's all.

MRS CASSIDY. How dare you talk of Caroline in such a way? *(After a pause.)* I wonder will she really marry him, though. Here she comes.
(Enter MISS CAROLINE *and* MISS ARABELLA DEAN.)*

ARABELLA. Oh it is always a sign that something is brewing in the family, when Belle Cassidy and Sarah Leech appear.

MRS LEECH. Caroline, what does she mean?

CAROLINE. Her remarks as a rule admit of no rational explanation.

MRS CASSIDY. Then you say, Caroline, that there is not likely to be a surprise for the family.

CAROLINE. Not that I am aware of –

MRS CASSIDY. Are you quite sure? Now think – because you know I expect – hem –

MRS LEECH. Belle, what are you beating about the bush in this way for?

MRS CASSIDY. Sarah, what do you mean? You forget the respect I have for Caroline and the family. You seem destitute of respect for either of them.

MRS LEECH. Ah – you are all down on me as usual.

353

ARABELLA. Sarah has spoiled the whole thing as usual.

CAROLINE. Belle, what affair of mine have you come to pry into?

MRS CASSIDY. I assure you, Caroline, you must not think such a thing for a moment.

CAROLINE. Well is it Jasper who excites your curiosity?

ARABELLA. Poor fellow, he is making so brave a stand.

CAROLINE. I call it disgraceful of him.

MRS CASSIDY. I am surprised, Caroline, that a woman of your sense should be upset by such a thing.

CAROLINE. You do not understand, Belle, the injury he will do us.

MRS LEECH. But, Caroline, he is not the only one. James and Michael are also in the movement.

MRS CASSIDY. Yes, I clearly see now it was James who ought to have taken the lead.

CAROLINE. Then, why on earth didn't he, Belle? I'm sure I wish he had. He had plenty of time to take the lead before ever Jasper joined the Corporation.

MRS CASSIDY. He may have felt, perhaps, that the movement might not, as you seem to think, conduce to the credit of the family.

CAROLINE. Just so – then why has he gone in for it at all?

MRS LEECH. But, Caroline, what do you mean? I thought you were regretting that he did not take the lead.

CAROLINE. Of course, I was. If the family must be disgraced by a member, I had rather it were some one else besides Jasper.

MRS CASSIDY. Caroline, do you realise the enormity of what you are saying? It is then comparitively an insignificant matter to you that my husband James should disgrace the family.

CAROLINE. It is a less calamity than that Jasper should go against his English friends. Even Alderman Foley now has begun to see Jasper's mistake.

MRS CASSIDY. Yes – Alderman Foley always sees his own interests very clearly.

MRS LEECH. Oh, so *you* have converted him, Caroline.

CAROLINE. He is a most estimable man.

MRS LEECH. When is it to be, Caroline? You needn't hide it from us any more.

CAROLINE. I don't understand your insinuations.

ARABELLA. Sarah now will give out the report through the town.

CAROLINE. I am sorry to say Sarah does not always confine her reports to truth.

MRS CASSIDY. Then do you pretend to deny the truth in this report Caroline?

354

CAROLINE. How dare you ask me such a question?

MRS CASSIDY. How dare you speak of James as you did?

CAROLINE. It does not matter what I say about him. He never was up to much.

MRS CASSIDY. He will very soon show you who is the real head of the family. (*Exit.*)

MRS LEECH. Poor James will now be driven to do something. (*Exit.*)

CAROLINE. I suppose she is going to make him oppose Jasper at the meeting. I wish some one would take Jasper's place.

ARABELLA. It will take a better man to do it than James.

CAROLINE. I suppose the meeting has already commenced its business.

ARABELLA. Yes – it must have. Do let us go and hear Jasper.

CAROLINE. Hear Jasper – my nephew, my benighted nephew, whom I have striven to educate with a sense of our family respectability – hear Jasper trail that respectability in the dust – ? Never – (ALDERMAN RALF KIRWAN *enters hurriedly.*)

KIRWAN. Oh – pardon me, Miss Dean. Good-day – where is your nephew?

CAROLINE. Isn't he at the meeting?

KIRWAN. No – where is he?

ARABELLA. Jasper not at the meeting – ? he hasn't been here since morning.

CAROLINE. We haven't a notion where he is now.

KIRWAN. Surely he knows that it is past the time. The meeting is impatient. I hurried across to bring him there.

CAROLINE. He is shirking the meeting.

KIRWAN. Oh this is impossible.

CAROLINE. His reputation is saved.

KIRWAN. You cannot be serious in what you are saying, Miss Dean.

ARABELLA. Jasper must have some reason for this.

KIRWAN. He will ruin us. Who is there now fit to lead us at the meeting?

CAROLINE. You – Alderman Kirwan –

KIRWAN. I – Miss Dean –?

CAROLINE. Yes you – why not?

KIRWAN. Oh – for several reasons –

CAROLINE. A man of your ability and character is just fitted for taking the chair. I wonder why you always keep yourself in the background.

KIRWAN. If I were to attempt any action it would at once excite several jealousies. There's Alderman Murphy. Then there's your cousin, Alderman Cassidy.

355

CAROLINE. Oh – James counts for nothing in a crisis like this. Alderman Murphy will not dare to create difficulties.

KIRWAN. I am not so sure about that.

CAROLINE. I tell you, you are the man, Alderman Kirwan. Do not miss the opportunity of your life. Just run across to the meeting. Explain matters. Rally the people; and no one will dare to oppose you.

KIRWAN. I am no leader, but I would risk anything to benefit our town.

CAROLINE. Of course you would. What – don't they all know you are such a clever man?

KIRWAN. I hope at least I am an honest one.

CAROLINE. Yes, and you have never taken that action in public affairs which was expected of you.

KIRWAN. Well – since your nephew has failed –

CAROLINE. Yes, – go and take his place.

ARABELLA. No one can take my Jasper's place. You will be on the losing side, Alderman Kirwan.

CAROLINE. Arabella, hold your tongue.

KIRWAN. I fear it is a hopeless task for me. I think I had better not attempt it.

CAROLINE. Ah – that is how people throw away their opportunities in life.

KIRWAN. Oh – if I could save our town from this disaster –

CAROLINE. What I advise is always the best.

KIRWAN. I will consider the matter.

CAROLINE. There is no time to consider. Go, do it at once.

ARABELLA. Perhaps you will find Jasper at the meeting, when you return there.

KIRWAN. Perhaps I may. I will go anyhow and do my best. There is no time to be lost. (*Exit.*)

CAROLINE. We are saved. We are saved.

ARABELLA. But if he succeeds in leading after all, and Hardman is defeated –

CAROLINE. Oh what do I care so long as it is not Jasper who defeats him, and we are safe with our English acquaintants. (THE MAID *enters followed by* ALDERMAN VALENTINE FOLEY. *Exit* THE MAID)

FOLEY. Isn't your nephew here, Miss Dean?

CAROLINE. No, where is he?

FOLEY. Ah – I see he doesn't intend to go to the meeting. The meeting will be a failure.

CAROLINE. So much the better –

FOLEY. Yes – so much the better –

CAROLINE. Then you are really and truly converted, Alderman Foley.

356

FOLEY. Madam, I am beginning to discern the charms of a refined and domestic private life.

ARABELLA. You won't be allowed much money for yourself, Alderman Foley.

CAROLINE. Arabella, you are a spiteful thing. (ALDERMAN JASPER DEAN *enters*.)

ARABELLA. Oh Jasper is that you?

CAROLINE. Where have you been?

DEAN. In my room –

CAROLINE. We thought you had gone out.

DEAN. No, I have not been out to-day.

ARABELLA. Do you know, Jasper, that they are waiting for you at the meeting?

DEAN. Are they?

CAROLINE. It is much too late to go now.

DEAN. I never intended going.

CAROLINE. Jasper, I see you have been hiding from them.

DEAN. Nothing of the sort – what makes you say that?

CAROLINE. Then why didn't you come down and tell Alderman Kirwan that you weren't going?

DEAN. I did not wish to have an argument with him. You know I have had serious doubts as to the justice of our agitation.

FOLEY. Quite so – I perfectly understand.

DEAN. Yes – I don't feel justified in going on any further with it.

CAROLINE. Well – for the sake of yourself and us all it's fortunate that your courage failed you.

DEAN. That is not true. I have followed my conscience in the matter.

ARABELLA. Yes, he has clearly done so. He told me he had serious doubts about his position, Caroline, after his interview at the hotel with Mr Hardman.

DEAN. Of course, Aunt Arabella – you remember I told you how Mr Hardman's figures and arguments influenced me. That money, you know, given by Anglebury towards public works in this town –

CAROLINE. I don't believe it. Your courage failed you. That was all. You didn't care about disgracing your family or alienating our respectable friends from us. It was only your want of courage detained you.

FOLEY. Anyhow, madam, *you* have a splendid courage.

CAROLINE. I am the only one of the family who has shown any through this miserable affair. (*A sound of tumult is heard outside in the street,*) Oh mercy, what is that?

FOLEY (*rushes to the window*). Hallo, there's Kirwan among a furious mob.

CAROLINE. Police, police, police –

FOLEY. He's laying about him with a stick.

CAROLINE. Police, police, police –

ARABELLA (*going towards the door*). I must run down and let him in –

CAROLINE. (*getting before her*). What are you doing, you lunatic? Do you want to draw the fury of the mob on the house?

FOLEY. Madam, he will be murdered.

CAROLINE. Do you want me to be murdered? I am terrified. (*She screams with fright and attended by* FOLEY, *sinks into a chair.*)

DEAN. Here, I will go and let him in.

CAROLINE. Don't allow him, Foley. Don't allow him, Foley. (*She screams.*)

ARABELLA. The mob will attack you, Jasper. They can't bear anyone on the losing side.

DEAN. Yes – I have lost everything now – everything – except Millicent.

ARABELLA (*looking out of the window*). The police are coming.

CAROLINE. Police, police, police –

DEAN. I have nowhere to go now but to Millicent. (*Exit.*)

ARABELLA. The police have dispersed the mob. Jasper is safe.

CAROLINE (*recovering*). I knew he hadn't courage, or he would have gone sooner.

FOLEY (*to* CAROLINE). Upon my honour and conscience, madam, I never saw anyone behave with such magnificent courage as you. (ALDERMAN RALF KIRWAN *hurriedly re-enters carrying a great stick.*)

KIRWAN. Hah, I think I have cracked a few skulls. I met your nephew rushing out of the house just now. Where was he?

ARABELLA. Here all the time –

KIRWAN. Oh dear – he opened the hall door for me and then hurried away towards the hotel. Well – I certainly have been a fool for my trouble.

FOLEY. Why, what have you done?

KIRWAN. I – fancy I of all others to have been persuaded by a woman's advice into this – well it serves me right.

ARABELLA. I told you, you'd be on the losing side. Pity you didn't take the right woman's advice, Alderman Kirwan.

FOLEY. Tell us what happened to you.

KIRWAN. Oh, dear, I have scarcely any breath left. Well, foolishly following Miss Caroline's advice against my own better judgment, I will admit, I went to try and unite those various sections at the meeting, in place of Jasper Dean who failed –

ARABELLA. Why do you say he failed? He will return again and take the lead in his town.

KIRWAN. Lead again? – never – he has lost his opportunity. It will never come to him again. He was the man for the movement. He might have been famous. A new movement will call forth a new man.

FOLEY. Tell us what happened at the meeting. (*Distant tumult is heard outside, which grows louder and louder during the following.*)

KIRWAN. When I addressed the meeting, and said that Dean couldn't be found, there was a yell of disappointment and rage as horrible as if it came out of hell. I tried to appease the excitement. I exhorted all parties still to keep united. I said I would lead them to victory. No sooner had I spoken of leading than Murphy started up, and denounced me in the most outrageous language. He even accused me of having prevented Dean from coming to the meeting, so that I might usurp his position as leader. Just think that I should be accused of such a thing – I who never wanted to lead at all, except to save the situation. Thereupon his party in the hall raised fresh uproar, and gave him such courage that he actually sat in the chair and declared *himself* leader of the whole town. This was the signal for a free fight. His party were soon beaten and driven out by the majority. In the storming of the platform he himself would have been torn to pieces but for the arrival of the police. When I left, they had nearly cleared the hall. Then it was, as the last of the people were being cleared out, that I saw Alderman Cassidy sit in the chair and declare himself leader. (*They all laugh.*)

CAROLINE. That is just like James Cassidy

FOLEY. After the storms of public life, how grateful to look down on the peaceful vista of domesticity – ! (*Furious tumult now outside, and sounds of glass breaking – stones are flung in through the window-panes from the street.*)

KIRWAN (*looking out of the window*). There are the Corporation running before the mob.

CAROLINE. Mercy – we shall be murdered. Where are the police? (*There is a loud knocking at the street door.*) Oh – they are breaking into the house.

FOLEY. Madam, while I am at your side, you need not fear the incursion of a million!

CAROLINE. Police, police, police – (*She faints and is supported by* FOLEY.)

FOLEY (*to the others who volunteer assistance*). Stand off, if you please. This lady belongs to me. (*He places her in an armchair and attends to her.*)

359

KIRWAN. The mob have chased the Corporation up the street.

ARABELLA. Who are those coming in here? (*Enter* ALDERMAN THOMAS MURPHY *torn and bleeding,* ALDERMEN JAMES CASSIDY, *and* MICHAEL LEECH.)

MURPHY. Whew – safe at last – well – anyhow it's a consolation that if I couldn't be leader myself, I have successfully prevented anybody else from being so.

CASSIDY. You did not prevent me.

MURPHY. You – ?

ARABELLA. Oh won't you let me bring you some refreshment, Alderman Murphy? You are in a dreadful plight. (*Exit.*)

LEECH. James was in the chair; and we passed a vote of censure on the whole proceedings.

KIRWAN. Yes – Cassidy and the family are strong when it is a question or censuring anybody. (MISS ARABELLA DEAN *re-enters followed by* THE MAID *who carries a tray with liquor, glasses etc. which she sets on a table and exit.*)

ARABELLA. Take a glass of something, Alderman Murphy.

CASSIDY (*mixing for himself a stiff glass and drinking*). It's well there was at least one of the family to take the necessary step. (*He drinks deeply, and fills another glass.*)

MURPHY. Confound Jasper Dean – if he only had the pluck to stick to his guns, I shouldn't be in this state. But I knew he was no good after yesterday. Oo – I'm sore. An organised band of the greatest blackguards in the town bludgeoned the meeting when the parties were all at loggerheads. I don't know who was leading those ruffians, but I believe they were sent there by Lawrence, although he didn't dare to appear himself. (*Cheers are heard outside, then the voice of* LAWRENCE *addressing the crowd.*)

KIRWAN. Faith, he dares to appear now at all events. Oh that big intolerable optimistic voice – ! (*A loud knocking is heard at the street door.* CAROLINE *is roused and screams.*)

MURPHY. Ugh – we're going to have him in here too.

CASSIDY (*who has all along been helping himself to the liquor*). Hic – a remarkably level-headed fellow Lawrence – hic – especially when his own interests are concerned – hic –

LEECH. Come over here James and sit down. I am afraid you are not very well, James. (*He puts him into an arm chair.*) (ALDERMAN DANIEL LAWRENCE *enters.*)

LAWRENCE. Ah – I thought Mr Hardman was here. But he will come directly. How do you do ladies? What, Alderman Murphy here – ? I am glad to see you, Alderman Murphy. How well you are looking.

I never –

MURPHY. I won't be long well, if I keep looking at you, Daniel Lawrence, you brute. (*Exit.*)

ARABELLA. Oh call him back. He will be murdered in the street.

LAWRENCE. There is no danger of that, my dear Miss Dean. The police have now arrived in force to protect the leaders of the people. (*Enter* MRS BELLE CASSIDY *and* MRS SARAH LEECH.)

MRS CASSIDY (*excitedly*). Where is my husband? Where is my husband?

MRS LEECH. Where are our husbands?

MRS CASSIDY. We were unable to get into the meeting. (*Perceives* CASSIDY.) James, James, what has come over you? James, you brute –

LEECH. Rouse yourself James. The eyes of the family are upon you.

CASSIDY (*huskily*). Go away. Go away.

MRS CASSIDY. You are all murdering my husband. You have done this, Caroline Dean, out of jealousy because he took the lead.

CAROLINE. Belle Cassidy how dare you say I am the cause of your husband's intemperance? You don't expect me to watch him when you are away.

MRS LEECH. Indeed Belle I told you it was a great risk letting him out of your sight to-day. Consider all the excitement –

LAWRENCE. Oh ladies his condition is pardonable, when so many had to fly before the people. (*More cheers outside.*) Ah! there is Mr Hardman.

KIRWAN. I would like to know how you and he have become so suddenly popular?

LAWRENCE. I said I had arranged with him to have a tramway constructed from our market square to that poor and congested suburb which has always been a source of difficulty to the political economists of our town. (*Enter* GEORGE HARDMAN, MISS MILLICENT FELL, ALDERMAN JASPER DEAN, *and* MRS COSTIGAN, *who waves her sweeping brush with the Union Jack tied like a flag to its handle.*)

MRS COSTIGAN. Hooray for the wedding – three cheers for Lawrence and Hardman the friends of the people –

KIRWAN. So the people like an ass in a field, has allowed itself to be caught by a handful of oats.

HARDMAN. No man who speaks like that, can love his town.

KIRWAN. Not love my town – ? I am the only one who loves her. I have done my poor best for her – yes – I alone among you all – and the only thanks I get is to have it believed I do not love her.

MRS COSTIGAN. You have insulted her people, you ruffian Ralf Kirwan.

361

KIRWAN. Of course – if we don't always beslaver them with flattery, we are insulting the people.

HARDMAN. I must say there is something divine about the judgment of the people.

MRS COSTIGAN. Thank you, Mr Hardman – because you said that, the people will follow you.

KIRWAN. What divine judgment – !

LAWRENCE. Tut-tut, that useful elderly woman is an incarnation of the voice and majesty of the people.

MRS COSTIGAN. Hooray! – we'll cheer any show, no matter what it is. And now we're going to have the wedding of Jasper Dean. There's nothing like a wedding after all.

HARDMAN. Yes, my brilliant friend Jasper has followed the dictates of his conscience and refused to join the immoral conspiracy against Anglebury.

LAWRENCE. A nefarious conspiracy that could have only ended, as it has, in deserved confusion –

KIRWAN. Of course it is now a conspiracy, because it has failed.

CAROLINE. And you have done all this Mr Hardman!

HARDMAN. Gentler influences were at work, my dear Miss Dean. True love instinctively guarded Jasper's best interests. That is the advantage of marrying an English girl. The greatness of England is founded on marriages of true love!

MILLICENT. Jasper dear, you are now a free man. We shall have abundant opportunities, after we are married, for congenial political activities.

DEAN. Dear Millicent, you always had a sympathetic way of putting things.

CAROLINE. He will now be able to remain respectable while he takes the lead.

KIRWAN. As if leaders are ever respectable –

ARABELLA. At all events he can be on the winning side.

LAWRENCE. Peace peace – it is time to merge everything into the harmony which Hymen has brought into our midst. Gentle influences have made more than one of us the wiser. If I mistake not, my respected colleague, Alderman Foley –

FOLEY (*leading* CAROLINE *forward*). Your surmise is correct. This lady has consented to be my wife.

KIRWAN. Hallo – what about your mission, Foley?

FOLEY. I am not going to stultify myself by –

LAWRENCE. The highest mission of any man is to look after his private interests.

KIRWAN. Anyhow this marriage can't possibly lessen his reputation for austerity.

CAROLINE. Alderman Kirwan, how dare you insult me?

DEAN. Aunt Caroline, are you mad? Such a marriage –

MILLICENT. Miss Dean I beg of you to pause before you make yourself and all of us ridiculous. I could tell you – (FOLEY *looks terrified.*)

CAROLINE. I will listen to no one. Do you think you are the only pair who have a right to marry?

MRS COSTIGAN. Certainly ma'am, the more weddings the better for the people – (FOLEY *triumphantly leads* CAROLINE *aside.*)

MRS LEECH. Ha – wasn't I right about Caroline?

ARABELLA. Yes the family always knew that Caroline had great common sense.

KIRWAN. Hers is the poetry of common sense!

LAWRENCE. Bless her – may she be happy! May happiness result to all from the harmony and prosperity that has supervened in our midst. I declare, when I see this charming young lady who is shortly to be the bride of my friend Jasper Dean, and when I think how much I – how much others with prospective appointments owe to her, I can scarcely suppress my enthusiasm. She is worthy of a statue in our town. I would subscribe a pound to it; for no woman has done such sound political service to her fellow citizens since Joan of Arc –

HARDMAN. Oh! come Alderman Lawrence, much as I admire and appreciate my niece, I think you are inclined to view her in the too dazzling sunshine of your prosperity.

LAWRENCE. Prosperity – ah what a wonder worker it is to be sure! We can bear much public calamity so long as our individual appointments are safe. Let a man but draw his salary and look after himself and his family, and, believe me, public affairs can very well look after themselves. This is the best for the public, and, you see, it tends to make the public man himself more popular. And now that I think of it, my dear Mayor, you should really have a residence in this town. If the Mayor of Anglebury were to live here occasionally, and to mix and converse with our townspeople. they would be so flattered by his presence among them, that they would cease to molest him by their grievances.

KIRWAN. Never – we want no ruler's residence. We only want justice.

LAWRENCE. Tut-tut – we are far too popular now to consider such trifles. Come, my dear Mayor, come, let us stand at the open window and enjoy our popularity.

MRS COSTIGAN. Let the people see their benefactors. Hooray –

LAWRENCE (*throws open the window, and is greeted with loud cheers*

363

from outside). Come, my dear Mayor. (HARDMAN *joins him at the window. The cheers now increase. The English national anthem is heard on a band outside.* HARDMAN *and* LAWRENCE *grasp each others' hands and bow their thanks. The ladies wave their handkerchiefs.* MRS COSTIGAN *cheers and waves her Union Jack. All, except* KIRWAN, *are intent upon what is going on in the street.*)

KIRWAN (*comes to the footlights*). For us this is always The Tale of a Town.

CURTAIN

SELECTED CHECKLIST OF THE WRITINGS OF GEORGE MOORE AND EDWARD MARTYN

COMPILED BY
COLIN SMYTHE

A. THE WRITINGS OF GEORGE MOORE

For the most part only the first editions of Moore's works are listed here, but many were revised each time they were republished. For a complete listing of Moore's publications, therefore, see Edwin Gilcher, *A Bibliography of George Moore* (Dekalb, Illinois: Northern Illinois University Press, 1970), and Edwin Gilcher, assisted by the shared expertise of Robert S. Becker and Clinton K. Krauss, *Supplement to A Bibliography of George Moore* (Westport, Connecticut: Meckler Corporation, and Gerrards Cross, Buckinghamshire: Colin Smythe, 1988). My thanks to Edwin Gilcher for his advice in the preparation of this list.

Plays
Worldliness, London [c. 1874]. No copy is known to exist, or to have existed, the sole reference to it being in *Confessions of a Young Man* and in I.A. Williams' 1921 bibliography of Moore's works.
The Fashionable Beauty (with Henry Glover), produced by Violet Melnot at the Avenue Theatre, London, on 7 April 1887. Unpublished.
It is often stated that Henry Paulton was Moore's collaborator on this play, but Glover's name is given in contemporary references to the play and on the manuscript preserved in the Lord Chamberlain's papers now in the British Library.
The Honeymoon in Eclipse (dramatisation of story by Mrs G.W. Godfrey), presented at St George's Hall, London by 'The Strolling Players' on 12 April 1888. The production was not licenced by the Lord Chamberlain. Unpublished.
The Three Lovers (with John Oliver Hobbes, pseud. of Mrs Pearl Craigie), also called *The Peacock's Feathers*, not performed, Unpublished. (Rewritten by Moore as *Elizabeth Cooper*).
Thérèse Raquin (revision of Moore's translation of Zola's play by Teixeria de Mattos), produced by the Independent Theatre at the Royalty Theatre, London on 9 October 1891. Unpublished.
A Manuscript of the play is preserved among the Lord Chamberlain's papers.
The Minister's Call (dramatisation of Frank Harris' *A Modern Idyll*, by

Arthur Symons collaborating with Moore), produced by the Independent Theatre at the Royalty Theatre on 4 March 1892.

Only Symons was listed as author. No manuscript of the play seems to have survived.

The Strike at Arlingford (three-act version), London: Walter Scott, 1893.

Originally a five-act version, reduced to three with the assistance of Arthur Kennedy. Produced by the Independent Theatre at the Opera Comique, in the Strand, London, on 21 February 1893, and three nights later at Manchester.

The Fool's Hour, Act 1 only, (by John Oliver Hobbes and Moore), in *The Yellow Book*, London, 1894. Apparently never completed. Never produced.

Le Sycomore (French translation of W.S. Gilbert's play *Sweet-hearts*, by Moore and Paul Alexis) produced by the Comedie Française, Paris, on 20 September 1894.

A copy of the script is preserved in Archives de France, Dossier F18 727, No. 17223 at the Bibliotheque Nationale, Paris.

Martin Luther (with Bernard Lopez), London: Remington & Co., 1897.

The Bending of the Bough, London: T. Fisher Unwin, 1900 (Rewritten version of Edward Martyn's *The Tail of a Town*), produced by the Irish Literary Theatre at the Gaiety Theatre, Dublin on 20 February 1900.

Diarmuid and Grania (with W.B. Yeats) produced for the Irish Literary Theatre by the F.R. Benson Company at the Gaiety Theatre, Dublin, 1901. Published in April-June 1951 issue of *The Dublin Magazine*, and as a limited edition of 25 copies with an introductory note by William Becker, in April 1951. The song by Yeats 'There are Seven that Pull the Thread' published in 1902 with music by Edward Elgar does not appear in this version, which appears to be a later one than that used for the production.

Journeys End in Lovers Meeting (with John Oliver Hobbes).

Printed in an unlocated pamphlet in 1894, and without listing Moore as co-author in her *Tales about Temperaments*, London: T. Fisher Unwin, 1902.

Based on a play by Caraquell. Played from time to time by Ellen Terry as a curtain raiser, starting 5 June 1895.

The Apostle, Dublin: Maunsel & Co., 1911.

Scenario published to protect the idea later developed in his novel, *The Brook Kerith*, 1916. Expanded edition, based on the unpublished *The Brook Kerith, A Spiritual Drama*, written in collaboration with John Lloyd Balderston, further revised, and published by William Heinemann in 1923; rewritten as

The Passing of the Essenes, London: William Heinemann, 1930.
    Produced in a slightly revised version at the Arts Theatre, London, on 1-5 October 1930, and published by Heinemann the following year.

Esther Waters (with Lennox Robinson), London: William Heinemann, 1913.
    A dramatization of part of his novel of the same name. As early as 1906 Moore had been working with Edward Knoblock and Robinson on a version. Produced by the Stage Society at the Apollo Theatre, London, on 10 December 1911.

Elizabeth Cooper, Dublin and London: Maunsel & Co., 1913.
    Produced by the Incorporated Stage Society at the Haymarket Theatre, London on 22 June 1913. Adapted by Edouard Dujardin and translated as *Clara Florise*, produced at the Comédie Royal, Paris, in 1914, and serialised in *L'Afrique du Nord Illustrée* in 1920. English version rewrite and re-titled as

The Coming of Gabrielle, London: privately printed for subscribers only by the Society of Irish Folklore, 1920.
    A revised version was first produced by Leon Lion at the St James's Theatre, London on 17 July 1923.

The Making of an Immortal, New York: The Bowling Green Press, and London: Faber & Gwyer Ltd., 1927. Edited for publication by John Eglinton. Produced on 1 April 1928 at the Arts Theatre, London (with incidental music by Sir Thomas Beecham, Sybil Thorndike as Queen Elizabeth, and Charles Laughton as Jonson).

Prose

A Modern Lover, London: Tinsley Bros., 1883. Rewritten as *Lewis Seymour and Some Women*, New York: Brentano, and London: William Heinemann, 1917.

A Mummer's Wife, London: Vizetelly & Co., 1884.

'Preface' to Émile Zola's *Piping Hot!* London: Vizetelly & Co. 1885.
    The translation of *Pot-Bouille* was possibly by Moore himself.

Literature at Nurse, London: Vizetelly & Co., 1885.

A Drama in Muslin, London: Vizetelly & Co., 1886.
    Rewritten as *Muslin*, London: William Heinemann, 1915.

A Mere Accident, London: Vizetelly & Co., 1887.
    Rewritten and condensed to form the 'John Norton' section of *Celibates*, 1895.

Confessions of a Young Man, London: Swan, Sonnenschein, Lowrey & Co., 1888.

Spring Days, London: Vizetelly & Co., 1888.

Mike Fletcher, London: Ward & Downey, 1889.

Impressions and Opinions, London: David Nutt, 1891.

Vain Fortune, London: Henry & Co., 1891.

'Our Dramatic Critics', in *The Pall Mall Gazette*, 9 and 10 September 1891.

'Why I Don't Write Plays', in *The Pall Mall Gazette*, 7 September 1892, p. 3.

Modern Painting, London: Walter Scott, 1894.

Esther Waters, London: Walter Scott, 1894.

'Introduction' to *Poor Folk*, by F. Dostoievsky, London: Elkin Mathews and John Lane; Boston: Roberts Brothers, 1894.

The Royal Academy, London: The New Budget Office, 1895.

Celibates, London: Walter Scott, 1895.

Evelyn Innes, London: T. Fisher Unwin, 1898.

'Is the Theatre a Place of Amusement?', in *Beltaine*, 2 (February, 1900), p. 9.

'The Irish Literary Renaissance and the Irish Language', in *The New Ireland Review*, XIII, 2 (April 1900), pp. 65-72.

'Literature at the Irish Language' in *Ideals in Ireland*, edited by Lady Gregory. London: At the Sign of the Unicorn, 1901.

'A Plea for the Soul of the Irish People', in *The Nineteenth Century*, February 1901, pp. 285-95.

Sister Teresa, London: T. Fisher Unwin, 1901.

'The Irish Literary Theatre', in *Sumhain*, 1 (1901), pp. 11-13

'On the Thoughtlessness of Critics', in *The Leader*, 9 November 1901.

The Untilled Field, London: T. Fisher Unwin, 1903.

The Lake, London: William Heinemann, 1903.

Reminiscences of the Impressionist Painters, Dublin: Maunsel & Co., 1906.

Memoirs of My Dead Life, London: William Heinemann, 1906.

Hail and Farewell!, 3 volumes, London: William Heinemann, 1911 (*Ave*), 1912 (*Salve*), 1914 (*Vale*).
  There are various subsequent editions, but presently most useful is the single volume edition, introduced, annotated and indexed by Richard Allen Cave, Gerrards Cross: Colin Smythe, 1976.

The Brook Kerith, A Syrian Story, Edinburgh: T. Werner Laurie, 1916.

A Story-Teller's Holiday, London: privately printed for subscribers only by the Society for Irish Folklore, 1919.

Avowals, London: privately printed for subscribers only by the Society for Irish Folklore, 1919.

369

Héloïse and Abélard, London: privately printed for subscribers only by the Society for Irish Folklore, 1921.
Revised sections were published as *Fragments from Héloïse and Abélard* privately printed for subscribers only by the Society, 1921.
In Single Strictness, London: William Heinemann, 1922. Rewritten as *Celibate Lives*, 1927.
Conversations in Ebury Street, London: William Heinemann, 1924.
The Pastoral Lives of Daphnis and Chloe, London: William Heinemann, 1924.
Daphnis and Chloe. Perronik [sic] *the Fool*, New York: printed for subscribers only, Boni & Liveright, 1924.
Peronnik the Fool, New York: William Edwin Rudge, 1926.
Ulick and Soracha, London: The Nonesuch Press, 1926.
Celebate Lives, London: William Heinemann, 1927.
Aphrodite in Aulis, London: William Heinemann, 1930.
A Flood, New York: Groff Conklin at the Harbor Press, 1930.
The Talking Pine, Paris: The Hours Press, 1931.
A Communication to my Friends, London: The Nonesuch Press, 1933.
In Minor Keys. The Uncollected Short Stories, edited with an introduction by David B. Eakin and Helmut E. Gerber, London: Fourth Estate, 1985.

Poetry
Flowers of Passion, London: Provost & Co., 1878.
Pagan Poems, London: Newman & Co., 1881.
Les Cloches de Corneville, lyrics by George and Augustus Moore, for private circulation, c. 1883.
La Ballade de l'Amant de Coeur, Burges [Augustus Moore] et Pot [Pot Stephens], c. 1886.

Collected Editions
The Collected Works of George Moore, Carra Edition, New York: Boni & Liveright, 1922-1924, 21 vols. for subscribers only.
The Uniform Edition, London: William Heinemann, 1924-1933, 20 vols. Reprinted as
The Ebury Edition, London: William Heinemann, 1936-1938, 20 vols.
Brentano Uniform Edition, New York: Brentano, 1912-1917, 10 vols.
(11 announced but *The Untilled Field* not published in the series).

Letters
Moore versus Harris, Detroit, Michigan: privately printed for subscribers, 1921.

Letters from George Moore to Edouard Dujardin, 1886-1922, selected, edited and translated by John Eglinton (pseud. of W.K. Magee), New York: Crosby Gaige, 1929.

George Moore in Quest of Locale, two letters to W.T. Stead, London: The Harvest Press, 1931.

Letters of George Moore (to John Eglinton), edited and with an introduction by the recipient, Bournemouth, 1942.

George Moore on Authorship, Cherry Plain, NY: ELG Press, 1950.

George Moore: Letters to Lady Cunard, 1895-1933, edited with an introduction and notes by Rupert Hart-Davis, London: Rupert Hart-Davis, 1957.

George Moore in Transition, Letters to T. Fisher Unwin and Lena Milman 1894-1910, edited with commentary by Helmut E. Gerber, Detroit, Michigan: Wayne State University Press, 1968.

George Moore's Correspondence with the Mysterious Countess, edited by David B. Eakin and Robert Langenfeld, Victoria, BC: University of Victoria, 1984.

'Gabrielle' was the Baroness Franzi Ripp.

George Moore on Parnassus. Letters (1900-1933) to Secretaries, Publishers, Printers, Agents, Literati, Friends and Acquaintances, edited with notes and critical-biographical commentary, by Helmut E. Gerber, with the assistance of O.M. Brack, Jr., Newark, Delaware: University of Delaware Press, 1988.

Books wholly or partly about George Moore

George Moore, by Susan L. Mitchell, Dublin and London: Maunsel & Co., 1916.

A Portrait of George Moore in a Study of his Work, by John Freeman, London: Privately printed for subscribers only, by T. Werner Laurie, 1922.

Conversations with George Moore, by Geraint Goodwin, London: Ernest Benn, 1929.

George Moore: 'A Disciple of Walter Pater', by Robert Porter Sechler, Philadelphia: privately printed, 1931.

George Moore, by Humbert Wolfe, London: Thornton Butterworth, 1931.

Das religiöse Gefuhl bei George Moore, by Herbert Weferling, Bottrop: Wilhelm Postberg, 1932.

The Influence of Flaubert on George Moore, by Walter D. Ferguson, Philadelphia: University of Pennsylvania Press, and London: Oxford University Press, 1934.

Epitaph on George Moore, by Charles Morgan, London and New York:

Macmillan, 1935.

The Life of George Moore, by Joseph [Maunsell] Hone, London: Victor Gollancz, 1936.

The Moores of Moore Hall, by Joseph Hone, London: Jonathan Cape, 1939.

George Moore's Naturalistic Prose, by Sonja Nejdefors-Frish, Uppsala: University of Uppsala Irish Studies, 1952.

The Critic's Alchemy: A Study of the Introduction of French Symbolism into England, by Ruth Zabriskie Temple, New York: Twayne, 1953.

George Moore: A Reconsideration, by Malcolm Brown, Seattle: University of Washington Press, 1955.

GM: Memories of George Moore, by Nancy Cunard, London: Rupert Hart-Davis, 1956.

George Moore et la France, by Georges-Paul Collet, Geneva: Droz, and Paris: Minard, 1957.

George Moore, by A. Norman Jeffares, London: Longmans, Green & Co., 1965.

George Moore: L'Homme et l'Oeuvre, by Jean C. Noel, Paris: Didier, 1966.

George Moore's Mind and Art, compiled and edited by Graham Owens, London: Oliver & Boyd, 1968.

The Man of Wax: Critical Essays on George Moore, edited by Douglas Hughes, New York: New York University Press, 1971.

George Moore: The Artist's Vision, The Storyteller's Art, by Janet Egleson Dunleavy, Lewisburg, PA: Bucknell University Press; Cranbury, NJ: Associated University Presses, 1973.

A Study of the Novels of George Moore, by Richard Allen Cave, Gerrards Cross: Colin Smythe, and Totowa, NJ: Barnes & Noble, 1978.

George Moore, by Anthony Farrow, Boston, 1978.

The Way Back: George Moore's The Untilled Field & The Lake, edited by Robert Welch, Dublin: Wolfhound Press, 1982.

George Moore in Perspective, edited by Janet Egleson Dunleavy, Gerrards Cross: Colin Smythe, and Totowa, NJ: Barnes & Noble Books, 1983.

George Moore and German Pessimism, by Patrick Bridgwater, Durham: University of Durham, 1988.

George Moore and the Autogenous Self: The Autobiography and Fiction, by Elizabeth Grubgeld, Syracuse, NY: Syracuse University Press, 1994.

For a detailed listing of books and articles wholly or partly about Moore, see *George Moore: An Annotated Secondary Bibliography of Writings About Him*, by Robert Langenfeld, New York: AMS Press, 1987.

B. THE WRITINGS OF EDWARD MARTYN

Plays

The Heather Field and *Maeve*, with an introduction by George Moore, London: Gerald Duckworth, 1899.

Published separately by Duckworth in 1917.

The Tale of a Town and *An Enchanted Sea*, Kilkenny: Standish O'Grady, and London: T. Fisher Unwin, 1902.

The Place-Hunters, in *The Leader* 26 July 1902.

Romulus and Remus, or *The Makers of Delights*, in Christmas supplement to *The Irish People*, 21 December 1907.

Grangecolman, Dublin: Maunsel & Co., 1912.

The Dream Physician, Dublin: Talbot Press, 1914.

The Privilege of Place, performed Dublin 1915, unpublished.

Regina Eyre, performed Dublin 1919, unpublished.

Prose

Morgante the Lesser, (under the pseudonym 'Sirius') London: Swan Sonnenschein, 1890.

'The Use of a Provincial Feis', in *The Daily Express* (Dublin), 17 September 1898.

'The Modern Drama in Germany' in *The Daily Express* (Dublin), 11 February 1899, p. 3.

'A Comparison Between English and Irish Theatrical Audiences', in *Beltaine*, 2 (February 1900), pp. 11-13.

'Two Irish Artists', in *The Leader*, 26 October 1901, pp. 141-42.

'A Plea for a National Theatre in Ireland', in *Samhain* 1 (1901), pp. 14-15.

Letter to the Editor, in *The United Irishman*, 19 April 1902, p. 1.

Ireland's Battle for her Language, Dublin: Gaelic League, 1910.

'*Little Eyolf* and *The Lady from the Sea* at the Theatrical Club', in *The Irish Review*, II, 23 (February 1913), p. 611.

'Wagner's Parsifal, or the Cult of Liturgical Aestheticism', in *The Irish Review*, II, 34 (December 1913), p. 538.

'The Recent Performance of Ibsen's *Rosmersholm*', in *The Irish Review*, III, 36 (February 1914), p. 660.

'A Plea for the Revival of the Irish Literary Theatre' in *The Irish Review*, IV, 38 (April 1914), pp. 79-84.

Books wholly or partly about Edward Martyn

Hail and Farewell!, by George Moore, in 3 volumes, London: William Heinemann, 1911, 1912, 1914.

Single volume edition, introduced, annotated and indexed by Richard Allen Cave, Gerrards Cross: Colin Smythe, 1976.

Edward Martyn and the Irish Revival, by Denis Gwynn, London: Jonathan Cape, 1930.

Edward Martyn and the Irish Theatre, by Sr. Marie-Thérèse Courtney, New York: Vantage Press, 1956.

Ibsen and the Beginnings of Anglo-Irish Drama, Vol. II: Edward Martyn, by Jan Setterquist, Uppsala: A.B. Lundequistska, and Dublin: Hodges Figgis, 1960.

Drama in Hardwicke Street. A History of the Irish Theatre Company, by William J. Feeney, Rutherford, Madison, Teaneck: Fairleigh Dickinson University Press, and London & Toronto: Associated University Presses, 1984.

IRISH DRAMA SELECTIONS
ISSN 0260-7962

1. SELECTED PLAYS OF LENNOX ROBINSON
Chosen and introduced by Christopher Murray
Contains *Patriots, The Whiteheaded Boy, Crabbed Youth and Age, The Big House, Drama at Inish, Church Street,* bibliographical checklist.

2. SELECTED PLAYS OF DENIS JOHNSTON
Chosen and introduced by Joseph Ronsley
Contains *The Old Lady Says 'No!', The Moon in the Yellow River, The Golden Cuckoo, The Dreaming Dust, The Scythe and the Sunset,* bibliographical checklist.

3. SELECTED PLAYS OF LADY GREGORY
Chosen and introduced by Mary FitzGerald
Contains *The Travelling Man, Spreading the News, Kincora, Hyacinth Halvey, The Doctor in Spite of Himself, The Gaol Gate, The Rising of the Moon, Dervorgilla, The Workhouse Ward, Grania, The Golden Apple, The Story Brought by Brigit, Dave,* Lady Gregory on playwriting and her plays, bibliographical checklist.

4. SELECTED PLAYS OF DION BOUCICAULT
Chosen and introduced by Andrew Parkin
Contains *London Assurance, The Corsican Brothers, The Octoroon, The Colleen Bawn, The Shaughraun, Robert Emmet,* bibliographical checklist.

5. SELECTED PLAYS OF ST. JOHN ERVINE
Chosen and introduced by John Cronin
Contains *Mixed Marriage, Jane Clegg, John Ferguson, Boyd's Shop, Friends and Relations,* prose extracts, bibliographical checklist.

6. SELECTED PLAYS OF BRIAN FRIEL
Chosen and introduced by Seamus Deane
Contains *Philadelphia, Here I Come, Translations, The Freedom of the City, Living Quarters, Faith Healer, Aristocrats,* bibliographical checklist.
This edition is only for sale in North America. Published by Faber & Faber in Great Britain.

7. SELECTED PLAYS OF DOUGLAS HYDE
   Chosen and introduced by Janet Egleson Dunleavy and Gareth Dunleavy
   Contains *The Twisting of the Rope, The Marriage, The Lost Saint, The Nativity, King James, The Bursting of the Bubble, The Tinker and the Sheeog, The Matchmaking, The Schoolmaster*, bibliographical checklist.
   The original Irish language texts are published with Lady Gregory's translations.

8. SELECTED PLAYS OF GEORGE MOORE AND EDWARD MARTYN
   Chosen and introduced by David B. Eakin and Michael Case
   Contains Moore's *The Strike at Arlingford, The Bending of the Bough, The Coming of Gabrielle, The Passing of the Essenes;* and Martyn's *The Heather Field, Maeve, The Tale of a Town*, bibliographical checklist.

9. SELECTED PLAYS OF HUGH LEONARD
   Chosen and introduced by S.F. Gallagher
   Contains *The Au Pair Man, The Patrick Pearse Motel, Da, Summer, A Life, Kill*, bibliographical checklist.

10. SELECTED PLAYS OF T.C. MURRAY
   Chosen and introduced by Richard Allen Cave
   Contains *Autumn Fire, Sovereign Love, Maurice Harte, The Briery Gap, The Pipe in the Fields, Birthright*, bibliographical checklist.

11. SELECTED PLAYS OF MICHEÁL MACLIAMMÓIR
   Chosen and introduced by John Barrett
   Contains *Where Stars Walk, Ill Met by Moonlight, The Mountains Look Different, The Liar, Prelude in Kazbeck Street*, 'On Plays and Players', bibliographical checklist.

2889

Moore, George, 1852-1933.

Selected plays of George
Moore and Edward Martyn